Stretching for Functional Flexibility

Stretching
for Functional
Flexibility

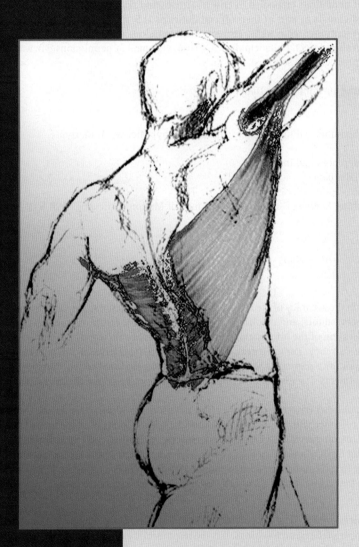

Phil Armiger, MPT
Licensed Physical Therapist
G-2 Sports Therapy
Seattle, Washington

Michael A. Martyn
Illustrator and Fitness Professional
Martyn Illustration
Renton, Washington

 Wolters Kluwer | Lippincott Williams & Wilkins
Health

Philadelphia · Baltimore · New York · London
Buenos Aires · Hong Kong · Sydney · Tokyo

Acquisitions Editor: Emily Lupash
Managing Editor: Andrea M. Klingler
Development Editor: David R. Payne
Marketing Manager: Christen D. Murphy
Production Editor: Beth Martz
Senior Designer: Joan Wendt
Compositor: Circle Graphics
Artwork: Michael Martyn

351 West Camden Street   530 Walnut Street
Baltimore, MD 21201   Philadelphia, PA 19106

Printed in the People's Republic of China

Library of Congress Cataloging-in-Publication Data

Armiger, Phil.
 Stretching for functional flexibility / Phil Armiger ; [illustrated by] Michael A. Martyn.
    p. ; cm.
 Includes bibliographical references and index.
 ISBN 978-0-7817-6792-7 (alk. paper)
 1.   Stretching exercises.   2.   Joints—Range of motion.   I. Title.
 [DNLM: 1.   Muscle Stretching Exercises—methods.   2.   Range of Motion, Articular.   WB 541
A729s 2010]
 RA781.63.A76 2010
 613.7'1—dc22

                   2008033728

DISCLAIMER

Care has been taken to confirm the accuracy of the information present and to describe generally accepted practices. However, the authors, editors, and publisher are not responsible for errors or omissions or for any consequences from application of the information in this book and make no warranty, expressed or implied, with respect to the currency, completeness, or accuracy of the contents of the publication. Application of this information in a particular situation remains the professional responsibility of the practitioner; the clinical treatments described and recommended may not be considered absolute and universal recommendations.

The authors, editors, and publisher have exerted every effort to ensure that drug selection and dosage set forth in this text are in accordance with the current recommendations and practice at the time of publication. However, in view of ongoing research, changes in government regulations, and the constant flow of information relating to drug therapy and drug reactions, the reader is urged to check the package insert for each drug for any change in indications and dosage and for added warnings and precautions. This is particularly important when the recommended agent is a new or infrequently employed drug.

Some drugs and medical devices presented in this publication have Food and Drug Administration (FDA) clearance for limited use in restricted research settings. It is the responsibility of the health care provider to ascertain the FDA status of each drug or device planned for use in their clinical practice.

To purchase additional copies of this book, call our customer service department at **(800) 638-3030** or fax orders to **(301) 223-2320**. International customers should call **(301) 223-2300**.

Visit Lippincott Williams & Wilkins on the Internet: http://www.lww.com. Lippincott Williams & Wilkins customer service representatives are available from 8:30 am to 6:00 pm, EST.

RRS0810

To my mother, Carole Armiger, who gave everything she had to see that her children had everything they needed.
She'll have to read the book and stretch in heaven, and I'll have to remember to put a coat on before going out in the cold—all by myself.
—Phil Armiger

To my best friend, Tim Burris, who at the beginning of every phone conversation asked, "Is it done yet?" I wish I could have told you, "Yes, Timmy, it's finally done."
—Mike Martyn

Preface

Stretching for Functional Flexibility is intended as a reference guide for the safe, effective, and efficient application of stretching exercises to improve range of motion and movement potential. It is organized to be useful both for the clinical professional and, ultimately, for the end user. Based on the most current research and on the clinical experience of the author and his colleagues in the field of physical therapy, Stretching for Functional Flexibility will be a valuable reference for physical, occupational, and massage therapists, athletic trainers, fitness trainers, coaches, sports and orthopedic physicians, doctors of chiropractic, and many other professionals dealing with the health and performance of the musculoskeletal system.

Stretching for Functional Flexibility was inspired by the need for consistent, research-based, and/or clinically based information regarding stretching. Widely varying theories and protocols seemed to beg for an accurate, easy-to-use, scientifically based work on the pursuit of flexibility. This book provides the "user" or lay person with clear, easy-to-use information, which will help improve the appropriate ranges of motion and, ultimately, improve movement.

With this goal in mind, all stretching directions are written in the second person, directly addressing lay people who are seeking to improve their flexibility. However, as noted above, this book also addresses the needs of healthcare professionals who may be recommending or even instructing their clients in stretching exercises. In this case, the directions are already in a format in which professionals can pass on to their clients. Furthermore, professionals are encouraged to practice the stretches themselves before teaching them to their clients.

This book is designed not only to improve flexibility and range of motion, but also to help the reader understand which muscles and joints need attention in the larger context of human posture and biomechanics. In this regard, information is provided that will help the reader understand how the need for range of motion fits into the scheme of efficient movement. This text provides simple tests to help determine which muscles need to be stretched and which do not. It also provides information about the muscles in question, including what the muscle does (action), its origin, and its insertion. In this manner, the clinician may become re-acquainted with particular muscles and their function and make better decisions about the prescription of individual exercises.

FOR THE CLINICIAN

An excellent quick reference for both general muscle groups and individual muscles, this text also provides clear artwork and text, detailing the stretching exercises. It also provides the origin, insertion, innervation, and action of each muscle covered.

FOR THE EDUCATOR

This book can be used as required or as a supplemental text for many programs that cover the topic of stretching. In addition to the details mentioned above, it includes stretching protocols, as well as the research behind them.

Also included are chapters on injury prevention and rehabilitation, determining which muscles need to be stretched, and an appendix with suggestions for further reading.

FOR THE INDIVIDUAL

This book provides all of the information necessary to allow the lay person to design and implement a safe and effective stretching program. Posture and work-related concerns and interventions are each covered in their own chapters. Chapter 6 outlines basic stretching programs that may be completed in 10, 20, or 30 minutes.

UNIQUE FEATURES

Below are some of the features of this book that make it unique:

1. Science: The information in this text is based on the most up-to-date research available on each particular topic of discussion. Older and classic research is included, in cases in which it is the most up-to-date research on a particular topic.

2. Proven Techniques and Principles: Techniques and principles are proven daily in a successful outpatient orthopedic physical therapy clinic. Information and protocols are based on the available, related medical literature. References are included. These practices are uncommon or non-existent in other works on stretching/flexibility.

3. Artwork: Clear, accurate drawings represent not only the relevant anatomy, but also clearly depict the positions necessary to perform the individual stretches. In Chapter 4, the individual muscles can be seen "through the body," *in* the stretching position.

4. Easy to Use: The organization of the text is straight forward and moves from the fundamentals necessary to understand stretching to basic stretches and finally into special applications. A "User's Guide" is provided below.

5. Stretch the Right Muscle: Chapter 3 provides a guide to help you choose which muscles to stretch and which to de-emphasize or leave alone completely. It includes a list of quick and easy tests to determine flexibility need for many of the major joints of the body.

6. General-to-Specific Stretches: General stretches for all major muscle groups are provided in Chapter 5, with the individual muscles involved listed, to provide a cross-reference to more detailed information in Chapter 4.

7. Muscle Function: As noted above, Chapter 4 will provide an excellent reference for muscle function, including the muscle's origin, insertion, innervation, action, and, of course, a description and illustration showing the muscle under stretch. In addition to the information listed above, it provides a picture of the target muscle under stretch.

8. Technical: For those who wish a more detailed understanding of the science behind flexibility, Chapters 1 and 2 discuss the "mechanics" of stretching as well as the scientific research that supports it.

9. At Work: Chapter 8 discusses the use of flexibility exercises to combat the aches and pains incurred in the workplace, whether they be due to prolonged positions, stress, or general ergonomics.

10. Prevention and Rehabilitation of Injuries: Chapter 10 discusses the basics of injury prevention and rehabilitation, then provides information regarding the use of stretching exercises to best address the given situation.

11. Caution!: Caution boxes are provided in any areas in which special considerations are needed in order to avoid injury. This "clinician's perspective" is particularly unique in books on stretching.

ADDITIONAL MATERIALS

Stretching for Functional Flexibility includes additional resources for students and instructors, available on the book's companion website at http://thePoint.lww.com/Armiger.

Instructors

Approved adopting instructors will be given access to an electronic image bank containing all the figures from the text.

Students

Purchasers of the text can access the searchable Full Text Online by going to the *Stretching for Functional Flexibility* website at http://thePoint.lww.com/Armiger. See the inside front cover of this text for more details, including the passcode you will need to gain access to the website.

User's Guide

This user's guide section is presented to help you derive the most efficient use of this book, while avoiding the time-consuming practice of flipping through pages or the laborious use of complicated indexes. It provides a useful guide, from goal setting through the actual performance of the exercise, helping you choose the most efficient pathway to suit your needs.

Some readers may wish to use *Stretching for Functional Flexibility* as a reference for stretches or basic muscle kinesiology. Others might wish to understand the science behind the pursuit of flexibility, while still others will want to "get right to it" and begin their stretching programs.

This user's guide provides a roadmap to allow you to get to the information you want most without wasting time or energy.

Below are some guidelines for efficient use:

1. First, read through this entire list.

2. Consider safety first. If you have any doubts, questions, or concerns, see your personal physician or other trusted healthcare practitioner before starting a program.

3. *Stretching for Functional Flexibility* is designed to give you all the information necessary to both understand the science behind flexibility *and* to perform the *appropriate* exercises safely and efficiently. It is therefore recommended that you read all of the chapters to get the best understanding of your program. If you wish to bypass the technical chapters in the beginning, it is recommended that you at least read Chapter 2 ("General Principles for Safe and Effective Stretching") and Chapter 3 ("Assessing Flexibility"). These two chapters will give you the basics of exercise protocol, help with description and movement terminology, and offer guidance regarding which muscles need stretching and which may be better left alone.

4. Establish goals first. Do you want to stretch a particular body part to improve a particular movement pattern? Or, do you just want a general stretching program? Is your stretching program to help with rehabilitation of an injury or for a particular sport? See the general categories below:
   a. Non-specific stretching programs designed to last 10, 20, and 30 minutes are outlined in Chapter 6.
   b. Stretches for major muscle groups, such as those muscles that "abduct" or lift out from the side or the shoulder, are addressed in Chapter 5. This chapter is linked to its more detailed partner, Chapter 4. Please see Figure P.1.
   c. Specific stretches of individual muscles, including origin, insertion, and action, are covered in Chapter 4. Note: This chapter is linked to its more general partner, Chapter 5. Please see Figure P.1 on the next page.
   d. Injuries, their prevention, and rehabilitation are covered in Chapter 10.
   e. Posture and flexibility are covered in Chapter 7.
   f. The science behind the pursuit of flexibility is covered in Chapters 1 and 2.

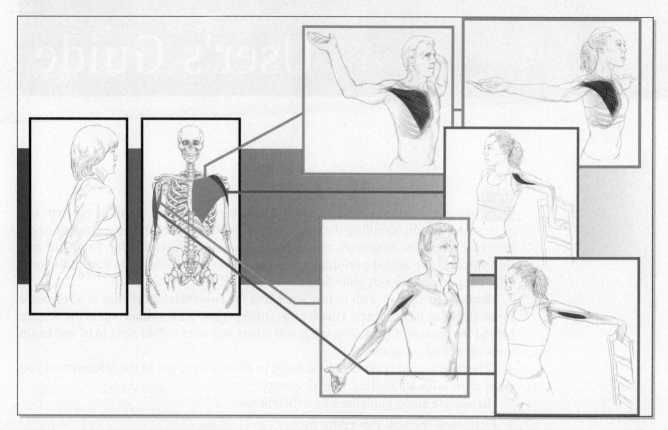

FIGURE P.1 Diagram showing the relationship of one of the particular muscles involved in a Chapter 5 "muscle group" to its specific stretch in Chapter 4, so that the reader easily understands the connection and its significance.

g. Advanced techniques for those experienced "stretchers" are discussed in Chapter 11.

SUMMARY

This book provides the latest information regarding the safe, efficient application of stretching exercises to help promote appropriate levels of flexibility for the enhancement of human movement and performance. The artwork and organization of the text make it an easy-to-use guide for the health/fitness professional and the individual user.

Phil Armiger, MPT
Licensed physical therapist,
specializing in biomechanics and
orthopedic physical therapy
G-2 Sports Therapy (www.G2sports.net)
Seattle, Washington

Michael Martyn
Illustrator and Fitness Professional
Martyn Illustration
Renton, Washington

Acknowledgments

It is difficult to accomplish anything meaningful in life without the help of others. Likewise, the realization of this book would not have been possible without the efforts of many generous and talented individuals. Though I will inevitably forget someone, and for this I apologize in advance, I would like to thank the many people who helped make this book a reality.

Thanks to the many professionals who took precious time from their already busy lives to help review the manuscript and give valuable feedback at various stages of the project. Thanks to Jim Stutzman, English professor at the University of Washington, who read my first draft and did not burst into laughter at my command of the English language (my only language). Thank you, Dan Swinscoe, MPT; Gil Schoos, MA, PT, OCS; Ali Schoos, PT, OCS; Gary Gussel, PT, ATC; Melissa Wolfe-Burke, MS, PT, ATC; Craig Davidson, MD; Rick Griffin MS, ATC; and Chris Cunninghan for your detailed reviews and excellent feedback of my original proposal.

Special thanks to Robyn Stuhr, MA, not only for your review, but also for always supporting me and for the hot tip—Lippincott Williams & Wilkins! Thanks, Neil Pratt, PhD, PT, for being an inspiration and never letting work get in the way of a good joke. I would also like to acknowledge the kindness and generosity of Mark Guthrie of the University of Washington's Physical Therapy Program, who generously donated his time, opened his facility, and connected me with his talented physical therapy staff even though I was never a student of physical therapy at the UW. Thank you, Tamara Hlava, for your professional and thoughtful contributions to the yoga section.

Thanks to Talina Marshall, LMT, and Annette Dong, for gracing the book as models. Thanks to Candace Ito, MPT, and Julie A. Vanni, DPT, for being models, helping with the photography, and being supportive co-workers. Special thanks to Martina Jambrichova for being a model and helping with the photography, not to mention being supportive and putting up with me during this seemingly endless process. I'd also like to thank my wonderful family of friends who supported me and continued to ask, "How's the book coming?" even though it had been going on for years and they must have been tired of it.

I am especially indebted to G. Kelley Fitzgerald, PhD, PT, not only for his valuable time spent during various parts of the proposal and the review processes, but also for his inspiration and "tough love" approach during the creation of this book and during my physical therapy education at Hahnemann University. It's quite likely that, without Kelley Fitzgerald's help, I would not have become a physical therapist in the first place.

This project would not have been possible if it were not for the talents and efforts of Mike Martyn, illustrator and owner of Martyn Illustration, whose excellent illustrations added tremendous value to the ideas expressed within the book.

Of course, the final product would not have been possible without the hard work of our colleagues at Lippincott Williams & Wilkins. Thanks to LWW's acquisitions editor, Pete Darcy, for not only giving me the chance to have my ideas become a reality, but for taking me to one of the Orioles ball games and allowing me to have a crab sandwich (where else but in Baltimore). Thanks to Robyn Alvarez for not changing professions, but rather maintaining a professional attitude when reviewing my first drafts.

Thanks to Andrea Klingler for taking on the project somewhere midstream and assuring a direct course to the finish. Thanks to Emily Lupash, Beth Martz, and the many others whom I did not have the pleasure to meet at LWW, but were instrumental in this book's production.

I'd also like to thank all of the professional reviewers for their detailed, objective, and sometimes critical reviews that have immensely improved the quality of this book. Thank you Laura Bonazzoli for doing an amazing job of taking my original manuscript and managing to integrate the feedback from *twelve* different professional reviewers. I am sure to have gone crazy if I had been charged with this task myself.

I'd even like to thank a particular reviewer of my original proposal (who should probably remain nameless), who provided a particularly personal attack devoid of any objective or useful feedback and gave me the additional incentive necessary to carry on when the project seemed insurmountable.

And finally, a huge thanks to David Payne and Kristen Spina for taking on the monumental task of making sure the final product was truly ready to go on the market.

Phil Armiger, MPT

Thanks to the models who gave their time and energy to this project. Your wonderful diversity has made this project even more enjoyable for me and surely for the readers. Thank you so much.

I would like to thank my better half, Jodie, and my in-laws for their patience and understanding during my absence; my mother, for first showing me how to draw; my brother, Kent, for letting me do the anatomical renderings for his pre-med projects ("Look what came of it!"); and my sister Laura and my brother Glen for their constant, loving support.

I would like to thank the teachers who have been instrumental in my career: Mr. Iverson, Mr. John Montelongo, and Mr. William Cumming. Your guidance, instruction, and wit have been invaluable.

I would also like to thank all the staff at LWW for their professionalism and kind support in the production of this book.

Michael A. Martyn

Reviewers

CARRIE ABRAHAM, PT, MPH, OCS
Clinical Assistant Professor
Wheeling Jesuit University
Wheeling, WV

LAURA ALLEN, NCTMB
Owner
THERA-SSAGE
Rutherfordton, NC

JONATHAN H. ANNING, PhD
Assistant Professor
Slippery Rock University
Slippery Rock, PA

NINA BEAMAN, MS, RNC-AWHC, CMA (AAMA)
Director of Nursing and Allied Health
Bryant & Stratton College
Richmond, VA

LORI DEWALD, EdD, ATC, CHES
Athletic Training Program Director
University of Minnesota Duluth
Duluth, MN

G. KELLEY FITZGERALD, PT, PhD, OCS
Associate Professor, Department of Physical Therapy, School of Health and
    Rehabilitation Sciences
University of Pittsburgh
Pittsburgh, PA

MICHAEL KRACKOW, PhD, ATC, PTA, CSCS
Associate Professor, Director, ATEP
College of Health Sciences
Roanoke, VA

STEPHEN M. PERLE, DC, MS
Professor of Clinical Sciences
Adjunct Professor of Mechanical Engineering
University of Bridgeport
Bridgeport, CT

MATT RADELET, MS, ATC, CSCS
Associate Athletic Trainer
University of Arizona
Tucson, AZ

ROBERT RUHLING, PhD
Professor
George Mason University
Manassas, VA

DEREK SURANIE, MEd, ATC
Assistant Professor
ATEP Director
North Georgia College & State University
Dahlonega, GA

GORDON WILCOX, MSc, CSEP, CEP
Professor
Algonquin College
Ottawa, Ontario
Canada

Contents

PART THREE
Special Stretches and Stretching Programs

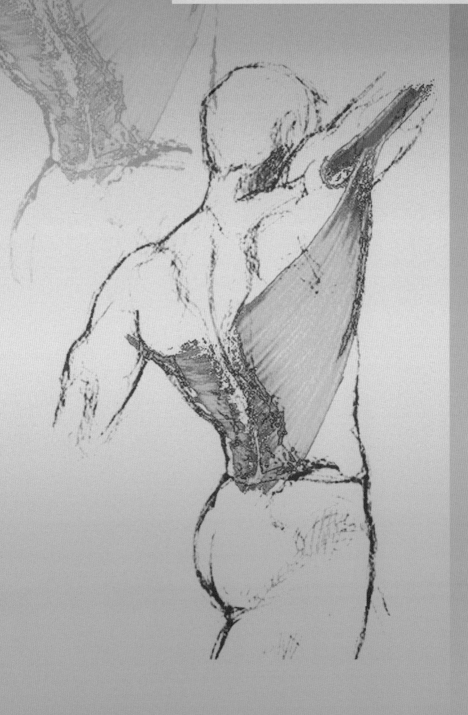

PART ONE

Stretching
Fundamentals

Introduction to Stretching

S tretching is the application of force to musculotendinous structures in order to achieve a change in their length, usually for the purposes of improving joint range of motion, reducing stiffness or soreness, or preparing for activity. Stretching is generally achieved by exercises that place muscles in a lengthened position for a prescribed period of time. There are many different methods purported to achieve this end, though few are supported by the literature. *Stretching for Functional Flexibility* combines the related scientific literature with proven clinical techniques in order to outline the safest and most effective means of stretching possible.

The opening section of this chapter describes the benefits of stretching that have been supported by valid research, as well as situations in which stretching is not advised. This discussion is followed by a description of a number of the more popular types of stretches. The chapter then identifies the mechanics of stretching, including a discussion of the involved tissues and the likely mechanisms for their lengthening. Finally, we explore the role of stretching within a full physical fitness program.

WHY STRETCH: THE BENEFITS OF STRETCHING

Our society has become ever more sedentary, with automation replacing many tasks that once caused us to move through, and thereby help maintain, our range of motion (ROM). Clinicians may prescribe stretching programs for many reasons, including improving performance, decreasing risk of injuries, rehabilitating after injury, improving posture, reducing aches and pains, and promoting relaxation. Additionally, as society has become ever more sedentary, with automation replacing many tasks that once caused us to move through, and thereby maintain our range of motion, the need for maintaining or improving our flexibility has become ever more pertinent. This chapter examines the known benefits of stretching and also calls into question a few very popular claims. In most, if not all, of the possible applications listed above, the primary goal is to improve, or at least maintain, range of motion.

Maintains and Improves Range of Motion

Maintenance or improvement in available ranges of motion is a fundamental benefit of the proper flexibility program. Limitations in ROM may interfere with activities of daily living, as when an individual with restricted knee flexion has difficulty ascending or descending stairs. These restrictions can also have indirect or secondary effects. For example, an individual with significantly shortened calves and a resultant lack of dorsiflexion (ankle bend) will likely compensate with increased hip flexion (lifting the knee higher) to allow the toes to clear the ground during the swing phase of gait (Fig. 1.1). The side effect of this chronic, excessive hip flexion may well be hip pain. Stretching to lengthen the restricted tissues may help resolve these limitations in function by improving the individual's ROM.

Stretching can also improve the performance of particular movements or movement patterns required by an individual's occupation or sport. It is hard to imagine anyone seriously pursuing any range-challenging sport or performing art without an integral flexibility program. Baseball, basketball, volleyball, track, tennis, soccer, and many others possess particular patterns of flexibility needs, demanding appropriate range of motion at many joints. Even more challenging from a flexibility perspective are sports or pursuits such as ballet, martial arts, or gymnastics in which athletes with "normal" levels of flexibility are challenged to attain "super-normal" levels.

Obviously, as particular levels of flexibility are important to success in many sports or activities, effective training programs must include appropriate strength, conditioning, functional, *and* flexibility training.

Research supports the connection between stretching and improvements in ROM. De Weijer et al found an 8-degree improvement in range that lasted for 24 hours following a single 30-second static stretch of the hamstring.[1] Winters et al found both

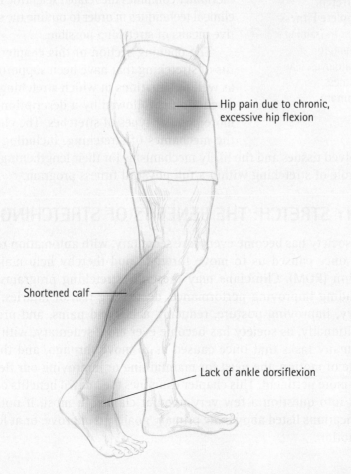

Hip pain due to chronic, excessive hip flexion

Shortened calf

Lack of ankle dorsiflexion

FIGURE 1.1 Significantly shortened calves and a resultant lack of dorsiflexion (ankle bend), resulting in increased hip flexion (lifting the knee higher) to allow the toes to clear the ground during the swing phase of gait.

active and passive stretching to be beneficial in reducing hip flexor tightness.[2] Nelson and Bandy showed a 12-degree gain in hamstring flexibility after a 6-week stretching program.[3]

While there is much evidence to support that ROM improves with stretching, there remains much debate about the magnitude of these gains and about the most effective means to achieve them.

Prevention of Injuries

Though there is little evidence linking the performance of stretching programs alone to the reduction of injury rates, most medical and training professionals will attest to the value of a flexibility program as a necessary and integral part of an overall training program. Most, if not all, athletic or health and fitness training programs include a stretching component. Further research is needed to investigate how flexibility programs fit into overall training programs and how their inclusion affects injury risk. Moore suggested that the implementation of workplace stretching programs may benefit employees with improved flexibility and possibly decreased risk of injuries.[4]

There is evidence that athletes with restricted ROM may be more likely to be injured than their more flexible counterparts. Witvrouw et al found that soccer players with more limited flexibility in their quadriceps or hamstrings were more likely to be injured during the soccer season.[5] Dadebo et al showed a significant correlation between the use of stretching programs and the decreased incidence of hamstring injuries in professional soccer players.[6] Stretching can improve flexibility in those individuals with ROM limitations.

Recent evidence has shown that stretching *before* competition is unlikely to reduce injury risk and appears to decrease performance in a number of tasks. This will be discussed later.

Injury Rehabilitation

Injuries generally fall into two major categories: acute or chronic. Acute injuries are those that have occurred relatively recently, as opposed to chronic injuries that seem to remain symptomatic well beyond their expected phase of healing. Acute injuries can be either traumatic or repetitive in origin. Whether acute or chronic, all injuries involve damaged tissue, usually to bone, muscle, ligament, tendon, nerve, vascular, lymphatic, or connective tissue. Most often, the injury will involve a combination of the above. In any case, there will usually be some loss of motion, strength, and function due to the resulting pain, inflammation, and scar tissue formation. Stretching is an essential and fundamental component of rehabilitation as it promotes restoration of normal joint function. Carefully controlled stretching may improve ROM via limiting excessive or inappropriate scar tissue formation. Malliaropoulos et al showed a significantly shorter time period required to regain normal ROM, as well as a significantly shorter period of time required in rehabilitation, in the stretching versus the control groups.[7] Determining the extent of these losses and designing a program to address them is a major challenge of successful rehabilitation. The application of a stretching exercise (i.e., frequency, intensity, duration) must be carefully modified to meet the needs of the injured tissue. Details of this will be discussed in Chapter 10.

Additionally, research suggests that stretching may also promote rehabilitation from injuries because of its effects at the cellular level. There is evidence that the mechanical elongation and the increased tensile forces applied during stretching increase the metabolic processes of cell proliferation, differentiation, and matrix formation, and may therefore be beneficial to tendon and ligament healing.[8] Bosch et al showed increases in fibronectin and collagen type I and III as a response to cyclic stretching.[9] A study by Squier suggested that the application of mechanical tension may increase the formation of myofibroblasts, the precursors to muscle cells, but more research on this effect is needed.[10] Skutek et al suggests that mechanical stretching activates intracellular signaling pathways, which in turn induce cellular apoptosis, and may essentially effect tendon remodeling.[11] However, while stretching seems to promote cellular-level changes compatible with tissue healing, research also indicates the need for care in dosage and application to avoid producing excessive inflammatory responses and the formation of scar tissue,[8] as well as to avoid overstretching tissues that can result in reduced length–tension relationships.[12]

As just noted, stretching is a key component of successful rehabilitation programs. Stretching, however, must be applied at the appropriate stage in the healing process. Traumatic joint injuries may require joint mobilization in which pressure is applied to the appropriate joint structures while carefully protecting others. Often, after successful joint mobilization, stretching exercises can be safely applied to lengthen the muscle tendon unit and further increase the joint's ROM. In cases of chronic overuse, the individual's exercise or other activity pattern should first be modified, and the movement mechanics corrected if necessary.

In either case a reduced ROM at a particular joint or joints may be the result. These restrictions may be effectively treated with careful stretching programs. Stretching is very important in regaining normal ROM, but its application parameters should be carefully controlled. Timing is also very important. *Painful tissue should never be aggressively stretched,* though in most cases careful motion through the "pain-free" ranges may be quite beneficial. Aggressively stretching recently injured tissue will not help it heal and may actually increase the level of injury. This explains why many individuals discover that their injury finally heals shortly after they stop stretching it. Details regarding stretching and its use during recovery from injuries will be covered in Chapter 10.

Posture

From a biomechanical perspective, abnormally shortened or contracted muscles must affect the resting position of joints and therefore postural alignment. For example, tight chest, or "pectoralis," muscles promote forward shoulder posture, as tight hamstrings may promote a loss of lumbar lordosis (reduced low back curve). With this understanding, most clinicians would intervene to stretch shortened muscles (and hopefully strengthen those muscles that are abnormally weak and/or lengthened) and thereby improve postural alignment. The research is as yet inconclusive regarding the real effects of stretching exercise on posture. A study by Wang et al examined the effects of a 6-week stretching and strengthening program and found a decrease in thoracic anterior inclination, though no change was observed in resting scapular position.[13]

Does the lack of conclusive evidence preclude the recommendation of stretching for individuals with poor posture? Certainly not. Posture is the result of a number of factors including muscle length, resting muscle tone, muscle strength and, quite significantly, awareness and motivation. Obviously then, even if sufficient strength, awareness, and motivation are present, ideal postures cannot be attained without adequate muscle length to achieve these postures. Posture will be covered in more detail in Chapter 11.

Counteracts Sedentary Lifestyle

Achieving and maintaining an appropriate level of flexibility is especially important for people whose occupation requires long periods of time in a stationary position, such as standing or being seated in front of a computer. Such work reduces the frequency and the amplitude of motion of normal activities of daily living, like walking, reaching, and bending, that might help individuals maintain their flexibility and joint range of motion. Many "mysterious" chronic neck, shoulder, and back complaints are likely due, at least in part, to a lack of normal movement. Sjolie showed a link between lower back pain and excessive use of the television or computer. For these individuals, stretching may be a critical component of a healthy lifestyle.[14]

Relaxation

Following the initial discomfort during application, stretching generally results in a pleasant, relaxed feeling in the muscle immediately afterward. The mechanism for this is unclear; however, stimulation of the stretch receptors in muscle, tendon, and ligament tissue probably plays a part. Wiemann and Hahn showed a decrease in EMG following a 15-minute period of hamstring stretching.[15] In a review article on stretching, Shrier et al suggests that stretching may induce some level of anesthesia.[16] This may contribute to our perception that stretching "feels good." Certainly many practitioners of yoga and similar movement arts will attest to the benefits of stretching in promoting relaxation.

Treatment and Prevention of Lower Back Pain

About 80% of Americans will experience lower back pain at some point in their lives.[17] Lower back pain is a significant cause of lost work time, reduced productivity, and workers' compensation claims, not to mention the disruption of the individual's personal and recreational life. A lack of flexibility is often a factor in chronic back pain. Abnormally shortened muscles affect the resting and functioning positions of the spine. Sjolie showed a significant correlation between lower back pain and both below-average hip flexion and below-average hamstring length.[14]

Chronically contracted muscles can cause an imbalance from front to back or from side to side. For example, a shortened psoas, or hip flexor muscle, on the right side may cause a slight right side bending in the lumbar spine. This may result in increased compression of the facet joints on the right side and/or increased stretch or tension in the paraspinal musculature on the left side. It might also cause an increase in the anterior

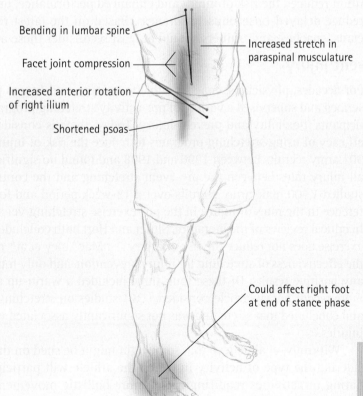

Bending in lumbar spine

Facet joint compression

Increased anterior rotation of right ilium

Shortened psoas

Increased stretch in paraspinal musculature

Could affect right foot at end of stance phase

FIGURE 1.2 Terminal stance with a shortened hip flexor, causing an anterior rotation of the right ilium.

(forward) rotation of the right ilium, which might be exacerbated at the end of the stance phase of the right foot (Fig. 1.2). While these mechanics may seen to be benign initially, the stress on the impacted soft tissues and joints can lead to significant micro-trauma, and hence injury, over time and repetition.

Reduces Age-related Declines in Health and Fitness

Declines in health and fitness with age are inevitable. Challenges in cardiovascular fitness, balance, strength, flexibility, and general function may be obvious in elderly adults. Ageing adults experience a loss of flexibility likely due to the stiffening of con-nective tissues such as cartilage, ligaments, and tendons. Muscle atrophy is also a major change associated with age, with a loss of both size and number of muscle cells. By age 80, there may be a 40% loss in the number of muscle fibers present at birth.[18]

These changes tend to be relatively small but are often complicated by inactiv-ity. However, the rate and magnitude of these changes are often very modifiable with appropriate exercise. Therefore, exercise programs promoting strength, flexibility, balance and coordination, and cardiovascular fitness become increasingly important as we age. For many elderly adults, old injuries and disorders such as arthritis may cause pain and stiffness further contributing to losses in ROM. Fortunately, seden-tary older adults have shown very significant gains in strength, flexibility and cardio-vascular fitness when participating in structured exercise programs.[19,20,21] As these declines progress with age, intervention with appropriate flexibility and condition-ing programs also become increasingly important as we age.

SITUATIONS IN WHICH STRETCHING IS NOT ADVISED

Although stretching confers numerous benefits substantiated by valid, reliable research, there are a number of once accepted applications that should be called into question. It was once commonly accepted that stretching before exercise or compe-tition reduced the risk of injury and enhanced performance, or that stretching helped reduce delayed-onset muscle soreness. Based on the latest research, prudent clini-cians, coaches, and trainers should at least reconsider these applications.

Pre-activity to Prevent Injury

For decades, physicians, coaches, athletic trainers, and fitness professionals have pre-scribed and supervised a variety of pre-activity stretching programs to improve the par-ticipants' flexibility and prevent injury. Today, there is considerable debate about the efficacy of using stretching programs to reduce the risk of injury. Amako et al studied 901 army recruits between 1996 and 1998 and found no significant difference in over-all injury rates between the pre-event stretching and the control groups.[22] Pope et al studied 1,500 male army recruits over a 12-week period and found no significant dif-ference in the rates of injury in the pre-exercise stretching versus the control groups.[23] In critical reviews of the literature, Shrier and Hart both concluded that stretching before exercise does not reduce the risk of injury.[24,25] MacAuley et al[26] reviewed 293 studies on the effectiveness of stretching for injury prevention, and only four of these studies found any positive results. Of these four, three included a warm-up as a co-intervention. A more recent review article considered 361 studies on stretching and sports-injury risk and concluded that stretching was not significantly associated with a reduction in total injuries.[27]

Witvrouw et al believe that some light might be shed on this controversy by con-sidering the type of activity in which the athlete will participate.[5] Athletes partici-pating in activities requiring rapid, more ballistic movements such as soccer and football (versus less-ballistic activities such as jogging, swimming, and cycling) may experience a reduced risk of injury with pre-event stretching because of the need for increased compliance in the muscle tendon unit required to perform these types of sports. While this is an interesting theory, more research is needed. It does, however, show the need to consider many variables, including the type of activity, when determining the best applications of stretching programs.

Based on the above discussion, the use of pre-exercise stretching solely for the purposes of injury prevention is without basis.

Pre-event to Improve Performance

There is also considerable debate about the advisability of pre-event stretching programs to improve athletic performance. Used for years to prepare athletes for competition, or the average jogger for a run, stretching before performance has met with some controversy. A number of recent studies have cast doubt on the usefulness of stretching programs performed immediately before activity. In a review article, Schrier[28] reviewed 23 studies of "acute" stretching (i.e., immediately before exercise) and concluded that most of the studies showed a reduction in performance. Fowles showed that muscle activation is slowed for roughly one hour following static stretch.[29] Evetovich et al showed a decrease in peak torque development as measured in the biceps brachii in young adults.[30] Fletcher et al showed a decrease in performance in the 20-meter sprint in the static stretching group.[31]

These findings have obvious implications in sports, especially those in which rapid activation of the muscle is key.

To Reduce Delayed-onset Muscle Soreness

Stretching has been prescribed and used for decades to combat delayed-onset muscle soreness (DOMS). Nevertheless, it is difficult to find any valid research that clearly shows a decrease in DOMS as a result of stretching.

DOMS usually occurs in response to a relatively intense bout of exercise to which the individual's body is not yet accustomed. Related soreness usually occurs about 24 hours post-exercise and may persist for up to two weeks. In addition to the soreness, there is generally an associated loss of strength.[32,33] It is thought to result from damaged muscle tissue and the consequent inflammatory response.[34]

Herbert and Gabriel concluded that stretching before or after exercise does not significantly limit post exercise soreness or reduce the risk of injury.[35] Though stretching has been prescribed for the relief of DOMS for many years, its lack of justification is not breaking news. Several older studies have found it ineffective. For example, a study of pre-exercise stretching with warm-up and a study of both pre-exercise and post-exercise stretching showed no significant effect.[32,36] Rodenburg et al studied the effects of warm-up and stretching before, and massage immediately following eccentric exercise, and was still unable to conclusively show any benefits to the experimental group.[37]

Interestingly, Smith et al compared the effects of static and ballistic stretching on DOMS and found that both actually produced DOMS in subjects unaccustomed to this type of exercise.[38] It also showed that static stretching produced significantly greater symptoms and levels of creatine kinase, than did ballistic stretching. Creatine kinase levels are an accepted marker for measuring DOMS.[32,34]

In light of the above research, it makes little sense to stretch aggressively to reduce muscle soreness. As mentioned earlier, stretching recently strained, painful tissue is never advisable. It may be therapeutic, however, to carefully move through available ROMs and to progress this range as symptoms decline and more motion returns, rather than attempt to "force" new ROMs. Active movement, emphasizing the antagonists as much as possible, will allow gentle passive motion of the injured agonist musculature and may enhance the healing process by facilitating blood flow.

TYPES OF STRETCHING

There are numerous stretching techniques including static, active, passive, proprioceptive neuromuscular facilitation (PNF), and ballistic. This section identifies the fundamental types of stretches and points out some of the merits, and possibly the limitations or possible risks, associated with each. Research has failed to conclusively identify the most effective method. Davis et al found that static stretching was more effective than PNF stretching,[39] while Sady et al and Etnyre et al suggested that PNF stretching may be more effective.[40,41] Webright et al showed active stretching equal in effectiveness to static stretching.[42]

"Stretching" generally refers to elongating by force. For the purposes of this discussion, stretching refers to applying sufficient force to lengthen musculotendinous structures to either maintain or improve the ROM at a particular joint or joints. ROM is generally self-explanatory; nevertheless, two subcategories deserve definition here. At a given joint, active range of motion (AROM) and passive range of motion (PROM) may be quite different, and understanding this difference is quite important to the clinician. AROM is the range of motion that a particular joint can be moved through via the action of the muscles alone. It is always less than or equal to PROM, which is the amount of motion available through application of outside forces. For example, an athlete lying prone can actively flex his or her knee to roughly 125 or 130 degrees. The application of outside forces, such as a therapist or trainer's hand pushing the athlete's heel toward his or her buttock, may result in 140 or 150 degrees of flexion. Understanding this difference may be critical in determining how to, or whether to, apply stretching forces in particular situations. For example, pain limiting PROM exercise (such as static stretching) will generally not preclude the use of active motion exercise throughout pain-free ranges. Details of this discussion will be covered in Chapter 10 (Stretching for Rehabilitation of Injuries).

Static

Probably the most widely accepted form of stretching, and method that will be recommended herein, static stretching is likely the safest, easiest to perform and at least among the most effective. It involves taking a muscle to its maximum length and then carefully applying a longitudinal force to achieve lengthened tissue.

The individual performing the stretch assumes a particular stretching position and generally applies the stretching force by himself or herself. A classic example is the typical hamstring stretch in which the individual places his or her heel on an elevated surface with a straight leg. He or she then leans forward at the waist (though in this text we will correct this) until a stretch is achieved at the hamstring. In this manner, the individual performing the stretch is under complete control of the intensity of the stretch and can make adjustments in position or tension immediately in response to the sensation of stretch. The details of performing static stretching will be covered in Chapter 3.

Active

Active stretching generally refers to stretching in which the application of force comes from the active contraction of muscles that are antagonistic (move in the opposite direction) to the muscle being stretched. In this way, there is excellent control of the stretching force, lessening the possibility of injury. Research shows active stretching yields improvements in range of motion roughly equal to that found with static stretching.[2,42] An example of this type of stretch might be extending your arm and hand out in front of you and then bending (flexing) your wrist and hand downward as far as possible. This should produce a stretching sensation in the top of your forearm. In this case, you are using your wrist and finger flexors (the antagonists) to affect a stretch in your wrist and finger extensors.

A possible drawback to this technique is the lack of stretching force available in many situations. Take for example a basic calf, or more specifically a gastrocnemius, stretch. To employ this technique, you would have to use the dorsiflexors of your ankle to impart enough force to effectively stretch your gastrocnemius. As a quick trial of this will show, there is insufficient force development for this to occur. Active stretching is, even in the case mentioned above, an excellent way to maintain or improve AROM and may be the preferred stretching modality in many injury-related or rehabilitation scenarios. These scenarios will be discussed in Chapter 10.

Proprioceptive Neuromuscular Facilitation (PNF)

PNF is a detailed science in itself and a basic discussion regarding it is covered in Chapter 11 (Advanced Stretching). In general, PNF stretching involves the coordinated use of neuromuscular reflexes to enhance stretching outcomes. An example would be the use of the reflex relaxation of a muscle brought on by contraction of the muscle's antagonist to prepare the target muscle, or agonist, for stretch. In a hamstring stretch for example, the clinician would first extend the client's hip and flex his or her knee to the end of range where resistance is felt. Next, the client would be asked to maximally contract his or her hamstring against the clinician's resistance, which would not allow any movement. This contraction might be held for 6 seconds, which would be immediately followed by relaxation of the muscle and the clinician's application of a stretching force, moving the hip into further flexion. Theoretically, the reflex relaxation in the muscle following its maximal contraction will allow for greater gains in hip flexion and, therefore, hamstring lengthening.

Ballistic

Taking a muscle to its maximum length and then applying a stretching force to it in a bouncing or repetitive manner is ballistic stretching. Most health and fitness professionals agree that ballistic stretching carries a higher risk of injury than static stretching. Bouncing may cause the intermittent application of excessive tension to the muscle-tendon unit causing microscopic (or worse) tearing of tissue. Additionally, since the muscle-tendon unit's natural response to the rapid application of tension is reflex contraction of the muscle under stress, repetitive stretching may cause repetitive contractions in the muscle. This reflex contraction is often referred to as the myotactic reflex and is described later. Based on this reflex contraction and the excess tension developed, ballistic stretching may not be the most productive or safest method to lengthen tissue. Most professionals will agree that it is necessary to relax a muscle before it can be effectively stretched.

Self-stretching Versus Partner or Clinician Stretching

Static, PNF, and ballistic stretches can be performed either by the individual or another person. Though popular in the world of professional athletics, the application of force by someone other than the individual undergoing the stretch immediately introduces an element of risk not present when the individual stretches himself or herself. Probably the most effective safeguard against injury is sensation of feel. The finely tuned sensation of stretch is imperative for both effective and safe stretching. It is not possible for even the most skilled clinician to feel what the individual being stretched feels; therefore, the clinician cannot make the appropriate adaptations with the same level of acuity as the individual.

This is not to say that partner or clinician stretching is never appropriate, as there are many cases, particularly in the rehabilitation of injuries, in which it may be the best choice. Anyone who has ever seen or experienced the scar-laden, range-restricted, post-surgical total knee replacement can attest to the value of stretching applied by a skilled and careful clinician. The value of a coach or athletic trainer stretching an uninjured, highly-skilled athlete may remain the subject of some debate.

MECHANICS OF STRETCHING

In order to better understand and make more informed decisions regarding the application of stretching programs, it is important to have some understanding of the actual tissues involved and the possible mechanisms responsible for their lengthening. The following section will investigate these basics.

Tissues Involved in Stretching

Human motion is possible because of a coordinated interaction between various tissues. These tissues that produce movement about a given joint in one direction also resist movement about that joint in the opposite direction. These tissues include bones, muscles ligaments, skin, fascia, fat, and vascular, lymphatic, and nervous tissues.

It seems clear that stretching lengthens soft tissues, but the changes it elicits at a neuromuscular level are still the subject of debate. Some discussion of the related tissue types is in order. We can then investigate the physiologic properties contributing to tissue lengthening.

A classic study by Johns and Wright described the relative contributions of various tissues to joint stiffness, attributing 47% to the joint capsule, 41% to the fascial component of muscle, 10% to the tendon, and 2% to the skin.[43] In exploring the pursuit of flexibility through stretching, therefore, we are primarily concerned with the resistance offered by the joint capsule and its associated ligamentous structures and the muscle-tendon unit and its associated fascia. Stretching the joint capsule generally requires specific forces applied to the joint in a gliding type motion roughly parallel to the surfaces of that joint. These techniques are usually performed by osteopaths, chiropractors, or physical therapists trained in joint mobilization or manipulation. In our pursuit of flexibility through stretching, it is primarily the fascial component of the muscle-tendon unit that we are trying to affect. In order to have a greater understanding of this, it may be helpful to review the general structure of muscle. While a detailed discussion of muscle structure and function are beyond the scope of this text, a basic overview may be helpful in understanding stretching theory.

Fascia may be described as a fibrous or "sheet-like" connective tissue used throughout the body to add structure and support to skin, bones, muscles, and organs. Figure 1.3 (next page) shows an example of fascia in the lower extremity. Fascia exists in two broad categories: superficial, and deep. Superficial fascia lies just below the skin and generally covers the entire body. Deep fascia covers each muscle and its tendon as well as being a major component of muscle tissue. Hence, fascia is often a primary limitation in ROM restrictions. As can be seen in Figure 1.3, each individual muscle cell, which contains the actual actin and myosin filaments that make contraction possible, is wrapped in fascia called an endomysium. A number of these cells, and the nerve cells that supply them, are bundled together to create a fascicle, which is wrapped in fascial tissue referred to as the perimysium. Several fascicles are bundled together with respective nerves, blood vessels, and muscle spindles (to be discussed later) by the epimysium, which is the fascial layer covering the entire muscle and blending with the tendon. The epimysium helps affix the entire structure to the bone.

Stretching the fascial component of muscle is the primary aim of static stretching, and differentiation of this tissue from others is critical in the safe application of stretching exercise.

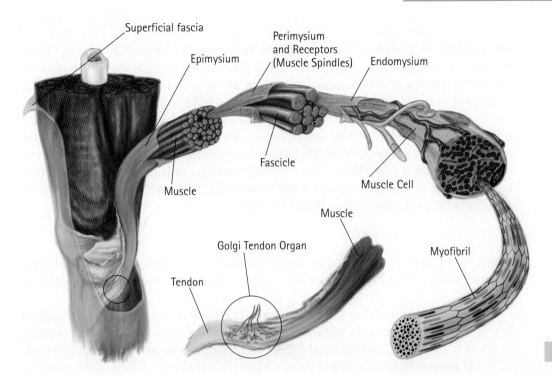

Superficial fascia

Epimysium

Perimysium and Receptors (Muscle Spindles)

Endomysium

Fascicle

Muscle Cell

Muscle

Muscle

Golgi Tendon Organ

Myofibril

Tendon

FIGURE 1.3 Muscle

In fact, when an individual shows notably restricted movement, and this restriction clearly does not originate within the muscle (i.e., there is an obvious restriction in movement and the implicated muscle-tendon unit seems to have no tension in it), he or she should be referred for medical diagnosis. This is especially true in cases when the motion is limited by (joint) pain.

Stretching applies forces to the joint that are quite different from those applied to the muscle. The forces applied to the joint are more perpendicular to the joint surfaces and usually include a combination of traction, compression, and shear depending on the particular part of the joint and on the particular stretch. The interested reader is referred to Appendix A for suggested readings on joint mechanics.

In certain circumstances, individuals will believe that they are stretching muscle when in fact they are stretching nervous or other tissues. For example, individuals frequently add dorsiflexion of their foot to a hamstring stretch because of the enhanced sensation they receive in their posterior thigh and knee. A quick review of basic anatomy will reveal that dorsiflexing the foot does not change the length of the hamstring; therefore, the resulting sensation must be from tension developed in another tissue which, in this case, is most likely additional tension placed on the sciatic/tibial nerve and or fascia. If the individual is experiencing lower back pain or related hamstring tightness or pain, stretching nervous tissue could exacerbate the pain or lead to further injury. The increased sensation of stretch caused by the addition of dorsiflexion will also likely decrease the amount of stretch applied to the hamstring, thereby decreasing the overall effectiveness of the stretch at its intended target. Use the information provided in this book to perform prescribed stretches appropriately to lengthen the target tissue and improve ROM safely.

Possible Mechanisms Contributing to Tissue Lengthening

It is easy to imagine lengthening a muscle. It is more difficult to understand what happens within the muscle itself. Does the tissue actually lengthen, or is more tissue added? Perhaps, increases in flexibility are merely increases in one's tolerance to stretch? Is the real answer a combination of the above?

HYPERPLASIA

Hyperplasia is the growth of muscle tissue by an increase in the number of cells versus an increase in the size of each individual cell (hypertrophy). There is some evidence that particular stretching scenarios actually result in an increase in the number of sarcomeres present in the muscle fiber. Tabary et al found significant increases in the number of sarcomeres in cat soleus muscles which were immobilized in lengthened positions.[44] Coutinho et al showed decreased atrophy and a decrease in the number of sarcomeres versus the control group in rat soleus muscles immobilized in shortened position but stretched every third day.[45] While more specific research needs to be done, the addition and subtraction of sarcomeres in response to stretching, or shortening, may be a possible contributor to observed tissue length changes.

PLASTIC DEFORMATION

To understand increases in flexibility that are attributable to actual changes in the length of tissue, it may help to first discuss the elastic, viscoelastic, and plastic properties of muscles.

An elastic substance is capable of changing length when an external force is applied to it. If this external force is released, this elastic material will return to its original length. In contrast, a plastic material can be deformed with an externally applied load, but it will not return to its original length. Viscosity may be described as the property of a fluid that causes it to resist flowing. For example, honey has a much greater viscosity than water, which is easily seen if you attempt to pour each. Most biologic tissue has both a viscous and an elastic component, and may therefore be described as having "viscoelastic" properties. Magnusson showed 30% viscoelastic stress relaxation (basically, a reduction in the amount of force needed to hold a muscle at a given length) in a muscle held in a static position of stretch for 90 seconds.[46] This may explain a major portion of the observed change in length occurring during a single stretch. Because muscle tissue has viscoelastic properties, tensile loads applied rapidly will be met with more resistance, initially limiting the elastic potential, whereas loads applied more gradually over longer periods of time will allow for greater elastic change. We can then see the importance of the rate of application of force when stretching muscle. Taylor et al investigated the viscoelastic properties of muscle and concluded that the risk of injury may be more related to the rate of force application than the actual technique involved.[47] Based on the above discussion it makes sense to apply stretching forces carefully, gradually increasing the tension as needed.

Plastic changes in length are those that occur as a response to sufficient tensile loads held for sufficient periods of time. "Sufficient" is obviously relative and depends on the particular tissue under load. In musculotendinous tissues, the load must be sufficient to first exhaust the elastic limit inherent in the muscle. The practical application of these loads will be discussed in Chapter 2.

OTHER POSSIBLE MECHANISMS

Increased tolerance to stretch, decreased muscular stiffness, and decreases in neuromuscular tone are additional proposed mechanisms for improvements in ROM. Increased tolerance to stretch implies no actual change in tissue length but rather a decrease in the amount of perceived stretch "sensation," allowing for movement throughout a greater ROM. Decreased muscle stiffness is thought to allow a given amount lengthening with a decreased amount of force. Laroche et al concluded that increases in ROM that occurred in response to both static and ballistic stretching was more likely due to an increase in stretch tolerance than to changes in muscle elasticity.[45] Halbertsma et al concluded that the measured improvements in

ROM were due primarily to increased stretch tolerance rather than decreased stiffness or changes in muscle elasticity.[49,50] A review article by Shrier et al also concluded that the decrease in stiffness is not as important as the increase in stretch tolerance.[16]

Finally, a decrease in neuromuscular tone may also play a part in the change in length of a muscle-tendon unit. As all skeletal muscle maintains a certain amount of activation, or tone even at "rest," an increase in the amount of this tone will restrict motion. Possible causes of increased tone include anxiety, pain, or any neurologic or neuromuscular disorder such as cerebral palsy, stroke, or head injury.

As we have seen, the properties contributing to tissue lengthening and the ultimate improvement in ROM are not yet fully understood. Suggestions for additional readings on the subject of tissue properties and proposed mechanisms of change are provided in Appendix A.

WHAT HAPPENS DURING A STATIC STRETCH?

Figure 1.4A shows a muscle-tendon unit at rest. From this point the joint is first moved through its ROM by a force created outside of the muscle itself. This force can be produced by the movements developed by the individual himself or herself or by a partner or clinician. During this period there is little change beyond the passive muscle lengthening that occurs as the actin and myosin filaments slide past one another. As the tissues reach their resting length, slack is taken up in the muscle-tendon unit. The wave-like orientation of the collagenous fibers within the tendon and other connective tissues begins to straighten (Fig. 1.4B), and after all of the slack is taken up in the system, the connective tissues, including the fascial layers comprising the muscle and the tendon, reach their elastic limit (Fig. 1.4C). Some research studies suggest that a majority of the lengthening that takes place is due to the change in length of the tendon.[35] Continuing to apply tension after this point should introduce plastic change in the connective tissues.

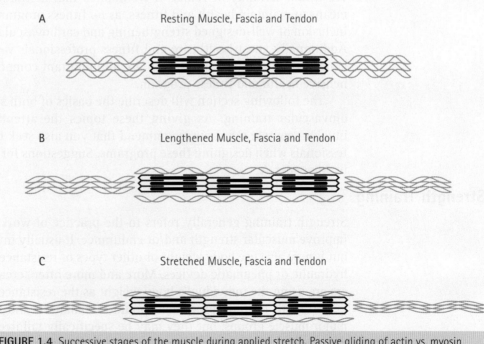

FIGURE 1.4 Successive stages of the muscle during applied stretch. Passive gliding of actin vs. myosin fibers, straightening of wave-like collagen, elastic limit of connective tissues.

In practical application, the stretching of tissues cannot take place independent of the neuromuscular control mechanisms inherent in human physiology. Two common reflexes play an important role in the pursuit of flexibility. The myotactic, or "stretch" reflex, is elicited whenever tension is applied to change the length of the muscle. Receptors known as muscle spindles are arranged within the perimysium (see Fig. 1.3). These receptors pass information on to the spinal cord, which responds by either causing contraction if the muscle is being stretched or relaxation if tension is being removed from it. The common knee-jerk reflex test is an example of the myotactic reflex (see Fig. 1.3). It is easy to see that excessive or rapid applications of stretching forces may result in muscle shortening rather than lengthening. This mechanism also calls into question ballistic stretching practices.

How then can a stretch occur? Holding a stretch with sufficient force will elicit another reflex, sometimes referred to as the inverse stretch reflex. This reflex involves the Golgi tendon organ (GTO). GTOs are arranged in series with the fascicles of the tendon, rather than within the muscle (see Fig. 1.3). These receptors respond to strong and sustained stretch by overriding the input of the muscle spindles and causing a reflex relaxation of the muscle. An individual performing a particular stretch may experience this the moment the muscle lets go and more range is achieved. It is likely that the actual plastic deformation can begin to take place some time after this.

The amount of tension applied, along with the frequency, intensity, and duration of its application, will be covered in Chapter 2.

Fortunately, from a clinical or practical perspective, a detailed understanding of tissue properties is not critical, as long as therapeutic outcomes are fairly well understood. Clinicians are much more concerned with the efficacy of stretching as a modality for improving flexibility to enhance health, fitness, performance, and general well-being. Meaningful outcomes can be achieved through careful attention to individual responses throughout the duration of the exercise programs.

COMPLETE FITNESS

We would certainly be remiss if we implied that flexibility alone was a sufficient means to maintain health and fitness, as no fitness program is complete without the inclusion of well-designed strengthening and cardiovascular conditioning programs. Additionally, most healthcare and fitness professionals would agree that nutrition, general health, and mental health are all important components in a truly comprehensive health and fitness program.

The following section will describe the basics of both strength training and cardiovascular training. As giving these topics the attention they deserve would involve separate texts, we recommend that you also seek the advice of trusted professionals when designing these programs. Suggestions for further reading are listed in Appendix A.

Strength Training

Strength training generally refers to the practice of working against resistance to improve muscular strength and/or endurance. It usually involves the use of weights, but it may also use body weight or other types of resistance such as that provided by hydraulic or pneumatic devices. More and more often, creative therapists and trainers are using the individual's body weight as the resistance.

Strength training programs should be balanced and work most of the body's major muscle groups, but they may be specifically tailored to emphasize that musculature most pertinent to the sport or activity at hand. They should also take into account individual strengths and weaknesses. Appropriate strength training is of obvious benefit to athletic performance, but it is also critical in the rehabilitation of injured tissues and joints. Improved strength should reduce the risk of injury in both athletic pursuits, and in activities of daily living. Strength training is also very important in moderating age-related injuries, declines in strength and fitness, and loss of function.[51] As mentioned earlier, the number of muscle fibers may decrease as much as 40% by age 80,[18] which depending on the individual's present state of training, could also amount to a very significant loss in overall muscle mass. In addition to the loss of mass there appears to be an increase in the amount of intramuscular fat with age.[52] Fortunately, research shows that proper strength training can help restore muscle mass in elderly subjects.[53]

Proper application of strength training programs is essential for all ages, not only for success, but to avoid injuries resulting from the training program. While detailed coverage of strength training is beyond the scope of this text, general guidelines will be discussed below.

Strengthening programs for beginners should emphasize low loads and correct movement patterns. It is better to begin with relatively lower loads and higher repetitions versus the relatively higher loads and decreased repetitions that may be necessary in more specific and advanced programs. This way, the beginner can focus on correct movement patterns and allows his or her tendons and joints to adapt to new loads. Choosing a weight that can be comfortably moved throughout the prescribed ROM for roughly 20 repetitions assures that the individual will not have to struggle with too heavy a weight and risk a strain injury. Beginners can do one set of 20–30 repetitions for their first month and then move into multiple sets of lower repetitions with higher resistance as they progress or as the specificity of their training demands. Doing only one set of exercises allows (time) for a greater variety of exercises and can provide for a more balanced and interesting workout. Additionally, experience suggests that those individuals who take on a more reasonable workout tend to stick with their program. This is in contrast to those who are worked so hard in the beginning that they find it difficult to return to their subsequent training sessions.

Training for Cardiovascular Fitness

Cardiovascular fitness generally refers to the ability of an individual's heart and lungs to provide oxygen to the working muscles via his or her vascular system. The benefits of cardiovascular fitness are well known and almost universally accepted. Appropriate levels of cardiovascular fitness may confer numerous health benefits including decreased risk of cardiovascular disease, hypertension, diabetes, and stroke. Appropriate training protocols yield successful results, even in ageing adults. Ades et al showed improvements in peak aerobic capacity after just 3 months of training.[21]

As with any exercise program, cardiovascular training programs should be begun and progressed conservatively. Most individuals would be well advised to have a general medical checkup before beginning an exercise program, especially if he or she has any suspicions regarding health issues.

After medical clearance, individuals can begin exercising and may wish to use the guidelines recommended by the American College of Sports Medicine (ACSM), which outlines a program 3–5× per week, consisting of 20–60 minutes of aerobic exercise.[54] Healthy individuals should exercise at a low intensity that elevates the heart rate to 50–85% of maximum (generally accepted as 220-age). This should allow the individual to carry on a conversation during the exercise. The ACSM also recommends a 5–10 minute warm-up before exercise and a cool-down period afterward.

SUMMARY

A well-designed flexibility program has many benefits. Stretching exercises can help individuals maintain or improve their ROM and, over the long term, improve performance, improve posture, recover from injuries, and improve other aspects of their general health. Recent research calls into question the long-standing practice of using vigorous stretching programs immediately before activities as this practice seems not only to be of no value in the prevention of injuries, it may also hamper performance in certain activities. The use of stretching programs to reduce delayed-onset muscle soreness seems universally without support in the related literature.

An appropriate flexibility program should be a part of an overall health and fitness program, which also includes strengthening and cardiovascular conditioning. Careful prescription and monitoring of all fitness programs is important to ensure continued, safe practice.

The following chapter discusses general principles for the safe and effective application of stretching programs.

REFERENCES

1. De Weijer VC, Gorniak GC, Shamus E. The effect of static stretch and warmup exercise on hamstring length over the course of 24 hours. J Orthop Sports Phys Ther December 2003;33(12):727–733.
2. Winters MV, Blake CG, Trost JS, et al. Passive versus active stretching of hip flexor muscles in subjects with limited hip extension: a randomized clinical trial. Phys Ther September 2004;84(9):800–807.
3. Nelson RT, Bandy WD. Eccentric training and static stretching improve hamstring flexibility of high school males. J Athl Train September 2004;39(3):254–258.
4. Moore TM. A workplace stretching program. Physiologic and perception measurements before and after participation. AAOHN J December 1998;46(12):563–568.
5. Witvrouw E, Danneels L, Asselman P, et al. Muscle flexibility as a risk factor for developing muscle injuries in male professional soccer players. A prospective study. Am J Sports Med January–February 2003;31(1):41–6.
6. Dadebo B, White J, George KP. A survey of flexibility training protocols and hamstring strains in professional football clubs in England. Br J Sports Med August 2004;38(6):793.
7. Malliaropoulos N, Papalexandris S, Papalada A, et al. The role of stretching in rehabilitation of hamstring injuries: 80 athletes follow up. Med Sci Sports Exerc May 2004;36(5):756–759.
8. Skutek M, van Griensven M, Zeichen J, et al. Cyclic mechanical stretching enhances secretion of Interleukin 6 in human tendon fibroblasts. Knee Surg Sports Traumatol Arthrosc September 2001;9(5):322–326.
9. Bosch U, Zeichen J, Skutek M, et al. Effect of cyclical stretch on matrix synthesis of human patellar tendon cells. Unfallchirurg May 2002;105(5):437–442.
10. Squier CA. The effect of stretching on formation of myofibroblasts in mouse skin. Cell Tissue Res 1981;220(2):325–335.
11. Skutek M, van Griensven M, Zeichen J, et al. Cyclic mechanical stretching of human patellar tendon fibroblasts: activation of JNK and modulation apoptosis. Knee Surg Sports Traumatol Arthrosc March 2003;11(2):122–129.
12. Flowers KR, McClure PW, McFadden C. Management of a patient with lacerations of the tendons of the extensor digitorum and extensor indicis muscles to the index finger. Phys Ther January 1996;76(1):61–66.
13. Wang CH, McClure P, Pratt NE, et al. Stretching and strengthening exercises: their effect on three dimensional scapular kinematics. Arch Phys Med Rehabil August 1999;80(8):923–929.
14. Sjole AN. Low-back pain in adolescents is associated with poor hip mobility and high body mass index. Scand J Med Sci Sports June 2004;14(3):168–175.
15. Wiemann K, Hahn K. Influences of stretching and circulatory exercises on flexibility parameters of human hamstrings. Int J Sports Med July 1997;18(5):340–346.
16. Shrier I. Stretching before exercise: an evidence based approach. Br J Sports Med 2000:34:324–325.
17. Jones GT, Macfarlane GJ. Epidemiology of low back pain in children and adolescents. Arch Dis Child March 2005;90(3):312–316.
18. McArdle WD, Katch FI, Katch VL. Essentials of Exercise Physiology. 2nd Ed. Baltimore: Lippincott Williams and Wilkins, 2000.

19. Delecluse C, Colman V, Roelants M, et al. Exercise programs for older men: mode and intensity to induce the highest possible health-related benefits. Prev Med October 2004;39(4):823–833.
20. Woods RH, Reyes R, Welsch MA, et al. Concurrent cardiovascular and resistance training in healthy older adults. Med Sci Sports Exerc October 2001;33(10):1751–1758.
21. Ades PA, Waldmann ML, Meyer WL, et al. Skeletal muscle and cardiovascular adaptations to exercise conditioning in older coronary patients. Circulation August 1, 1996;94(3):323–30.
22. Amako M, Oda T, Masuoka K, et al. Effect of static stretching on prevention of injuries for military recruits. Mil Med June 2003;168(6):442–446.
23. Pope RP, Herbert RD, Kirwan JD, et al. A randomized trial of pre-exercise stretching for prevention of lower-limb injury. Med Sci Sports Exerc 2000;32(2):271–277.
24. Shrier I. Stretching before exercise does not reduce the risk of local muscle injury: a critical review of the clinical and basic science literature. Clin J Sport Med 1999;9(4):221–227.
25. Hart. Effect of stretching on sport injury risk: a review. Med Sci Sports Exerc March 2004;36(3):371–378.
26. MacAuley D, Best TM. Reducing the risk of injury due to exercise. Br Med J August 2002;325:451–452.
27. Thacker SB, Gilchrist J, Stroup F, Kimsey CD Jr. The impact of stretching on sports injury risk: a systematic review of the literature. Med Sci Sport Exerc 2004;36(3):371–378.
28. Shrier I. Does stretching improve performance? A systematic and critical review of the literature. Clin J Sport Med September 2004;14(5):267–273.
29. Fowles JRF, Sale DG, MacDougall JD. Reduced strength after passive stretch of the human plantar flexors. J Appl Physiol September 2000;89(3):1179–1188.
30. Evetovich TK, Nauman NJ, Conley DS, et al. Effect of static stretching of the biceps brachii on torque, electromyography, and mechanomyography during concentric isokinetic muscle actions. J Strength Cond Res August 2003;17(3):484–488.
31. Fletcher IM, Jones B. The effect of different warm-up stretch protocols on 20 meter sprint performance in trained rugby union players. J Strength Cond Res November 2004;18(4):885–888.
32. Lund H, Vestergaard-Poulsen P, Kanstrup IL, et al. The effect of passive stretching on delayed onset muscle soreness, and other detrimental effects following eccentric exercise. Scand J Med Sci Sports August 1998;8(4):216–221.
33. Johansson PH, Lindstrom L, Sundelin G, et al. The effects of preexercise stretching on muscular soreness, tenderness and force loss following heavy eccentric exercise. Scand J Med Sci Sports August 1999;9(4):219–225.
34. Smith LL, Bond JA, Holbert D, et al. Differential white cell count after two bouts of downhill running. Int J Sports Med August 1998;19(6):432–437.
35. Herbert RD, Gabriel M. Effects of stretching before and after exercising on muscle soreness and risk of injury: systematic review. BMJ August 31, 2002;325(7362):468.
36. High DM, Howley ET, Franks BD. The effects of static stretching and warm-up on prevention of delayed-onset muscle soreness. Res Q Exerc Sport December 1989;60(4):357–361.
37. Rodenburg JB, Steenbeek D, Schiereck P, et al. Warm-up, stretching and massage diminish harmful effects of eccentric exercise. Int J Sports Med October 1994;15(7):414–419.
38. Smith LL, Brunetz MH, Chenier TC, et al. The effects of static and ballistic stretching on delayed onset muscle soreness and creatine kinase. Res Q Exerc Sport March 1993;64(1):103–107.
39. Davis DS, Ashby PE, McCale KL, et al. The effectiveness of 3 stretching techniques on hamstring flexibility using consistent stretching parameters. J Strength Cond Res February 2005;19(1):27–32.
40. Sady SP, Wortman M, Blanke D. Flexibility training: ballistic, static or proprioceptive neuromuscular facilitation? Arch Phys Med Rehabil June 1982;63(6):261–263.
41. Etnyre BR, Abraham LD. Gains in range of ankle dorsiflexion using three popular stretching techniques. Am J Phys Med August 1986;65(4):189–196.
42. Webright WG, Randolf BJ, Perrin DH. Comparison of nonballistic active knee extension in neural slump position and static stretch techniques on hamstring flexibility. J Orthop Sports Phys Ther July 1997;26(1):7–13.
43. Johns RJ, Wright V. Relative Importance of various tissues in joint stiffness. J Appl Physiol 1962;17(5):824–828.
44. Tabary JC, Tabary C, Tardieu C, et al. Physiological and structural changes in the cat's soleus muscle due to immobilization at different lengths by plaster casts. J Physiol July 1972;224(1):223–244.
45. Coutinho IL, Gomes AR, Franca CN, et al. Effect of passive stretching on the immobilized soleus muscle fiber morphology. Braz J Med Biol Res December 2004;37(12):1853–1861.
46. Magnusson SP. Passive properties of human skeletal muscle during stretch maneuvers. A review. Scand J Med Sci Sports April 1998;8(2):65–77.
47. Taylor DC, Dalton JD Jr, Seaber AV, et al. Viscoelastic properties of muscle tendon units: the biomechanical effects of stretching. Am J Sports Med 1990;18(3):300–309.

48. Laroche DP, Connolly DA. Effects of stretching on passive muscle tension and response to eccentric exercise. Am J Sports Med June 2006;34(6):1000–1007.

49. Halbertsma JP, van Bolhuis AI, Goeken LN. Sport stretching: effect on passive muscle stiffness of short hamstrings. Arch Phys Med Rehabil July 1996;77(7):688–692.

50. Halbertsma JP, Goeken LN. Stretching exercises: effect on passive extensibility and stiffness in short hamstrings of healthy subjects. Arch Phys Med Rehabil September 1994;75(9):976–981.

51. Hunt A. Musculoskeletal fitness: the keystone in overall well-being and injury prevention. [Review]. Clin Orthop Relat Res April 2003;(409):96–105.

52. Pahor M, Kritchevsky S. Research hypotheses on muscle wasting, aging, loss of function and disability. J Nutr Health Aging 1998;2(2):97–100.

53. Frontera WR, Meredith CN, O'Reilly KP, et al. Strength conditioning in older men: skeletal muscle hypertrophy and improved function. J Appl Physiol March 1998;64(3):1038–1044.

54. American College of Sports Medicine 2005. Available at http://www.acsm.org. Accessed October 2005.

General Principles for Safe and Effective Stretching

T his chapter provides the information necessary for performing a stretching program safely and effectively. We begin by reviewing the terminology necessary for describing position, location, and movement. We then discuss goal setting, factors to consider for safe and effective stretching, and how to evaluate progress. An understanding of the principles in this chapter will help you select and perform an appropriate stretching program from those described in Parts II and III of this book.

TERMINOLOGY OF MOVEMENT: A BRIEF REVIEW

The *anatomical position* is a reference position for the human body used by professionals in healthcare, fitness, and the life sciences. A person in the anatomical position is standing straight up, with the arms hanging by the sides and the palms facing forward (Fig. 2.1). The lower extremities are also straight with the knees and feet facing forward. To ensure correct and consistent communication, we will use the anatomical position as a reference point when describing the location of muscle attachments, joint positions, and other aspects of anatomy, as well as when defining movement.

Reference Directions

With the anatomical position as the foundation, we will use the following terms to precisely locate structures and define movements, which will ultimately allow for the accurate description of the stretching exercises (Fig. 2.2).

MEDIAL/LATERAL

Medial describes a position closer to the vertical midline of the body than something else. For example, the scapula is medial to the humerus, and the tibia is medial to the fibula. In contrast, *lateral* means farther away from the center of the body than the reference point. For example, the scapula is lateral to the thoracic spine.

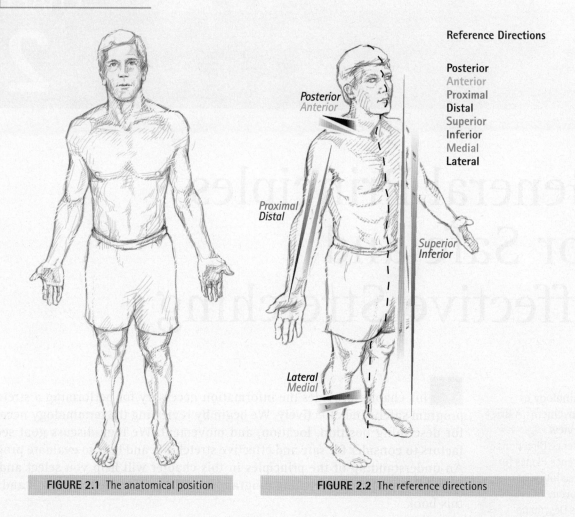

Reference Directions

Posterior
Anterior
Proximal
Distal
Superior
Inferior
Medial
Lateral

FIGURE 2.1 The anatomical position

FIGURE 2.2 The reference directions

PROXIMAL/DISTAL

Proximal describes a position closer to the middle of the body than something else. For examples, the hip is proximal to the knee, and the knee is proximal to the ankle. *Distal* refers to farther away from the middle of the body than some reference points. Therefore, we say that the knee is distal to the hip, and the ankle is distal to both the knee and the hip.

ANTERIOR/POSTERIOR

Anterior refers to the front of the body, whereas *posterior* refers to the back. These terms may also refer to reference directions; for example, the stomach is anterior to the spine, or the calcaneus is posterior to the metatarsals. A view in which you are looking straight on, toward the front of the body, may be referred to as an anterior-posterior (AP) view, and a posterior-anterior (PA) view looks at the back of the body toward the front.

SUPERIOR/INFERIOR

Superior describes a position above something else. For example, the cervical spine is superior to the thoracic spine. *Inferior* means below; thus, in the anatomical position, the tibia is inferior to the femur.

In many cases, body parts or regions may be described with more than one directional term. For example, the radius is both lateral to the ulna and distal to the humerus when the body is in the anatomical position; the head of the humerus is both lateral to the scapula and superior to the shaft of the humerus; and so on.

Reference Planes for Description of Movement

A shared terminology for the basic planes of the body is also helpful when communicating about body positions and movements (Fig. 2.3). The *frontal* (or *coronal*) *plane* divides the body vertically into anterior and a posterior sections. The *sagittal* (or *median*) *plane* also divides the body into two vertical sections, but the division is at a 90° angle to the frontal plane and splits the body into a left and a right side. The *transverse plane* divides the body horizontally into upper and lower sections and is perpendicular to both the frontal and sagittal planes.

Terms Describing Functional Relationships

Muscles produce action at joints by shortening (or pulling) one bone toward another. A muscle producing such a shortening is referred to as an *agonist* (or *prime mover*) and a muscle opposing that action is referred to as an *antagonist*. You can easily determine how a particular muscle functions by noting which side of the joint it is on and then imagining what motion a shortening of this muscle might produce. A muscle on the opposite side of that particular joint would produce the opposite movement. For example, the contraction of the biceps muscle produces elbow flexion, making it the agonist, whereas the triceps muscle would serve in this case as the antagonist, producing extension at the elbow.

In general, the point of musculotendinous attachment on the stationary bone is referred to as the *origin,* and the point of attachment on the moving bone is referred to as the *insertion.* Note that the same bone can be moving for one action and stationary for another, making these terms occasionally ambiguous. For example, when an individual in a seated position straightens his or her leg, the quadriceps shorten

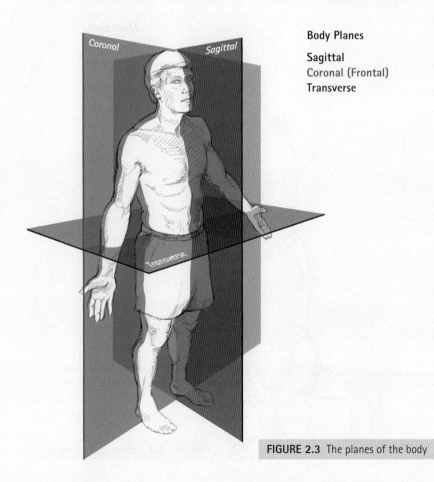

Body Planes

Sagittal
Coronal (Frontal)
Transverse

FIGURE 2.3 The planes of the body

to pull the tibia forward and extend the knee. In this case, the tibia is the moving bone and the quadriceps' point of insertion is the tibial tuberosity. In contrast, when the same individual rises from a chair, the tibia remains relatively stationary while the quadriceps straighten the femur. In this case, the tibial tuberosity is the origin, and the femur is the insertion. To avoid confusion, most clinical texts designate the more proximal attachment as the origin, and the more distal attachment as the insertion. Chapter 4 identifies the origin, insertion, action, and stretch for all of the muscles addressed in this book.

Movements Allowed by Joints

Movements allowed by joints are usually described with one of the following terms: flexion, extension, abduction, adduction, internal (or medial) rotation, and external (or lateral) rotation. Some joints, however, have other terms associated with movements occurring *only* at those joints such as "dorsiflexion" or "plantarflexion" of the ankle, or pronation or supination of the forearm. In the descriptions of these movements below, notice that we identify one body plane in which the movement generally occurs. In reality, movement is rarely limited to one plane and instead occurs in some combination of all three.

Flexion is any movement at a joint that decreases the angle between the two or more bones. An example is elbow flexion, which brings the hand toward the shoulder and decreases the angle between the ulna and the humerus. Flexion of the spine bends the head and torso forward. Flexion generally occurs in the sagittal plane (Fig. 2.4).

Extension is any movement at a joint that increases the angle between the bones. It is in the opposite direction of flexion at any given joint. For example, the

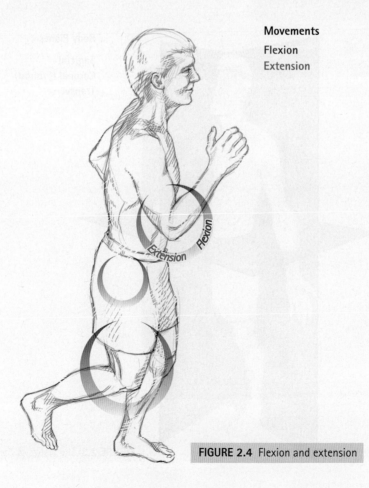

Movements
Flexion
Extension

FIGURE 2.4 Flexion and extension

elbow joint allows for extension to 180° between the upper and lower arm. Extension of a joint beyond straight (0 degree flexion or 180 degrees extension) is termed *hyperextension*. Like flexion, extension generally occurs in the sagittal plane (see Fig. 2.4).

Abduction is any movement that takes the moving bone away from the (usually) vertical centerline of the body. This movement generally occurs in the frontal plane. For example, the abduction of the hip moves the leg laterally (Fig. 2.5).

Adduction is any movement that takes the moving bone toward the (usually) vertical centerline, in the opposite direction of abduction. This motion also generally occurs in the frontal plane. An example is the adduction of the hip, which moves the leg medially (see Fig. 2.5).

Internal (medial) rotation generally occurs around the long axis of the moving bone and is in the transverse plane. The direction is toward the vertical midline of the body. An example is the internal rotation of the humerus, which would cause the hand to turn inward as seen in Figure 2.5.

External (lateral) rotation also generally occurs around the long axis of the moving bone and is in the transverse plane. The direction is lateral, away from the vertical midline of the body. An example is the external rotation of the humerus, which would cause the hand to turn outward as seen in Figure 2.5.

Pronation and *supination* refer to motion both at the forearm and at the foot. Supination of the forearm turns the palm up from a position in which the elbow is flexed 90 degrees. Pronation of the forearm turns the palm downward from a neutral or supinated position. This motion occurs predominantly in the sagittal plane if the elbow is bent to 90 degrees with the hands in front of the body (Fig. 2.6).

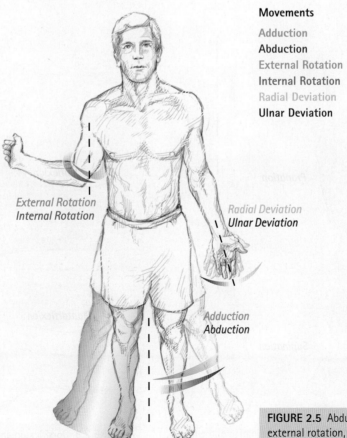

Movements

Adduction
Abduction
External Rotation
Internal Rotation
Radial Deviation
Ulnar Deviation

External Rotation
Internal Rotation

Radial Deviation
Ulnar Deviation

Adduction
Abduction

FIGURE 2.5 Abduction/adduction, internal/external rotation, and ulnar/radial deviation

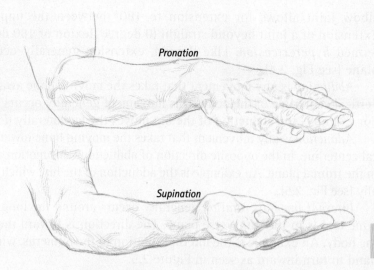

FIGURE 2.6 Pronation and supination of the forearm

Pronation at the foot generally refers to a lowering of the arch. It is generally associated with eversion (a tilting inward) of the calcaneus. Supination of the foot is generally associated with an inversion of the calcaneus (tilting outward) and an increasing arch height. As these motions are quite complex and involve multiple joints, it is difficult to describe them as moving predominately in one plane. However, pronation and supination may be described as moving *predominately* in the frontal and transverse planes (Fig. 2.7).

Dorsiflexion generally refers to motion at the ankle joint. It occurs mostly in the sagittal plane and decreases the angle between the foot and the shin (Fig. 2.8). *Plantarflexion* also generally refers to motion occurring at the ankle joint and in the

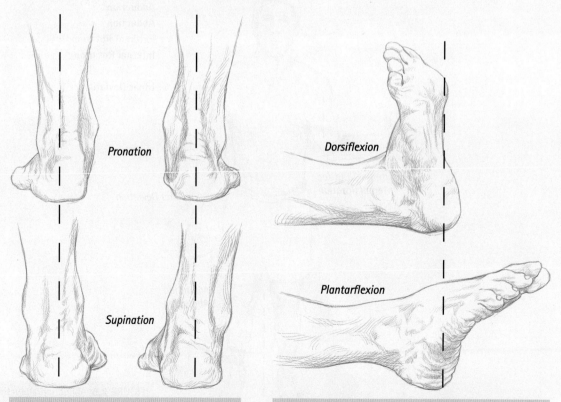

FIGURE 2.7 Pronation and supination of the foot

FIGURE 2.8 Dorsiflexion and plantarflexion of the ankle

sagittal plane, but describes motion moving in a plantar direction or in the direction of the bottom of the foot. This increases the angle between the foot and the shin (Fig. 2.8).

Ulnar deviation is the movement of the wrist/hand in the frontal plane in the direction of the ulna, or toward the body when in anatomical position (Fig. 2.5). *Radial deviation* is movement of the wrist/hand in the frontal plane in the direction of the radius, or away from the body when in anatomical position (Fig. 2.5).

SETTING GOALS

Before undertaking any stretching program, it makes sense to first create a clear vision of what we are trying to achieve. Establishing reasonable, measurable, flexibility goals will not only help monitor progress, but will provide the feedback necessary to modify the program if progress is not sufficient. Is the goal of the program to improve range of motion (ROM) at one or several joints? Is it to improve the motion of joints in which injury or disuse has led to some limitation? Perhaps a student athlete wants to improve his or her overall conditioning prior to the beginning of the fall sports season. We should first determine what we hope to accomplish in the wider context, and then work to identify more specific goals, such as actual ROM measurements to be attained.

After considering the needs and concerns based on lifestyle or activity demands, we should incorporate other possibly influential information, such as general health, history of injury, occupation, or time restraints, into the goal development process.

We should develop both general and specific goals and document them in a way that makes progress measurable. For example, an athlete may report that he wishes to improve his general flexibility, as well as his hamstring and adductor flexibility specifically to improve his performance in hurdling. As part of goal setting for this individual, a clinician would conduct a complete assessment of ROM to establish baseline data. (Assessment of joint ROM is the subject of Chapter 3.) For example, the clinician might determine that this individual's ankle (talocrural) ROM is 15 degrees and agree that his goal will be 20 degrees. In many cases, consultation with professionals knowledgeable with the particular sport or activity may prove quite helpful in the development of accurate flexibility goals. This may also be true when dealing with the limitations caused by specific disease processes or injuries, as the insights gained from one's physician may prove invaluable in choosing appropriate and realistic goals. With measurable goals and baseline data in place, you will be able to monitor progress and make any necessary modifications in the program early on, thus avoiding poor outcomes.

In many cases, the demands of a particular athletic pursuit or occupation determine the target joints and the related muscles that deserve the most attention. For example, maintaining the length of the hamstrings may be very important to a competitive sprinter based on the shear demands placed on this muscle group during this activity. In this case, maintenance of length may be the goal, unless it is determined by careful analysis that the length should be increased. This may be quite different from the needs of a hurdler who must significantly improve his or her adductor flexibility to effectively clear the hurdles.

When setting goals, bear in mind that a joint may be restricted in its ROM for several reasons not involving the muscle-tendon unit. As discussed in Chapter 1, for normal, healthy joints, about 47% of the resistance to movement originates in the joint capsule, 41% in the muscle, 10% in the tendon, and 2% in the skin.[1] An injured joint may offer resistance before any tension is put on the muscle-tendon complex. It is important to be able to discern between the familiar sensation of "stretch" and other sensations such as pain, pressure, or undue resistance buildup in the *joint,* or pain, numbness, burning, or tingling in the muscle or tendon. Symptoms such as these may indicate the need for physician screening before designing a flexibility program.

Finally, when setting goals, refer to the preface of this book, which identifies the stretching programs described in each chapter of Parts II and III. For example, Chapter 7 provides stretches for those who wish to improve their posture. If the individual is stretching to prepare for a particular sport or activity, one should first refer to Chapter 9 to see if the particular sport is listed. If not, one should determine which muscles or body regions are most critical to the activity and then refer to Chapter 5 for stretches of major muscle groups.

FACTORS TO CONSIDER FOR SAFE AND EFFECTIVE STRETCHING

Once general and specific goals have been established, you can use the information in the rest of this chapter to help ensure safe and effective performance of the exercises.

Cautions and Contraindications

In general, the stretches described and illustrated in this book are safe and unlikely to cause injury if performed correctly. Nevertheless, as with any exercise program, individuals with significant pain, physical challenges, or disease should be referred to their primary care provider before proceeding. Disorders that require medical clearance include all significant musculoskeletal conditions, such as a history of acute injury, chronic injury, rheumatoid or osteoarthritis, fibromyalgia, and neuromuscular diseases such as multiple sclerosis and Parkinson's disease. Cardiovascular disease, including hypertension and/or a history of heart attack or stroke, should also prompt medical referral, as should other possibly debilitating diseases such as cancer.

As discussed in Chapter 1, limitations in joint ROM are predominantly caused by either the length of the muscle tendon unit or by the restriction of the joint itself. When the primary restriction is within the joint, stretching may not be helpful or even safe. If there is pain or resistance to movement well before normal joint ROM is attained, physician referral is essential. Joint limitations might be caused by damaged or irregular joint surfaces, shortened ligamentous or joint capsular tissues, excessive inflammation, or loose bodies within the joint. These conditions might be caused by trauma, repetitive stress, inflammatory conditions such as arthritis, or other disease processes such as malignancy.

If applied thoughtfully and if the guidelines set forth in this book are followed, stretching can be safely utilized by all healthy people, large and small, young and old, active and sedentary. Though responses to stretching exercise may vary, paying careful attention to the sensations experienced during and after the stretch should allow safe, successful application by almost everyone. As with any exercise program, pain should be a red flag and should prompt medical clearance, especially if the pain is unexplained or severe. As mentioned in Chapter 1, one should never aggressively stretch acutely painful tissue.

When to Stretch

As there seems no clear consensus regarding the best time to stretch, combined with the knowledge that time constraints can become an excuse for failing to maintain any exercise program, the time should be determined based on what is best for the individual in terms of his or her schedule, habits, and lifestyle. In this way, the chances for actual performance of the stretching program are maximized, whether it be done in the morning, afternoon, or evening.

Warming Up

Most health and fitness professionals, including physicians and athletic trainers, would agree that a warm-up is a necessary first step for any program of physical activity, which includes stretching.

Though widely accepted and practiced, the use of warm-up before stretching has only limited support in the literature and its need before stretching is, at best, controversial. The majority of related research shows no significant benefit to warming up before stretching,[2,3,4,5,6,7] though the study of Wenos et al[8] did show a significant improvement in hip ROM versus the control group. MacAuley et al reviewed 293 articles on stretching and injury prevention and found that, without exception, those indicating a positive effect included a warm-up as a cointervention.[9] Safran et al suggest that the combination of active warm-up and stretching may allow the muscle to temporarily assume longer lengths via increases in tissue temperature and the elasticity of connective tissues.[10] Though this supports the common sense notion that warming up increases the pliability of tissues in the short term, it seems as though the majority of the research shows that this effect is temporary and does *not* lead to overall improved outcomes in the ultimate pursuit of flexibility.

Warming up before an activity is supported by a number of researchers who have shown improved performance of certain activities following a warm-up.[11,12,13]

As the research is as yet inconclusive regarding the effectiveness of using a warm-up before stretching,[14] it has not shown to be harmful or detrimental, and while we can no longer adamantly imply its necessity, we can still recommend its use. It may be particularly beneficial in colder conditions, though these details have not yet been carefully studied. Its use does seem to be of benefit in increasing blood flow and preparing for activity, so we will consider its use below. While we will continue to suggest the use of a warm-up before stretching, we will no longer suggest that stretching should *not* be performed without adequate warm-up.

A *warm-up* may be defined as any activity vigorous enough to raise the body's core temperature to produce a light sweat. Walking, jogging, or light calisthenics would qualify as a warm-up, as would gentle aerobics, cycling, or stair climbing. The intensity of the warm-up also seems to be an important factor in its application. Stewart et al found that a 15-minute warm-up at about 60–70% $VO2_{max}$ was beneficial to enhance subsequent anaerobic performance.[12] ($VO2_{max}$ is a measure of one's maximal ability to transport oxygen to working muscles; it is often used as a measure of fitness.) For our purposes, however, we will consider a warm-up of about 3 to 5 minutes at an intensity producing a light sweat to warm the body and prepare its tissues for stretching.

Intensity

Intensity is a subjective experience and is therefore a difficult parameter to measure precisely. Obviously, an appropriate load must be placed on the muscle-tendon unit to stimulate change; however, determining this load outside of the laboratory can be difficult. Because of this, the development of an acute sense of "stretch" becomes critical.

The sensation of "stretch" is possible because of a variety of sensory receptors located in joints, muscles, tendons, and ligaments. These receptors gather information regarding everything from light touch to position sense to pain. Proprioceptors are specialized receptors that collect information regarding the joint's position, movement direction and velocity, tension in the muscle, or pain and transmit that information to the spinal cord and/or brain. A detailed discussion of each of these receptors is beyond the scope of this book; however, two deserve mention here (both were discussed in Chapter 1). Muscle spindles are located within the muscle belly and respond to rapid changes in muscle lengthening by causing reflex *contraction* of the muscle via a message sent to the spinal cord. Golgi tendon organs, by contrast, are located within the tendon and respond to significant applications of force by causing a reflex *relaxation* of the muscle, likely to prevent tearing.

Feedback from these receptors allows us to define the sensation of stretch. Paying attention to the details of this feedback will allow clients to refine the amount of tension developed and assure a safe, yet effective stretch.

How much force to use? While the force to be used is difficult to quantify, the best results should come from applying force carefully and paying particular attention to the sensations involved, while avoiding a level of intensity that elicits pain. Begin new stretching programs by "under-doing" it. Individuals can increase the loads as needed as they develop an appropriate sense of "stretch" and carefully monitor their progress toward established goals. A gradual approach also allows time for the muscle-tendon units to adapt to newly applied loads over weeks and months rather than being subjected to a potentially injurious level of tension at the outset of the stretching program. A summary of guidelines to help individuals use the appropriate amount of tension follows:

1. Stretching should elicit the feeling of a "strong stretch" in the muscle belly. Avoid stretching to the point of pain. Stretching should not be painful at the muscle or associated joints.

2. Pay attention to what you are doing and feeling throughout the stretching program. If you maintain awareness, you will eventually develop a sense of the appropriate level of force to apply.

3. Monitor your progress. If your progress is not satisfactory, you may have to gradually and carefully increase the amount of tension that you apply.

4. Start easily. It is better to "under-stretch" early in the stretching program and then to gradually increase the applied tension after several weeks of stretching.

Rate and Application of Tension

It is important to understand not only the amount of tension to apply but also how to apply it. Slow, controlled stretches have a much lower risk of injury than rapidly applied stretches. Taylor et al showed that both peak tensile force and absorbed energy were dependent on the rate at which the tension was applied.[15] With more rapidly applied forces, the muscle-tendon unit is subjected to higher peak forces and higher levels of total force absorption and may therefore be more likely to ultimately sustain injury than with more slowly applied loads. As the authors suggest in their conclusion, many of the injuries sustained in stretching programs may be due, at least in part, to the rate at which the tension is applied, rather than on the actual technique employed. The possibility of attaining a more effective stretch is also enhanced by a more slowly applied tension, because this controlled application is less likely to elicit the stretch reflex which may cause reflex contraction of the muscle under tension. The stretch reflex was discussed in Chapter 1.

Slowly applying tension is important, but as we have seen in Chapter 1, the muscle-tendon unit behaves viscoelastically, exhibiting the properties of both viscous and elastic materials.

Stress relaxation is a mechanical property of viscoelastic tissues. It is defined as the decline in the level of force necessary to hold a given tissue at a constant (stretched) length. For a particular individual for example, holding a hamstring stretch might require 40 pounds of force initially, but over the ensuing 20 seconds, the force required might only be 35 pounds. Hewson et al studied the stress relaxation occurring in stretches held at a constant angle and concluded that the majority of the "relaxation" occurred in the first 15–20 seconds.[16] Stress relaxation is probably the reason we feel the muscle ease after about 15–20 seconds into the stretch. At this point, the amount of force that we need to apply to hold the stretch decreases. To affect the elastic component, we should maintain the original level of stretching force that will cause further lengthening of the muscle-tendon unit until it reaches its elastic limit. Continuing to hold the stretch at this point should allow for further changes in length to occur due to creep. Creep is the change in length in the muscle-tendon unit occurring in response to the constant application of force held over time.

So, apply tension slowly and carefully, maintaining that tension beyond the initial relaxation phase of the muscle. Hold times are discussed below.

Duration of Stretch

Studies have investigated the efficacy of hold times varying from just a few seconds to as long as hours. We will restrict this discussion to the parameters that make sense for the practical application of stretching for healthy individuals. Holding stretches for at least 20 seconds will probably assure that we have at least achieved the lengthening due to stress relaxation. For a more practical viewpoint, the following discussion considers the predominant literature investigating hold times and stretching outcomes.

Several investigators have compared the effects of different hold times in human subjects. Zito et al studied 19 healthy volunteers with limitations in ankle dorsiflexion to determine the lasting effects of two repetitions of a 15-second stretch.[17] They found no significant lasting gains. Bandy and Irion randomly assigned 57 men and women to one of four groups.[18] The control group did no stretching. The other three groups stretched 5 days a week for 15, 30, and 60 seconds, respectively. Data analysis revealed that both the 30- and the 60-second groups improved their ROM significantly more than either the 15-second or the control group. Additionally, there was no significant difference in the ROM gains in the 60-second versus the 30-second group. One older study may support the effectiveness of a 15-second hold. Madding et al found no difference in hip abduction ROM in response to static holds of 15, 45, and 120 seconds.[19] As Madding et al's study was of hip abduction, and the Bandy and Irion study was of the hamstrings, we must also consider the possibility of different muscle groups requiring different hold times. Additionally, we must consider other factors such as age, injury, and disease—stretching topics for which there has been little research. For example, in a study of elderly participants (>65 years of age), Feland et al showed significantly greater gains in hamstring flexibility in the group stretching for 60 seconds than in the group stretching for either 30 or 15 seconds.[20] This is in stark contrast to Bandy's study that showed no greater benefit in the 60- versus the 30-second groups.

Considering that the preponderance of research supports hold times of about 30 seconds, it seems a reasonable starting point. As there may be variability not only among different groups of subjects such as the diseased or elderly but also among different muscle groups, we should consider modifying hold times if results are poor. With hold times at or beyond 30 seconds, long-term beneficial lengthening of the muscle-tendon unit is more likely to occur. Again, because one of the principles of an effective flexibility program is to set goals and monitor progress, changes in hold times can be manipulated to meet certain needs or special conditions.

Frequency

The above discussion provides a rationale for a hold time of at least 30 seconds for each individual stretch. We now consider the number of sets and frequency of stretching exercises to perform to make progress.

Another study by Bandy et al compared the effects of stretching for 30 versus 60 seconds and performing one versus three repetitions.[21] They concluded that 30 seconds was an effective hold time for increasing hamstring flexibility, and that there were no further significant gains from either increasing the hold times or repeating the stretches three times per session. Therefore, for healthy individuals, performance of individual stretches once per day should be sufficient. Clearly more research is necessary to support this recommendation and to clarify differing needs in different populations such as those challenged by disease or injury. Most healthcare professionals agree that performance of careful stretching exercises more than once daily may be warranted in individuals with clearly defined limitations.

FREQUENCY: PER DAY AND WEEK

Godges et al studied the effect of passive hip-extension exercises on hip-extension ROM and found significant improvement with only *two* 6-minute stretching sessions per week.[22] In the Bandy et al study cited above, the program was repeated 5 days per week.[21] It is possible that some gains can be made if individuals perform their stretching program at least twice per week, especially if these individuals are not accustomed to this type of exercise. However, because most of the available research has shown progress based on three to five sessions per week, it seems reasonable to use this guideline as a starting point. Again, if weekly or monthly review shows less than desirable progress, the frequency can be modified to increase the number of days per week and/or the number of times per day.

Since research for specific populations is lacking, it is difficult to assign a frequency to individuals with specific challenges. It is probable that the scar tissue formation and subsequent adhesion of tissues that result from injury might warrant more frequent application of stretching techniques. Until there is conclusive research to help guide these decisions, the prudent individual may wish to start conservatively at one session per day, four to five times per week, closely monitor his or her progress, and then increase the frequency if needed. Most fitness and healthcare practitioners advise their clients to stretch two to three times per day at least daily, and we are unaware of any negative effects of this practice.

Cooling Down

Cooling down is an accepted practice following high-intensity exercise as it helps in restoring homeostasis, lowering elevated heart rates and blood pressure, and allowing redistribution of blood flow previously flooding the working muscles. Apparently, cooling down allows the body to make these changes with greater efficiency than merely stopping exercise. Takahashi et al found that the resting average heart rate following the 6-minute cool down period was significantly lower in the active cool down group versus the control group.[23] This may suggest a more rapid return to homeostasis after active cool down.

Cool down usually consists of lower intensity movement(s), which may or may not mimic the activity that it follows. It can be accomplished by easy jogging, walking, or cycling. In many cases, stretching will be included in the cool down period. Though wide variability exists, the cool down period is often in the range of 5–10 minutes.

Regarding stretching, however, there is no research showing benefit or detriment. Because there is little elevation of heart rate, blood pressure, or major redistribution of blood flow associated with stretching, cooling down would seem of little value following a stretching program. Nevertheless, it does make sense to perform a cool down after more vigorous exercise or activity and immediately before a stretching program. In this way, the cool down serves essentially as a transition to the stretching program.

EVALUATING PROGRESS

Earlier in this chapter, we recommended setting measurable goals and establishing baseline data. These are essential steps if one is to be successful in evaluating progress over time. If progress is not satisfactory, one should first consider increasing the number of times per week and then the number of times per day that the individual performs the program. If the desired progress is still not being met, one should consider increasing the amount of tension applied.

Careful monitoring of progress will assure the greatest chances for success with the least chance of injury. A written diary including dates, protocol details, and progress toward goals provides excellent feedback regarding the success, or failure, of any stretching program. It also provides the necessary detail to be able to make the best decisions regarding appropriate changes in frequency and/or intensity. A sample stretching diary is provided in Table 2.1.

Duration of Stretching Program

How long should stretching programs be continued? To answer this question, we will first consider the effects of stretching in both the short and long term. It is important to understand the effects immediately following individual stretches as well as the effects of a dedicated stretching program occurring over weeks, months, or longer. We can then discuss the ultimate duration of stretching programs.

SHORT-TERM GAINS

The short-term ROM gains from a single bout of stretching exercise have been shown to last for as long as 24 hours.[3] Unfortunately, other researchers have reached different conclusions, as Spernoga et al found that the gains made from applying of a single bout of a PNF technique to remain significant for less than 8 minutes.[24] Depino et al found lasting effects for only 3 minutes.[25] Obviously, more research needs to be done in this area before we can draw conclusions regarding the short-term effects of stretching. Because we are not recommending the use of stretching programs immediately *before* activity (see Chapter 1), we are less concerned with the short-term gains in range and more interested in the long-term gains achieved and maintained following weeks of stretching.

TABLE 2.1 **SAMPLE STRETCHING DIARY**

Joint/Motion/ Protocol	Protocol (×/day/×/wk)	Initial	Goal/wk	Week #					
				1	2	3	4	5	6
elbow/flex*	1×/3×	45	80/4wk	55	55	57	62		
ankle/d-flex**	1×/5×	4	20/6wk	10	14	14	18	22	22**

From the above sample diary we can see that the individual was monitoring progress of the ROM of two different joints, elbow flexion, and ankle dorsiflexion.

*In the first example, a review of progress shows that stretches performed to increase elbow flexion were performed once per day, 3 days per week, over a 4-week period. We can see that some progress was made; however, it fell short of the 4-week goal of 80 degrees. In this situation, it may make sense to modify the program to increase the number of days per week to 5 or 6, and then recheck in another 4 weeks.

**In the second example, stretches for ankle dorsiflexion performed once per day, 5×/week proved sufficient to attain the dorsiflexion goal of 20 degrees in 6 weeks.

To safely achieve positive results, we recommend that you take time to set realistic, measurable goals.

LONG-TERM GAINS

It is generally accepted that proper stretching techniques can produce significant improvements in ROM, but we have yet to discuss how long these gains will remain after cessation of the stretching program. Knowing this will help us prescribe the ultimate duration of stretching programs. Brucker et al showed that gains achieved in ankle dorsiflexion over the course of an 18-day stretching program remained significant for 3 weeks following cessation of the program.[26] Willy et al showed *no* retention 4 weeks following the gains made in a 6-week stretching program.[27] Based on this information, it seems possible that we might get away without stretching for about 2–3 weeks before sacrificing our hard-earned flexibility gains.

Most of the research showing positive gains in ROM was based on studies taking place over 4 to 6 weeks. Based on this evidence, as well as on anecdotal and professional experience, we are suggesting that to achieve significant, long-term changes in ROM, it is necessary to commit to weeks of regular practice. While maintenance of these gains is likely easier than achieving them in the first place, the regular practice of stretching exercise should become a lifestyle, as hard-earned gains will be lost without regular practice.

SUMMARY

A common understanding and a shared terminology for descriptions of anatomy and movement allow for effective communication among healthcare providers and clients. Careful attention to the details of the stretching protocol will help individuals safely achieve useful gains in ROM. Monitoring this progress will help refine protocol to ensure continued success.

Below are principles for safe and effective stretching:

1. Carefully consider and design your flexibility program, assuring that it is well balanced and addresses your specific needs for ROM.

2. If not performing the stretching program after activity, consider warming up using calisthenics, walking, jogging, or other aerobic activity to increase muscle and core temperature. Achieving a light sweat is a good indicator of appropriate warm-up.

3. Assume the appropriate stretch position and carefully apply tension to the target tissue. Aim for the sensation of a "strong stretch" in the target muscle. Maintain your awareness during the stretching period, and be aware of sensations such as pain or joint restriction that may suggest either decreasing the intensity or changing or discontinuing the stretch.

4. Hold even tension (this may mean that you will need to move further into the stretch as the muscle relaxes) for 30 seconds. Longer hold times are okay, but they do not seem to provide any additional benefits except in injured or elderly populations. There is some question as to whether or not shorter hold times are of any value in the long-term improvement of ROM.

5. Repeat the program at least three times per week, or more often if the results are not satisfactory. It is likely that four or five times per week may yield better results if three times per week proves insufficient. This may be more likely the case when dealing with specific populations, such as those recovering from injury, those with abnormal tone, or the elderly.

6. Keep track of your progress toward your goals. In this way you will be able to make adaptations to your program as necessary. Common adap-

tations include increasing the amount of tension, increasing the number of sessions per week, or both.

7. Structure time into your workout program to be sure that flexibility is regularly included, as consistency will provide for the best results.

REFERENCES

1. Johns RJ, Wright V. Relative importance of various tissues in joint stiffness. J Appl Physiol 1962;17(5): 824–828.
2. Zakas A, Grammatikopoulou MG, Zakas N, et al. The effect of active warm-up and stretching on the flexibility of adolescent soccer players. J Sports Med Phys Fitness March 2006;46(1):57–61.
3. de Weijer VC, Gorniak GC, Shamus E. The effect of static stretch and warm-up exercise on hamstring length over the course of 24 hours. J Orthop Sports Phys Ther December 2003;33(12):727–733.
4. Knight CA, Rutledge CR, Cox ME, et al. Effect of superficial heat, deep heat, and active exercise warm-up on the extensibility of the plantar flexors. Phys Ther June 2001;81(6):1206–1214.
5. van Mechelen W, Hiobil H, Kemper HC, et al. Prevention of running injuries by warm-up, cool-down, and stretching exercises. Am J Sports Med September–October 1993;21(5):711–719.
6. Williford HN, East JB, Smith FH, et al. Evaluation of warm-up for improvement in flexibility. Am J Sports Med 1986;14(4):316–319.
7. Wiktorsson-Moller M, Oberg BL, Ekstreand J, et al. Effects of warming up, massage, and stretching on range of motion and muscle strength in the lower extremity. Am J Sports Med July–August 1983; 11(4):249–252.
8. Wenos DL, Konin JG. Controlled warm-up intensity enhances hip range of motion. J Strength Cond Res August 2004;18(3):529–533.
9. MacAuley D, Best TM. Reducing the risk of injury due to exercise. Br Med J 325:451–452.
10. Safran MR, Seaber AV, Garrett WE Jr. Warm-up and muscular injury prevention: An update. Sports Med 1989;8(4):239–249.
11. Bishop D. Warm-Up II: Performance changes following active warm-up and how to structure the warm-up. Sports Med 2003;33(7):483–498.
12. Stewart IB, Sleivert GG. The effect of warm up intensity on range of motion and anaerobic performance. J Orthop Sports Phys Ther February 1998;27(2):154–161.
13. Rosenbaum D, Hennig EM. The influence of stretching and warm-up exercises on Achilles tendon reflex activity. J Sports Sci December 1995;13(6):481–490.
14. Fradkin AJ, Gabbe BJ, Cameron PA. J Sci Med Sport June 2006;9(3):214–220.
15. Taylor DC, Dalton JD Jr, Seaber AV, et al. Viscoelastic properties of muscle tendon units: The biomechanical effects of stretching. Am J Sports Med 1990;18(3):300–309.
16. Hewson D, Dombroski E, McNair PJ, et al. Stretching at the ankle joint: Viscoelastic responses for different hold times. 5th IOC World Congress on Sport Sciences. 1999 November.
17. Zito M, Driver D, Parker C, et al. Lasting effects of one bout of two 15-second stretches on ankle dorsiflexion range of motion. J Orthop Sports Phys Ther 1997;26(4):214–221.
18. Bandy WD, Irion JM. The effect of time on static stretch on the flexibility of the hamstring muscles. Phys Ther 1994;74(9):845–852.
19. Madding SW, Wong JG, Hallum A, et al. Effect of duration of passive stretch on hip abduction range of motion. J Orthop Sports Phys Ther 1987;8:409–416.
20. Feland JB, Myrer JW, Schulthies SS, et al. The effect of duration of stretching of the hamstring muscle group for increasing range of motion in people aged 65 years or older. Phys Ther May 2001;81(5): 1110–1117.
21. Bandy WD, Irion JM, Briggler M. The effect of time and frequency of static stretching on the flexibility of the hamstring muscles. Phys Ther 1997;77(10):1090–1096.
22. Godges JJ, MacRae PG, Engelke KA. Effects of exercise on hip range of motion, trunk muscle performance, and gait economy. Phys Ther July 1993;73(7):468–477.
23. Takahashi T, Okada A, Hayano J, et al. Influence of cool-down exercise on autonomic control of heart rate during recovery from dynamic exercise. Front Med Biol Eng 2002;11(4):249–259.
24. Spernoga SG, Uhl TL, Arnold BL, et al. Duration of maintained hamstring flexibility after a one-time hold-relax protocol. J Athl Train March 2001;36(1):44–48.
25. Depino GM, Webright WG, Arnold BL. Duration of maintained hamstring flexibility after cessation of an acute static stretching protocol. J Athl Train January 2000;35(1):56–59.
26. Brucker JB, Knight KL, Rubley MD, et al. An 18-day stretching regimen, with or without pulsed, short-wave diathermy, and ankle dorsiflexion after 3 weeks. J Athl Train October–December 2005;40(4): 276–280.
27. Willy RW, Kyle BA, Moore SA, et al. Effect of cessation and resumption of static hamstring muscle stretching on joint range of motion. J Orthop Sports Phys Ther March 2001;31(3):138–144.

Assessing Flexibility

Not everyone has the same flexibility needs or flexibility potential. Our flexibility potential is affected by genetics, gender, age, lifestyle, medical history, occupation, and, of course, type and level of physical activity. It is therefore unwise to assume that all stretches are beneficial and safe for everyone.

For example, some individuals may have particularly tight hamstrings or pectoral muscles that deserve specific attention. These same individuals may also have a hypermobile lumbar spine that should *not* be stretched. This chapter is designed to help you construct an effective stretching program based on individual need.

As each individual has unique flexibility needs, the first step toward developing a specific flexibility program is to assess posture and available range of motion (ROM). We can then compare the available motion to the determined need to develop the most appropriate flexibility program. This chapter has been developed to help you perform this assessment. It provides a head to toe testing sequence to help determine if ROM is adequate, restricted, or excessive. Please keep in mind that these tests are meant as a guide and the ROM normative data are averages based on a healthy college age population. To determine useful ROMs at particular joints for particular athletic pursuits, the reader is encouraged to seek sources specific to that particular sport or activity. Additional sources are listed at the end of this chapter.

After a brief discussion of posture assessment (a more thorough discussion of posture is provided in Chapter 7), this chapter describes techniques for assessing movement at all major joints. A description of normal movement is followed by information on identifying the amount of motion expected. This information is provided as a guide to help determine if changes in ROM are necessary and generally to what degree. It should be used in concert with knowledge of both need and the individual's physiologic makeup. For more specific assessment, numerical data have been provided as a reference. In most cases, these numerical values are derived from the *Measurement of Joint Motion* by Norkin and White.[1] We have chosen to use this source as it was the only available source that offered ROM values throughout the body. Other sources found slightly different values for select joints; to include all of these sources would be extremely cumbersome, distracting, and of no real benefit to the intended use of this chapter, which is to provide general guidelines for ROM and how to assess it.

As Norkin and White have used a number of different references, we have chosen those values published by the American Academy of Orthopedic Surgeons (AAOS) to ensure consistency and avoid confusion with differing values. In cases where Norkin and White did not provide values (or these values were not useful for this specific application), we have chosen an alternative source. In these cases, alternative sources are listed. We have attempted to provide these ROM values in two basic forms: first in terms of a practical measurement as described in the "test" and then, more formally, in degrees. This format allows the text to be used as both a quick reference to expected motion and as a more detailed evaluation tool. The muscles that may be causing the restriction are listed under the headings "General Stretch" and "Specific Stretches," which identify a stretch for either the muscle group (from Chapter 5) or for each individual muscle (from Chapter 4). The techniques for performing the recommended stretches are detailed in Chapters 4 and 5.

The tests in this chapter may be used to make an initial evaluation and also to measure the progress of the prescribed stretching program. Consider recording the test "scores" obtained at the initial evaluation, and then again at regular intervals such as 6 or 12 weeks. In this way, you can track progress in particular "problem" areas.

> **CAUTION!** Please bear in mind that the information in this chapter is intended to be used only as a guide. Individuals with painful or particularly restricted or hyper-mobile movements should be referred to their primary care provider. While listing every possible restriction to joint movement that you should be aware of would necessitate a chapter on its own, we have denoted a couple of situations in which injuries are frequently encountered. These are identified by the "Caution!" symbol.

ASSESSING POSTURE

For the purposes of this discussion, we will define *posture* as the position in which the upright body is held. It is typically characterized by the relationship of skeletal regions, such as the head, spinal regions, pelvis, knees, and ankles, with one another. Posture results from the interaction of a number of factors including strength, flexibility, joint ROM, age-related factors, gender, and genetics. These components may be influenced throughout an individual's growth and development by activity level, types of physical activities pursued (including athletic pursuits, occupation, and avocation), medical history, and possibly even social factors such as self-esteem.

"Good" posture reflects a positioning of the skeleton that allows for optimal functioning of all of its individual components. It is generally described as a position in which the ear, shoulder, hip, and knee are aligned over a point just in front of the ankle joint (Fig. 3.1). In the spine, this is usually synonymous with the existence of three gentle curves—the concave cervical curvature, the convex thoracic curvature, and the concave lumbar curvature. These curves may be influenced by the amount of flexibility in the muscles that help control motion at these joints.

Posture is much more than aesthetic. Good posture allows for the optimal functioning of joints throughout the body. It also allows for the optimal function of the internal organs. In contrast, poor posture may cause excessive or abnormal stress on the vertebral column as well as on the muscles, tendons, ligaments, and connective tissues that support it. Increased pressures on intra-thoracic organs may also impair blood flow and compromise the functions of these organs.

Common postural abnormalities include forward head, rounded shoulders, increased thoracic curvature, increased lumbar curvature, and hyper-extended knees (Fig. 3.2). A flexibility program designed to help correct the components of this common "poor" posture should address the following:

- Forward head: Lower cervical and upper thoracic extensors may be overstretched. Lower cervical flexors and upper cervical extensors may need stretching.
- Forward and rounded shoulders: Spinal and thoracic extensors, scapular adductors, and shoulder external rotators may be overstretched. Spinal flexors, shoulder

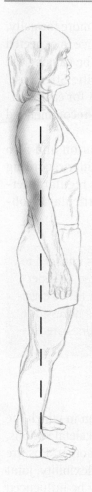

FIGURE 3.1 "Good" posture. Notice the three spinal curves: the concave cervical curvature, the convex thoracic curvature, and the concave lumbar curvature. Notice the vertical line drawn from ear, through shoulder, hip, and knee and ending just in front of the ankle.

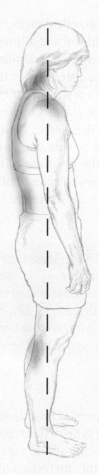

FIGURE 3.2 "Poor" posture. Notice the forward head, forward and rounded shoulders, hyper-extended lower back, and hyper-extended knees.

flexors, horizontal flexors, internal rotators, and scapular protractors may need stretching.

- Hyper-extended lower back: Abdominal muscles, lumbar joints, and anterior hip ligaments may be overstretched. Lower spinal extensors and hip flexors may need stretching.
- Hyper-extended knees: Knee joint capsule and ligaments may be overstretched. Ankle plantar flexors may need to be stretched.

ASSESSING RANGE OF MOTION

The following guide is arranged to help you easily identify possible problem areas. The movement in question is described first, followed by the quick test, average motion available, and then the stretch or stretches recommended to treat any restriction. (The muscles listed are also the possible muscular restrictions to movement.) Again, the techniques for stretching the muscle groups are listed in Chapter 5, and those for the individual muscles are listed in Chapter 4.

Please note that the tests included here are not exhaustive but should be appropriate for use with most individuals. See the end-of-chapter references for sources to consult if you need additional information on testing ROM for specific needs.

For a number of movements, "subtests" are provided to help distinguish between two or more muscles that perform the same general movement (and therefore restrict the same antagonistic movement). A few subtests address the differences between restrictions caused by multi-joint muscles (muscles that cross more than one joint) versus those caused by single-joint muscles, as these are often important distinctions to make.

Cervical Spine

Below are flexibility tests for the cervical spine.

> ⚠ **CAUTION!** Please be aware that restrictions in movement at the cervical spine that cause light-headedness, dizziness, local or referred pain, tingling, or numbness may indicate potentially hazardous injury to joint, nerve, or blood vessel. These cases should be thoroughly evaluated by a professional specializing in spinal dysfunction before continuing.

CERVICAL FLEXION: UPPER

TEST POSITION. Standing with head, shoulders, back, and heels against the wall. Both hands are placed behind the cervical curvature to maintain the curve and ensure that motion occurs above this level.

TEST. Nod the head attempting to isolate movement to the upper vertebrae. Check for 10–20 degrees of "nod" with no change in position of lower cervical vertebrae (Fig. 3.3).

AVERAGE MOTION AVAILABLE. 15 degrees (total flexion/extension at the atlanto-occipital joint)[2]

GENERAL STRETCH. Cervical extensors

SPECIFIC STRETCHES. Rectus capitus posterior major and minor, and obliquus capitus superior and inferior

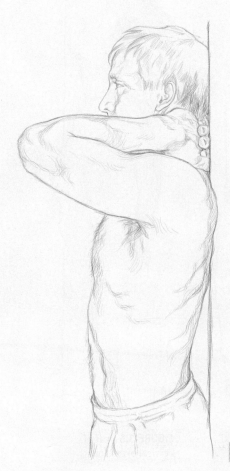

FIGURE 3.3 Test of cervical flexion: upper

CERVICAL FLEXION: LOWER

TEST POSITION. Standing with head and shoulders against the wall

TEST. Flex the head, moving chin toward chest. Chin should come within one inch of the sternum (Fig. 3.4).

AVERAGE MOTION AVAILABLE. AAOS 45 degrees

GENERAL STRETCH. Cervical extensors

SPECIFIC STRETCHES. Longissimus capitus, semispinalis capitis, and splenius capitus

CERVICAL EXTENSION

TEST POSITION. Standing, facing a wall, nose touching wall

TEST. Place the fingers of one hand just beneath the occiput. Look up toward the ceiling by lifting the chin up along the wall, encouraging a lengthening along the front of the neck while *carefully* guiding the motion up and back (Fig. 3.5). There should be 1–2 finger widths (½–1 inches) between the occiput and the seventh cervical vertebra (prominent bump at the bottom of neck/upper shoulders).

AVERAGE MOTION AVAILABLE. AAOS 45 degrees

GENERAL STRETCH. Cervical flexors

SPECIFIC STRETCHES. Longus coli, sternohyoid, omohyoid, platysma

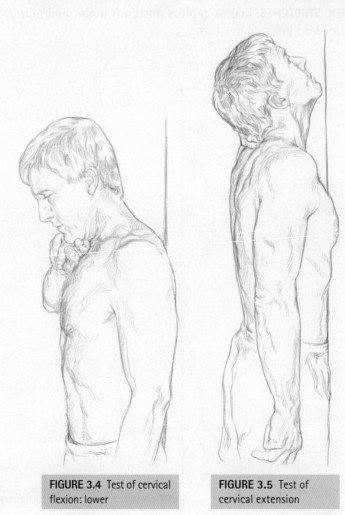

FIGURE 3.4 Test of cervical flexion: lower

FIGURE 3.5 Test of cervical extension

CERVICAL ROTATION

TEST POSITION. Standing with back of head and shoulders against a wall

TEST. Rotate the head toward the wall, being careful not to side-bend (laterally flex) the neck (Fig. 3.6). Check for 2–3 finger widths (1–2 inches) between the cheekbone and the wall.

AVERAGE MOTION AVAILABLE. AAOS 60 degrees

GENERAL STRETCH. Cervical rotators

SPECIFIC STRETCHES. Sternocleidomastoid, upper trapezius, obliquus capitus inferior, splenius capitus

CERVICAL SIDE-BENDING

TEST POSITION. Standing with back of head and shoulders against a wall

TEST. Tilt the head directly to the left without allowing rotation (i.e., ear toward shoulder) (Fig. 3.7). Use the number of finger widths of the right hand as measurement. Three or 4 finger widths (1.5–2.0 inches) is normal.

AVERAGE MOTION AVAILABLE. AAOS 45 degrees

GENERAL STRETCH. Cervical side-benders (lateral flexors)

SPECIFIC STRETCHES. Upper trapezius, splenius capitus, longissimus capitus, obliquus capitus superior, obliquus capitus inferior

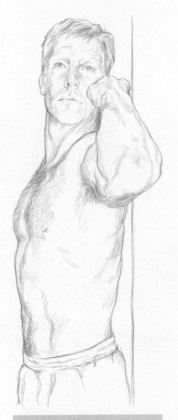

FIGURE 3.6 Test of cervical rotation

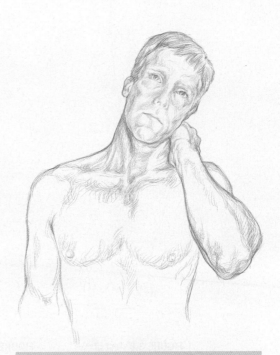

FIGURE 3.7 Test of cervical side-bending

Shoulder

Below are flexibility tests for the shoulder region.

SHOULDER FLEXION

TEST POSITION. Standing in doorway, arms overhead, palms against inside of doorway.

TEST. Keeping spine straight, move forward in doorway (Fig. 3.8). Arms should extend vertically.

AVERAGE MOTION AVAILABLE. AAOS 180 degrees

GENERAL STRETCH. Shoulder extensors

SPECIFIC STRETCHES. Posterior deltoid, latissimus dorsi, teres minor, teres major, triceps brachii-long head

SHOULDER EXTENSION

TEST POSITION. Standing, hands held together behind back

TEST. Lift hands behind back, keeping elbows straight (Fig. 3.9). Arms should extend about 12 inches behind back.

AVERAGE MOTION AVAILABLE. AAOS 60 degrees

GENERAL STRETCH. Shoulder flexors

SPECIFIC STRETCHES. Anterior deltoid, pectoralis major–clavicular portion, biceps brachii–long head, coracobrachialis

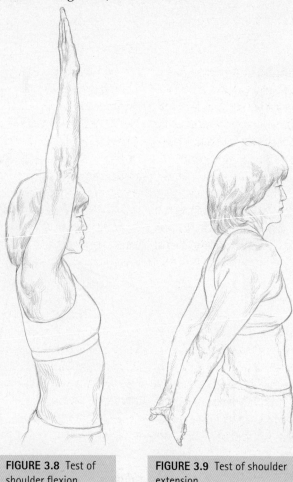

FIGURE 3.8 Test of shoulder flexion

FIGURE 3.9 Test of shoulder extension

SHOULDER ABDUCTION

TEST POSITION. Standing with back against the wall, arms extended horizontally from shoulders, palms facing up

TEST. Abduct both arms, keeping them flat against the wall (Fig. 3.10). Hands should come together and upper arms should come in contact with the head.

AVERAGE MOTION AVAILABLE. AAOS 180 degrees

GENERAL STRETCH. Shoulder adductors

SPECIFIC STRETCHES. Pectoralis major, latissimus dorsi, teres major, rhomboids major and minor

SHOULDER INTERNAL ROTATION

TEST POSITION. Lying supine with left shoulder abducted to 90 degrees, left elbow bent to 90 degrees, forearm pronated

TEST. Keep the left shoulder stable by applying a firm downward pressure with the palm of the right hand while bringing the palm of the left hand toward the floor (Fig. 3.11). The left wrist should come within 4 to 6 inches of the floor. Repeat the test on the right shoulder.

AVERAGE MOTION AVAILABLE. AAOS 70 degrees

GENERAL STRETCH. Shoulder external rotators

SPECIFIC STRETCHES. Posterior deltoid, infraspinatus, teres minor

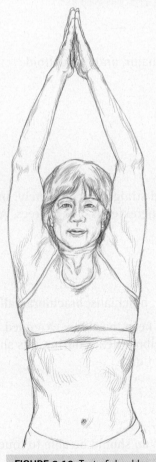

FIGURE 3.10 Test of shoulder abduction

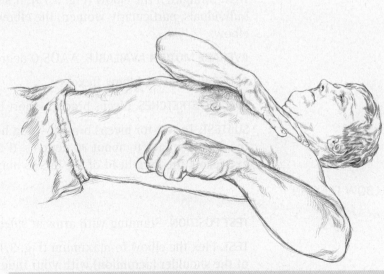

FIGURE 3.11 Test of shoulder internal rotation

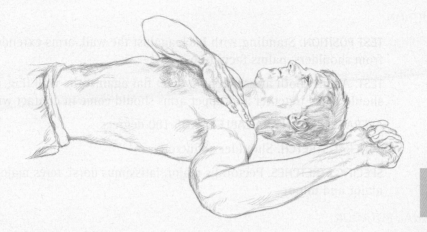

SHOULDER EXTERNAL ROTATION

TEST POSITION. Lying supine with left shoulder abducted to 90 degrees, left elbow bent to 90 degrees, forearm pronated

TEST. Keep the left shoulder stable by applying a firm downward pressure with the palm of the right hand while moving the left forearm and hand back toward the floor (externally or laterally rotating the shoulder) (Fig. 3.12). The back (posterior) of the left wrist should come within 1 to 2 inches of the floor. Repeat the test on the right shoulder.

AVERAGE MOTION AVAILABLE. AAOS 90 degrees

GENERAL STRETCH. Shoulder internal rotators

SPECIFIC STRETCHES. Subscapularis, pectoralis major, anterior deltoid

Elbow

Below are flexibility tests for the elbow region.

ELBOW EXTENSION

TEST POSITION. Standing, arms relaxed at sides

TEST. Straighten the elbow (Fig. 3.13). It should straighten completely. In many individuals, particularly women, the elbow hyperextends 2–5 degrees. Assess both elbows.

AVERAGE MOTION AVAILABLE. AAOS 0 degrees

GENERAL STRETCH. Elbow flexors

SPECIFIC STRETCHES. Biceps brachii—short head, brachialis, brachioradialis

SUBTEST. To test for biceps brachii—long head, keep the elbow extended and extend the shoulder back to about 30 degrees. If the elbow flexes during this shoulder extension, the long head of the biceps may be tight.

ELBOW FLEXION

TEST POSITION. Standing with arms at sides

TEST. Flex the elbow to maximum (Fig. 3.14). You should be able to touch the top of the shoulder (acromion) with your index finger. Assess both elbows.

AVERAGE MOTION AVAILABLE. AAOS 150 degrees

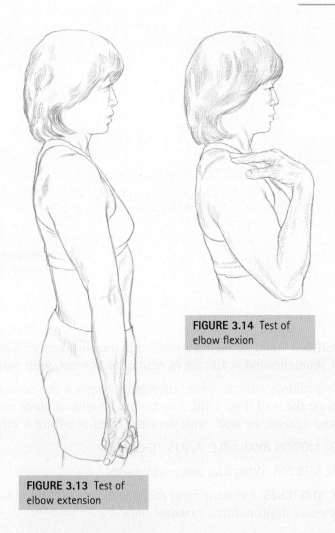

FIGURE 3.14 Test of elbow flexion

FIGURE 3.13 Test of elbow extension

GENERAL STRETCH. Elbow extensors

SPECIFIC STRETCHES. Triceps brachii—medial and middle heads, anconeus

SUBTEST. To test for triceps brachii—long head, hold end position achieved above with index finger on acromion, and raise elbow up overhead until upper arm is vertical. If this motion is difficult, the long head of the triceps may be tight.

Wrist, Hand, and Fingers

Below are flexibility tests for the wrist, hand, and fingers.

WRIST EXTENSION

TEST POSITION. Standing facing a wall with shoulders flexed to 90 degrees and arms outstretched, hands in front of shoulders, wrists in neutral alignment, with palms facing downward

TEST. Keep elbows straight while attempting to place hands flat on the wall (Fig. 3.15). Normal ROM will allow you to place your hands flat on the wall with your elbows straight.

AVERAGE MOTION AVAILABLE. AAOS 80 degrees

GENERAL STRETCH. Wrist and finger flexors

SPECIFIC STRETCHES. Flexor carpi radialis, palmaris longus, flexor digitorum profundus and superficialis, flexor carpi ulnaris

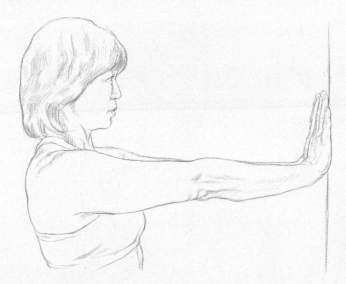

WRIST FLEXION

TEST POSITION. Standing facing a wall with arms outstretched, so that hands are in front of shoulders and wrists are in neutral alignment, with palms facing downward

TEST. Keep elbows straight while attempting to place the dorsum (back) of hands flat against the wall (Fig. 3.16). You should be able to place most of the back of your hand against the wall, with the wrist coming within 1 inch.

AVERAGE MOTION AVAILABLE. AAOS 70 degrees

GENERAL STRETCH. Wrist and finger extensors.

SPECIFIC STRETCHES. Extensor carpi radialis, extensor carpi ulnaris, extensor digitorum, extensor digiti minimi, extensor indicis

FINGER FLEXION

TEST POSITION. Standing with shoulders flexed to 90 degrees (arms outstretched in front of shoulders) with palms facing downward

TEST. Attempt to make a tight fist, and then flex the wrist 30–40 degrees (Fig. 3.17). Test both hands.

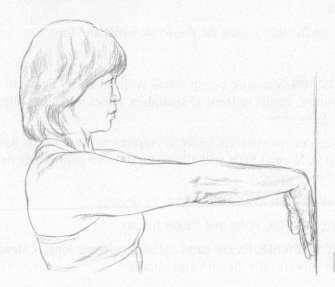

FIGURE 3.16 Test of wrist flexion

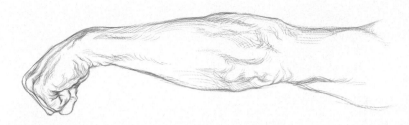

FIGURE 3.17 Test of finger flexion

AVERAGE MOTION AVAILABLE. References available are for each joint (metacarpophalangeal, interphalangeal) and beyond the scope of this text (see references in Appendix A for more information).

GENERAL STRETCH. Wrist and finger extensors

SPECIFIC STRETCHES. Extensor digitorum, extensor indicis, extensor digiti minimi

NOTE. If unable to make a fist with the wrist in neutral alignment (i.e., before flexing the wrist), a simple musculotendinous restriction is unlikely, and a joint restriction should be considered. If this restriction is significant and/or painful, consider referral to an appropriate hand specialist.

FINGER EXTENSION

TEST POSITION. Standing or seated with the elbow flexed and the forearm supinated (palm facing up)

TEST. Open the hand as wide as possible (Fig. 3.18). It should open to reveal a flat or slightly hyper-extended position. Test both hands.

AVERAGE MOTION AVAILABLE. References available are for each joint (metacarpophalangeal, interphalangeal) and beyond the scope of this text (see references in Appendix A for more information).

GENERAL STRETCH. Wrist/Hand/Finger flexors

SPECIFIC STRETCHES. Flexor pollicus brevis, abductor pollicus brevis, adductor pollicus, flexor digiti minimi, lumbricales

Thoracic and Lumbar Spine

Below are flexibility tests for the thoracic and lumbar spine regions.

THORACIC EXTENSION

TEST POSITION. Standing, back and shoulders against a wall

TEST. First, tilt the pelvis posteriorly, flattening the lower back (lumbar spine) against the wall (Fig. 3.19). Next, attempt to extend the mid/upper back (thoracic

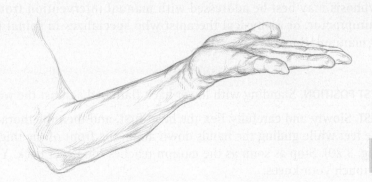

FIGURE 3.18 Test of finger extension

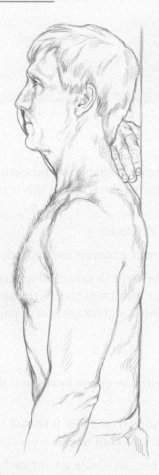

FIGURE 3.19 Test of thoracic extension

spine) and flatten it against the wall. You should observe no more than 2–3 finger widths (1.0–1.5 inches) between the spinous processes of the C7 to T1 vertebrae and the wall.

AVERAGE MOTION AVAILABLE. AAOS 25 degrees (combined motion between thoracic and lumbar spines)

GENERAL STRETCH. Lumbar and thoracic flexors

SPECIFIC STRETCHES. Rectus abdominus and, indirectly, via forward head postures: sternocleidomastoid, scalenes, platysma

NOTE. A significant lack of thoracic extension accompanied by a significantly flexed resting position is characteristic of kyphosis, a disorder that may be related to osteoporosis. Although stretching the thoracic and abdominal flexors is a useful intervention, severely restricted thoracic extension and clinical kyphosis may best be addressed with manual intervention from an osteopath, a chiropractor, or a physical therapist who specializes in spinal joint mobilization or manipulation.

THORACIC FLEXION

TEST POSITION. Standing with lower back flattened against the wall

TEST. Slowly and carefully flex the head first, and then the thoracic spine toward the feet while gliding the hands down along the front of the thighs for support (Fig. 3.20). Stop as soon as the motion reaches the lower back. You should be able to touch your knees.

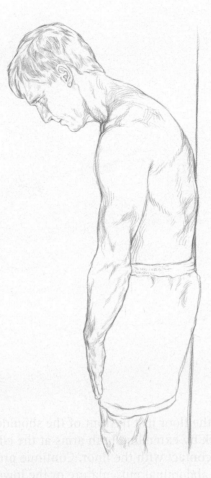

FIGURE 3.20 Test of thoracic flexion

AVERAGE MOTION AVAILABLE. AAOS 80 degrees (combined motion between thoracic and lumbar spines)

GENERAL STRETCH. Spine extensors

SPECIFIC STRETCHES. Spinalis thoracis, iliocostalis thoracis, longissimus thoracis

LUMBAR FLEXION

TEST POSITION. Lying supine

TEST. Begin by using the arms and hands to pull both knees toward the chest. While keeping head, neck, shoulders, and upper back flat on the floor, continue to pull the knees up toward the chest until a gentle curve is formed by the lower back (Fig. 3.21). There should be about and 4 or 5 finger widths (3–4 inches) between your coccyx (tailbone) and the floor.

AVERAGE MOTION AVAILABLE. AAOS 80 degrees (combined motion between thoracic and lumbar spines).

GENERAL STRETCH. Spine extensors

SPECIFIC STRETCHES. Erector spinae, multifidus, quadratus lumborum

CAUTION! Severe pain, or pain, numbness, and tingling in the leg or foot, brought on by this maneuver may be indicative of lumbar pathology. This test should be modified to eliminate these symptoms or discontinued altogether. Further evaluation by a specialist may be prudent at this point.

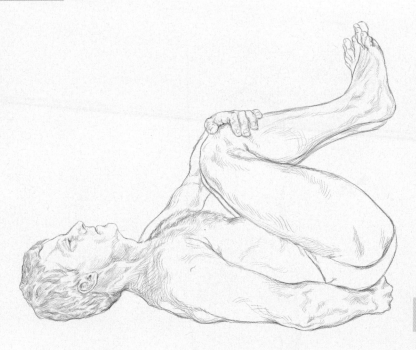

FIGURE 3.21 Test of lumbar flexion

LUMBAR EXTENSION

TEST POSITION. Lying prone

TEST. Place both hands on the floor just in front of the shoulders (Fig. 3.22). Press the upper body up and back by extending both arms at the elbows. Keep the front of the hip bones (ASIS) in contact with the floor. Continue pressing up until a mild tension is felt in either the abdominal musculature or the lower back. *Do not* press up through lower back pain. You should be able to extend your arms comfortably.

AVERAGE MOTION AVAILABLE. AAOS 50 degrees

GENERAL STRETCH. Lumbar flexors, hip flexors

SPECIFIC STRETCHES. Rectus abdominus, internal oblique, external oblique, psoas

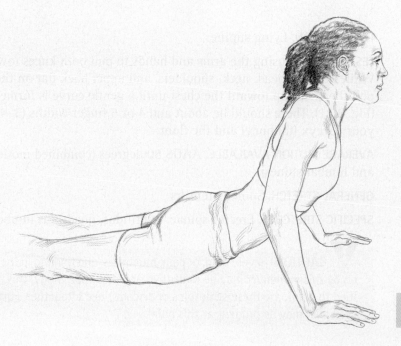

FIGURE 3.22 Test of lumbar extension

⚠ CAUTION! Severe pain, or pain, numbness, and tingling in the leg or foot, brought on by this maneuver may be indicative of lumbar pathology. This test should be modified to eliminate these symptoms or discontinued altogether. Further evaluation by a specialist may be prudent at this point. Individuals with spondylolisthesis should *not* perform this test.

Hip

Below are flexibility tests for the hip region.

HIP FLEXION

TEST POSITION. Lying supine, legs extended

TEST. Pull one knee up to the chest, allowing the hip to flex completely (Fig. 3.23). There should be contact between the thigh and abdominal area. Test hip flexion on both sides.

AVERAGE MOTION AVAILABLE. AAOS 120 degrees

GENERAL STRETCH. Hip extensors

SPECIFIC STRETCHES. Gluteus maximus, posterior fibers of gluteus medius

HIP EXTENSION

TEST POSITION. Supine with thighs and legs hanging off of plinth so that the lower back and buttocks are just supported, knees relaxed

TEST. Pull your left knee toward your chest until the lower back is flattened against the table (Fig. 3.24). The right thigh should hang below the level of the table about 20–30 degrees. Then test extension at the left hip.

AVERAGE MOTION AVAILABLE. AAOS 20 degrees

GENERAL STRETCH. Hip flexors

SPECIFIC STRETCHES. Psoas major, psoas minor, iliacus, rectus femoris

HIP ABDUCTION

TEST POSITION. Lying supine with buttocks against the wall and legs straight up, supported against the wall

TEST. Allow your legs to fall to their respective sides (abduction) while maintaining contact with the wall (Fig. 3.25). There should be at least a 90-degree angle between the legs.

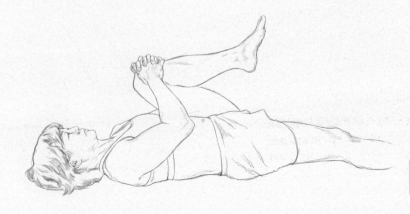

FIGURE 3.23 Test of hip flexion

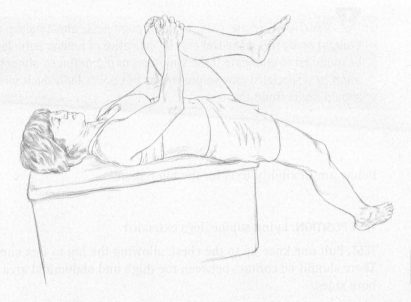

FIGURE 3.24 Test of hip extension

AVERAGE MOTION AVAILABLE. AAOS 45 degrees

GENERAL STRETCHES. Hip adductors

SPECIFIC STRETCHES. Pectineus, adductor longus, adductor brevis, adductor magnus, gracilus

HIP ADDUCTION

TEST POSITION. Lying on the left side on the plinth or other supportive surface so that the waist is supported, but the entire right leg is able to hang freely downward. Left thigh should be flexed forward, knee bent, and out of the way of the unsupported right leg.

TEST. Use your right hand to exert downward pressure on the right hip, flattening the left waist, hip, and torso against the table (Fig. 3.26). Then allow the extended right leg to hang down. The right leg should fall well below the plane of the upper body about 30 degrees. Also test adduction of left hip.

AVERAGE MOTION AVAILABLE. AAOS 30 degrees

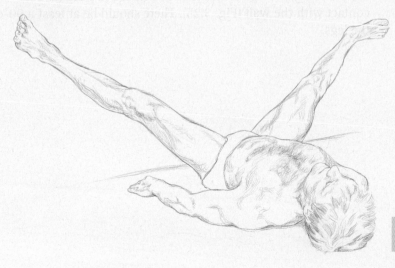

FIGURE 3.25 Test of hip abduction

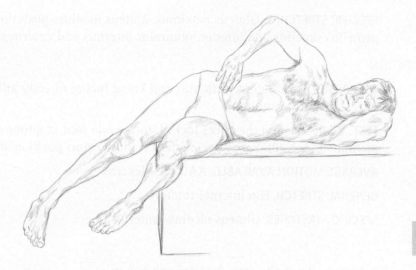

FIGURE 3.26 Test
of hip adduction

GENERAL STRETCH. Hip abductors

SPECIFIC STRETCHES. Gluteus minimus, gluteus medius, tensor fascia latae

HIP INTERNAL ROTATION

TEST POSITION. Standing, with hips and knees facing directly forward. Note position of feet at start position—they will likely be pointed outward 10–20 degrees.

TEST. Keeping the knees straight, rotate one foot at a time inward as far as possible (Fig. 3.27). Forty-five degrees from the start position should be available.

AVERAGE MOTION AVAILABLE. AAOS 45 degrees

GENERAL STRETCH. Hip external rotators

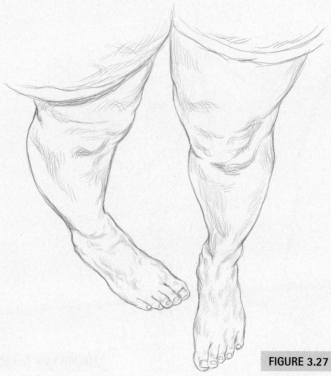

FIGURE 3.27 Test of hip internal rotation

SPECIFIC STRETCHES. Gluteus maximus. gluteus medius—posterior fibers, piriformis, gemellus superior and inferior, obturator internus and externus, quadratus femoris

HIP EXTERNAL ROTATION

TEST POSITION. Standing, with hips and knees facing directly anterior. Note position of feet at start position.

TEST. While keeping the knees locked, rotate one foot at a time outward as far as possible (Fig. 3.28). Forty-five degrees from the start position should be available.

AVERAGE MOTION AVAILABLE. AAOS 45 degrees

GENERAL STRETCH. Hip internal rotators

SPECIFIC STRETCHES. Gluteus medius—anterior fibers

Knee

Below are flexibility tests for the knee region.

KNEE EXTENSION

TEST POSITION. Lying supine, perpendicular to doorway with one leg through and the other (test leg) resting against the doorway, knee extended

TEST. Keep the knee of the test leg straight while moving the entire body as close to the doorway as possible (Fig. 3.29). This may require some assistance from the bent leg and the hands. The buttocks should come within 1 foot of the doorway for men and 6 inches for women. Test extension at both knees.

AVERAGE MOTION AVAILABLE. AAOS 10 degrees

GENERAL STRETCH. Knee flexors

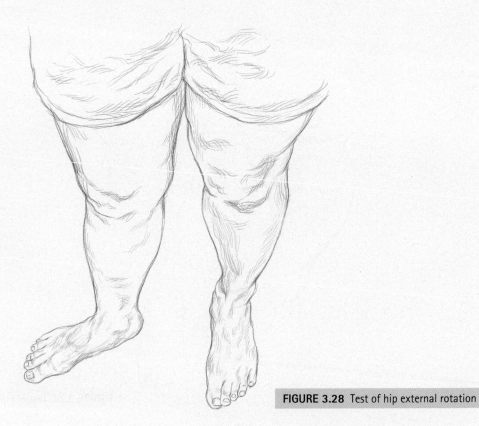

FIGURE 3.28 Test of hip external rotation

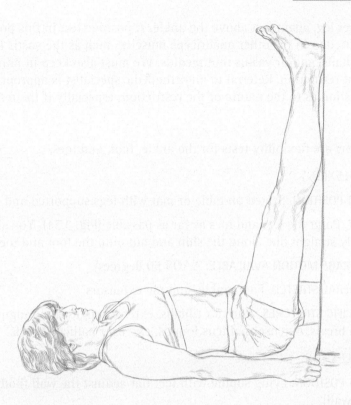

FIGURE 3.29 Test of knee extension

SPECIFIC STRETCHES. Semimembranosus, semitendinosus, biceps femoris–long head

NOTE. If the knee cannot be completely extended (i.e., straightened) even if both legs are extended on the floor, there may be a restriction in the knee joint itself. It is also possible, though uncommon, that this restriction is related to a severe shortness of the short head of biceps femoris, gastrocnemius, and popliteus.

KNEE FLEXION

TEST POSITION. Lying prone on table or mat with test leg flexed to about 90 degrees

TEST. Grasp the lower leg just proximal to the ankle and pull it toward the buttocks (Fig. 3.30). The heel should come within 2 inches of the buttocks. Test flexion of both knees.

AVERAGE MOTION AVAILABLE. AAOS 135 degrees

GENERAL STRETCH. Knee extensors

SPECIFIC STRETCHES. Rectus femoris

NOTE. If there is inappropriate knee flexion, try testing again in the supine position. Pull knee to chest and then attempt to pull heel to buttock via a firm grip on the

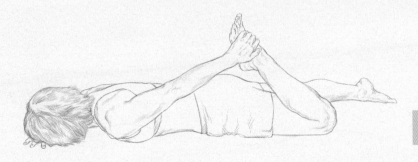

FIGURE 3.30 Test of knee flexion

lower leg, again just above the ankle. A positive test in this position may imply restriction in the other quadriceps muscles, such as the vastis lateralis, vastus medialis, and/or vastus intermedius. We must also keep in mind the possibility of a joint restriction. Referral to an orthopedic specialist is appropriate if there is any question as to the nature of the restriction, especially if the restriction is painful.

Ankle, Foot, and Toes

Below are flexibility tests for the ankle, foot, and toes.

ANKLE FLEXION (PLANTARFLEXION)

TEST POSITION. Seated on table or mat with legs supported and knees extended

TEST. Point the feet and toes as far as possible (Fig. 3.31). You should observe a relatively straight line along the shin and out onto the foot and toes. Check both sides.

AVERAGE MOTION AVAILABLE. AAOS 50 degrees

GENERAL STRETCH. Foot, ankle, and toe extensors

SPECIFIC STRETCHES. Anterior tibialis, extensor digitorum longus, extensor digitorum brevis, extensor hallicus longus, extensor hallicus brevis

ANKLE EXTENSION (DORSIFLEXION)

TEST POSITION. Lying supine with feet flat against the wall (body perpendicular to the wall)

TEST. Keep the heel in contact with the wall while attempting to pull the balls of feet and toes away from wall (Fig. 3.32). There should be a space of 1–2 inches between the ball of foot and the wall. Bear in mind that this test primarily emphasizes the gastrocnemius, while the alternative test below is more indicative of restrictions in the soleus, the other plantar flexors, and/or the ankle joint itself. Test both sides.

AVERAGE MOTION AVAILABLE. AAOS 20 degrees

ALTERNATIVE TEST. Stand facing a wall with the toes roughly 2–3 inches from the wall. Attempt to bend the knees and touch them to the wall while keeping the heels on the floor. If the knee(s) touch, move backward in increments of about half an inch until the point at which the knees can no longer touch the wall. At the last point in which the knee(s) can still touch the wall, the distance between the toes and the wall should be about 3 inches. An inability to touch the wall is a significant restriction, especially if occurring unilaterally (on one side only). As this alternative test is performed in full weight bearing, there may be considerably more than the 20 degrees of dorsiflexion suggested above.

GENERAL STRETCH. Foot, ankle, and toe flexors

SPECIFIC STRETCHES. Gastrocnemius, soleus, peroneus longus, peroneus brevis, posterior tibialis, flexor digitorum longus, flexor hallicus longus

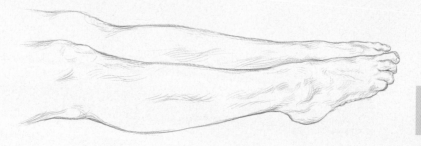

FIGURE 3.31 Test of ankle plantar-flexion

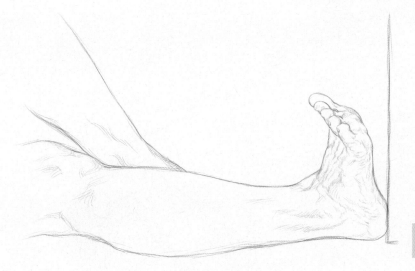

FIGURE 3.32 Test of ankle dorsiflexion

TOE FLEXION

TEST POSITION. Seated with right leg crossed over left knee

TEST. Place the left hand across the dorsum of the right foot and gently pull all of the toes toward the body (Fig. 3.33). The toes (proximal phalanges) should form a roughly 45-degree angle with the plane of the dorsal surface of the foot. Test both feet.

AVERAGE MOTION AVAILABLE. AAOS 40 degrees (45 degrees at great toe).[3] Notice that these measurements are for the metatarsophalangeal (MTP) joints.

GENERAL STRETCH. Toe extensors

SPECIFIC STRETCHES. Extensor digitorum longus, extensor digitorum brevis, extensor hallicus longus, extensor hallicus brevis

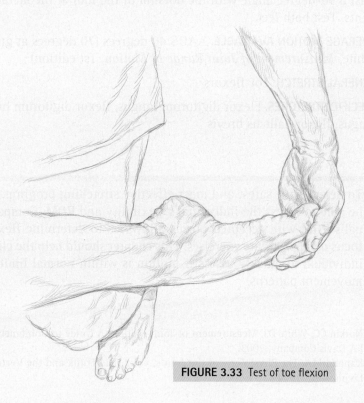

FIGURE 3.33 Test of toe flexion

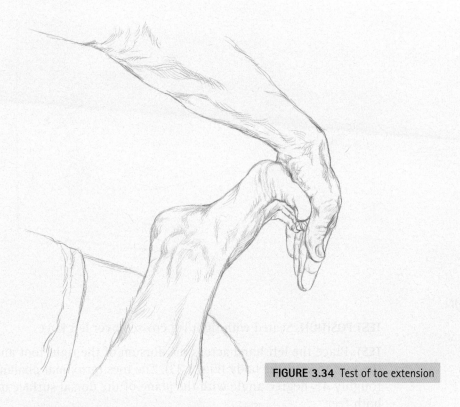

FIGURE 3.34 Test of toe extension

TOE EXTENSION

TEST POSITION. Seated, with test foot resting across opposite knee

TEST. Place the opposite left hand against the plantar surface of the right foot, so that the toes rest against the palm of the hand (Fig. 3.34). Use the palm of the left hand to push the toes into extension (toward the shin). The toes should form at least a 90-degree angle with the dorsum of the foot at the metatarsal-phalangeal joints. Test both feet.

AVERAGE MOTION AVAILABLE. AAOS 40 degrees (70 degrees at great toe) (Norkin and White, *Measurement of Joint Range of Motion,* 1st edition)

GENERAL STRETCH. Toe flexors

SPECIFIC STRETCHES. Flexor digitorum longus, flexor digitorum brevis, flexor hallucis longus, flexor hallucis brevis

SUMMARY

To develop the safest and most effective stretching program, it is necessary to be able to assess the individual's flexibility and ROM. Comparing the individual's ROM with accepted norms allows us to determine flexibility goals and focus on appropriate exercises. This chapter should help the clinician and/or the individual to quickly assess if motion is within normal limits for most useful movement patterns.

REFERENCES

1. Norkin CC, White DJ. Measurement of Joint Motion: A Guide to Goniometry. 3rd Ed. Philadelphia: FA Davis Company, 2003.
2. Kapandji IA. The Physiology of the Joints, vol 3, The Trunk and the Vertebral Column. Churchill Livingstone, 1974.

3. Norkin CC, White DJ. Measurement of Joint Motion: A Guide to Goniometry. 1st Ed. Philadelphia: FA Davis Company, 1985.

SUGGESTED READING

1. Palmer ML, Epler ME. Fundamentals of Musculoskeletal Assessment Techniques. 2nd Ed. Baltimore: Lippincott Williams and Wilkins, 1998.
2. Kendall FP, McCreary EK, Provance PG, et al. Muscles Testing and Function with Posture and Pain. 5th Ed. Baltimore Lippincott Williams and Wilkins, 2005.
3. Youdas YW, Garrett TR, Suman VJ, et al. Normal range of motion of the cervical spine: an initial goniometric study. Phys Ther 1992;72:770–780.

PART TWO

Basic Stretches
and Stretching
Programs

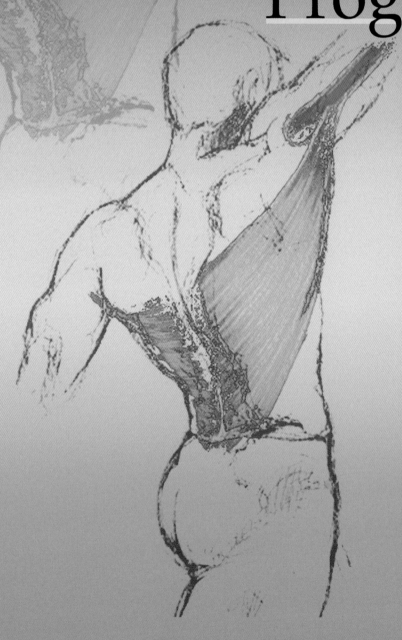

Stretches for Individual Muscles

T his chapter is intended for use by clinicians who, through careful evaluation, have determined a need to stretch particular muscles to improve function, restore balance, or relieve symptoms. Skilled clinicians may determine the need for addressing specific muscles, whether unilaterally or bilaterally, rather than more general "groups" of muscles. The chapter provides all of the information necessary to safely stretch almost all of the muscles producing human movement. It is intended for use as a detailed reference, not as a basic stretching program. For more general applications of stretching, see the table of contents.

In addition to the stretch technique, we have included the origin, insertion, primary action, and innervation for each individual muscle. This information may be useful for planning a general stretching program for client fitness or designing a program specific to a certain sport or activity. It may be particularly useful with clients rehabilitating from acute or chronic injury. The chapter also allows you to review basic muscle function without having to consult additional resources.

Although the chapter is comprehensive, it does not include the muscles responsible for facial expression, speech, mastication, swallowing, voice projection, digestion, primary respiration, etc. These are beyond the scope of this text. Please see Appendix A for further reading.

Every attempt has been made to provide stretching exercises that isolate the particular muscle discussed; however, even a shallow investigation of musculoskeletal anatomy will reveal that we are emphasizing, rather than isolating, each muscle. This is true because the complex arrangement of muscles that produce human movement necessitate that many of these muscles share common functions and occupy the same regions within the framework of the human skeleton.

ORGANIZATION OF STRETCHES FOR INDIVIDUAL MUSCLES

The stretches are presented from head to toe and grouped together by function within each area. For example, the muscles in the forearm producing motion at the wrist and hand are subdivided into flexors, extensors, and pronators/supinators. The individual stretches are described for either the right or the left side of the body, and, because of this, you may have to translate right to left or from left to right depending on the side you wish to stretch.

The terms origin and insertion were defined and discussed in Chapter 2. As noted there, origins and insertions will often reciprocate depending on the function of the system as a whole. In most human movement, there is no real fixed point because both the origin and the insertion are moving simultaneously. The terms *origin* and *insertion* are used in this chapter because they are consistent with most anatomy and physiology texts; however, you should be aware of their limitations.

Most muscles perform a number of functions, not all of which can be identified in this chapter. Instead, the chapter lists the function for each muscle that is generally accepted as the primary action produced by contraction of that individual muscle. As you work with this chapter, bear in mind that combinations of movement produced by one muscle are the norm, not the exception. In addition, the primary action of each muscle refers to the motion that would be generated in the open chain, that is, with the distal end of the bone free to move. For example, contracting your quadriceps muscle when you are in a seated position with your lower leg and foot free to move produces extension of your knee, thereby swinging your foot out and forward. In contrast, imagine standing with one foot on a step as if you were about to ascend a flight of stairs; contracting your quadriceps in this position would still cause your knee to extend, but instead of your foot moving, your body would move up over your foot. This is an example of a closed chain motion. The chapter lists each muscle's open chain function because it is generally easier to see and, again, it is consistent with most anatomy and physiology texts. But for much of the movement occurring in life, it would be more accurate to describe closed chain function or some combination of open and closed. Obviously, listing all of the possibilities would require an additional text.

The nerve supply to each of the muscles is also listed. This information should be useful in developing stretching programs to help aid in recovery from injuries which may, or may not involve nervous system structures. Knowledge of innervation may help identify the nerves which have been affected as well as predict other problem areas. For example, in the case of a herniated disc, which may be compressing nerve roots and causing functional losses or hyperactivity in particular muscles or groups of muscles, having easy access to innervations may aid in predicting other muscles or groups that may be affected and in making the ultimate diagnosis of the root problem.

Research on ideal hold times for stretches is discussed in detail in Chapter 2. As a brief guideline, hold each stretch for 30 seconds at an intensity sufficient to elicit a feeling of stretch, not pain.

HEAD AND NECK

Below are stretches for specific muscles of the head and neck.

> ⚠ **CAUTION!** Please be aware that restrictions in movement at the cervical spine that cause light-headedness, dizziness, local or referred pain, tingling, or numbness may indicate potentially hazardous injury to a joint, nerve, or blood vessel. These cases should be thoroughly evaluated by a professional specializing in spinal dysfunction before continuing.

Cervical Flexors

Below are stretches for the cervical flexors.

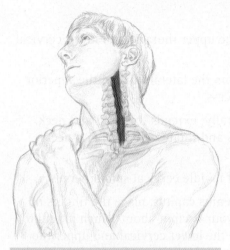

FIGURE 4.1

LONGUS CAPITUS AND LONGUS COLLI

ORIGIN. Anterior lateral aspects of vertebral bodies beginning at C1 (longus colli) and at the occiput (longus capitus)

INSERTION. Adjacent anterolateral aspect of adjacent vertebral bodies down to the upper thoracic levels

PRIMARY ACTION. Acting bilaterally, flexes the neck (and head) forward. Acting unilaterally, side-bends and rotates the vertebra above toward the working side.

INNERVATION. Longus capitus: anterior rami of C1–C3, longus colli: anterior rami of C2–C6

STRETCH. To stretch the longus capitus and longus colli on the left, first elevate your left shoulder by placing your left hand on top of your right shoulder so that the fingers of your left hand rest on the back of your right scapula (Fig. 4.1). Turn your head roughly 45 degrees toward the right and then side-bend it also toward the right. Carefully extend your head and neck.

OMOHYOID

ORIGIN. Superior, anterior aspect of the scapula, near the suprascapular notch

INSERTION. Hyoid bone

PRIMARY ACTION. Depresses, retracts, and stabilizes the hyoid bone. Acting bilaterally, may assist in flexion of the neck.

INNERVATION. Branch of ansa cervicalis (C1–C3)

STRETCH. To stretch your left omohyoid, first depress and retract your left scapula (Fig. 4.2). Place the fingers of your right hand on the left side of your hyoid bone (the crease where your neck meets your jaw). With the assistance of your right hand, move your head into right side-bending, then right rotation, finally lifting your chin and tilting your head back into extension.

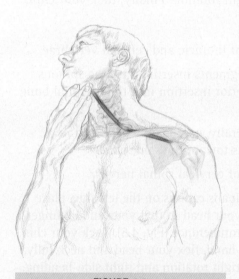

FIGURE 4.2

STERNOHYOID

ORIGIN. Posterior aspect of manubrium of the sternum

INSERTION. Hyoid bone

PRIMARY ACTION. Depresses the hyoid bone and larynx. May assist in flexion of the neck.

INNERVATION. Branch of ansa cervicalis (C1–C3)

STRETCH. To stretch your left sternohyoid, place the fingers of your right hand over your hyoid bone at the top of your throat, and the fingers of your left hand over your sternoclavicular joint (Fig. 4.3). With your right hand, carefully lift your head and neck back into extension while your left hand stabilizes your sternoclavicular joint. Now, carefully rotate your head toward the right.

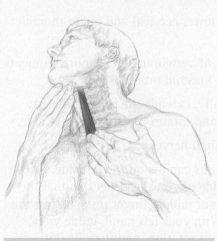

FIGURE 4.3

Cervical Extensors

Below are stretches for the cervical extensors.

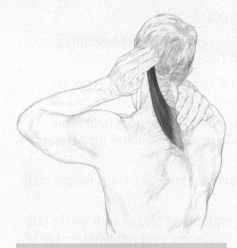

FIGURE 4.4

SPLENIUS CAPITUS

ORIGIN. Spinous processes of the upper thoracic and lower cervical vertebrae

INSERTION. Base of the skull from the lateral third of the superior nuchal line to the mastoid process

PRIMARY ACTION. Acting bilaterally, extends the head and neck. Acting unilaterally, side-bends and rotates the head and neck toward the same side.

INNERVATION. Posterior rami of middle cervical spinal nerves

STRETCH. To stretch the left splenius capitus, place the fingers of your left hand on the base of your occiput about 1 inch lateral to the midline (Fig. 4.4). Stabilize the lower cervical and upper thoracic vertebrae with pressure from the fingers of your right hand over the spinous processes of C6–T1 (prominence at the base of your neck). With your left hand, guide your head into right side-bending, then flexion, and right rotation. Finally, tuck your chin.

SEMISPINALIS CAPITUS

ORIGIN. Transverse processes of thoracic and cervical vertebrae

INSERTION. Spanning 4 to 6 segments inserting into the spinous processes above with the superior insertion into the occipital bone just lateral to the midline

PRIMARY ACTION. Acting bilaterally, extends the head and neck. Acting unilaterally, side-bends toward the same side.

INNERVATION. Posterior ramii of cervical spinal nerves

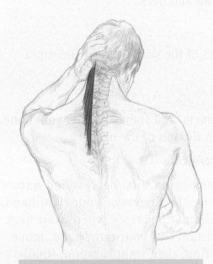

FIGURE 4.5

STRETCH. To stretch the semispinalis capitus on the left side, place your left hand on the back of your head so that your middle finger is on your external occipital protuberance (Fig. 4.5). Tuck your chin. With the guidance of your left hand, flex your head and neck fully, and then continue with slight right rotation and right side-bending.

LONGISSIMUS CAPITUS

ORIGIN. Transverse processes in lower cervical and upper thoracic areas

INSERTION. Transverse processes of vertebrae two or more segments above, finally inserting into the mastoid process of the skull

PRIMARY ACTION. Acting bilaterally, extends the head and neck. Acting unilaterally, side-bends and rotates toward the same side.

INNERVATION. Dorsal ramii of spinal nerves

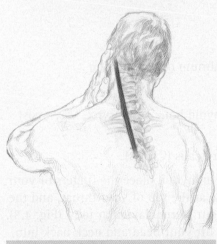

FIGURE 4.6

STRETCH. To stretch the longissimus capitus on the left side, place your left hand against the left side of your head/neck so that the distal interphalangeal joint of your middle finger rests against the left mastoid process (Fig. 4.6). With your left hand, guide your head into right side-bending, right rotation, and then flexion.

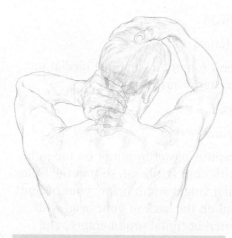

FIGURE 4.7

OBLIQUUS CAPITUS SUPERIOR

ORIGIN. Transverse process of C1 (atlas)

INSERTION. Occipital bone

PRIMARY ACTION. Acting bilaterally, extends the head backwards. Acting unilaterally, sidebends the head toward the same side.

INNERVATION. Dorsal ramii of spinal nerves

STRETCH. To stretch the obliquus capitus superior on the left side, grasp your neck just below your head, with your left hand stabilizing your neck (Fig. 4.7). Place your right hand on top of your head and tilt your head directly toward the right, minimizing the motion below the first cervical vertebra. Next, turn your head slightly toward the right with the assistance of your right hand.

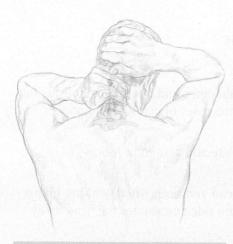

FIGURE 4.8

OBLIQUUS CAPITUS INFERIOR

ORIGIN. Spinous process of C-2 (axis)

INSERTION. Transverse process of C-1

PRIMARY ACTION. Acting bilaterally, extends C-1 on C-2. Acting unilaterally, produces side-bending and rotation toward the same side.

INNERVATION. Dorsal ramii of spinal nerves.

STRETCH. To stretch the obliquus capitis inferior on the left side, place your right hand on the back of your head with your index and middle fingers just below your occiput (Fig. 4.8). Place your left hand just below your right and tightly grasp your neck, minimizing the motion below C-2 as you use your right hand to help tilt your head into right side-bending and then into right rotation.

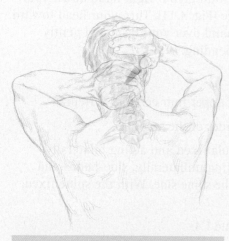

FIGURE 4.9

RECTUS CAPITUS POSTERIOR MAJOR

ORIGIN. Spinous processes of C-2

INSERTION. Occiput, just lateral to the insertion of the rectus capitus posterior minor

PRIMARY ACTION. Acting bilaterally, extends the head. Acting unilaterally, side-bends and rotates the head toward the same side.

INNERVATION. Dorsal ramii of spinal nerves

STRETCH. To stretch the rectus capitus posterior major on the right side, first grasp your neck from behind with your left hand, so that the little finger of your left hand is about 2 finger widths below your occiput (Fig. 4.9). Place your right hand above your left so that the index and middle fingers are just below your occiput. Using your right hand, guide your head forward into flexion, and then into left rotation and left side-bending, while minimizing the motion below C-2 with your left hand.

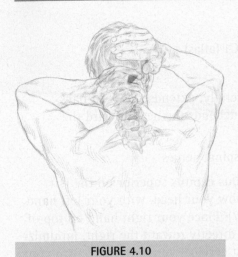

FIGURE 4.10

RECTUS CAPITUS POSTERIOR MINOR

ORIGIN. Spinous process of C-1 (atlas)

INSERTION. Occiput, slightly lateral to midline and just medial to the insertion of rectus capitus posterior major

PRIMARY ACTION. Extends the head

INNERVATION. Dorsal ramii of spinal nerves

STRETCH. To stretch the rectus capitus posterior minor on the right, grasp your neck from behind with your left hand, so that the little finger of your left hand is about 1 finger width below your occiput (Fig. 4.10). Place your right hand on the back of your head with your index finger over the external occipital protuberance, and carefully flex your head by tucking your chin. Then add slight left rotation and left side-bending, using your right hand as a guide and your left hand to stabilize below C-1.

Cervical Side-Benders

Below are stretches for the cervical side-benders.

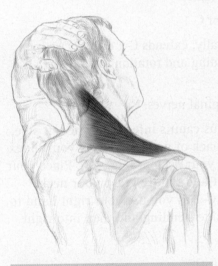

FIGURE 4.11

UPPER TRAPEZIUS

ORIGIN. External occipital protuberance and lateral third of nuchal line, nuchal ligament spinous processes of cervical and upper thoracic vertebrae

INSERTION. Lateral third of clavicle and acromion process of scapula

PRIMARY ACTION. Extends the head and neck when working bilaterally. Side-bends toward the same side and rotates the head away when working unilaterally.

INNERVATION. Spinal accessory nerve and C3 and C4 nerves

STRETCH. To stretch the upper trapezius on your right side, first depress your right shoulder by sliding your right hand down your right hip toward your right knee (Fig. 4.11). Turn your head toward the right, then place your left hand over your head and gently assist your head into left side-bending.

LEVATOR SCAPULA

ORIGIN. Transverse processes of upper four cervical vertebrae

INSERTION. Superior, medial border of the scapula

PRIMARY ACTION. With the scapula fixed and acting bilaterally, extends the head and neck. Acting unilaterally, side-bends and rotates head and neck toward the same side. With the spine fixed, elevates the scapula.

INNERVATION. Branches of C3 and C4

STRETCH. To stretch the levator scapula on your right side, reach your right hand down and away from your body about a 45-degree angle (Fig. 4.12). Turn your head to the left. Place your left hand on top of your head so that your fingers hook under the back of the right side of your head. Guide your head and neck forward and toward the left.

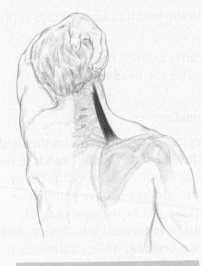

FIGURE 4.12

SCALENES, ANTERIOR, MIDDLE, AND POSTERIOR

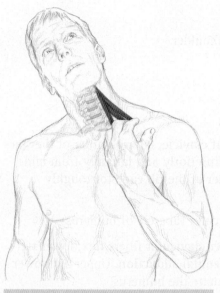

FIGURE 4.13

ORIGIN. Transverse processes of the second through seventh cervical vertebrae, the anterior from the third through the sixth, the middle from the second through the seventh, and the posterior from the fourth through the seventh

INSERTION. Anterior and middle to the first rib, and the posterior to the second rib, at the angle near midshaft

PRIMARY ACTION. Acting bilaterally, flexes the neck. Acting unilaterally, side-bends toward the same side, and rotates away.

INNERVATION. Branches of the cervical ventral ramii

STRETCH. To stretch the scalenes on the left side, first place the fingers of your left hand on your clavicle about midshaft (Fig. 4.13). Turn your head toward the left about 45 degrees, and then slowly and carefully lean it toward the right, while using your left hand to hold down your left clavicle.

Cervical Rotators

Below are stretches for the cervical rotators

STERNOCLEIDOMASTOID

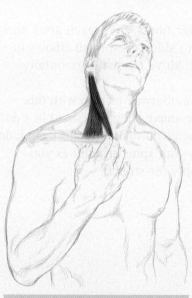

FIGURE 4.14

ORIGIN. Two heads of origin, one from the superior-anterior surface of manubrium of the sternum and the other from the medial end of the clavicle.

INSERTION. Mastoid process of temporal bone

PRIMARY ACTION. Acting bilaterally, flexes the head and neck. Acting unilaterally, side-bends the head toward the same side and rotates it away.

INNERVATION. Spinal accessory nerve and spinal nerves C2 and C3

STRETCH. To stretch your right sternocleidomastoid, first turn your head toward the right and place the fingers of your right hand on the medial end of your right clavicle (Fig. 4.14). Next, side-bend your head toward the left, and finally extend your head and neck carefully backward.

SHOULDER

Below are stretches for specific muscles of the shoulder.

Shoulder Flexors

Below are stretches for the shoulder flexors.

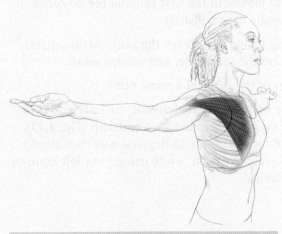

FIGURE 4.15

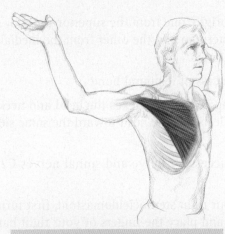

FIGURE 4.16

PECTORALIS MAJOR

ORIGIN. Medial third of clavicle, lateral border of the sternum, and diagonally inferiorly and laterally from midline along lower border of the rib cage for roughly 3–5 inches

INSERTION. Crest of greater tubercle of humerus

PRIMARY ACTION. Upper clavicular fibers flex; lower sternal fibers best at horizontal adduction. Upper and lower fibers also medially rotate the humerus.

INNERVATION. Medial and lateral pectoral nerves (C5, C6, C7, C8, T1)

STRETCH. To stretch the upper fibers bilaterally, reach both arms behind you and roll forearms out as far as possible (Fig. 4.15).

To stretch the lower fibers, first reach arms horizontally straight out to sides, then bend elbows to 90 degrees (Fig. 4.16). Move elbows horizontally backward.

You may also use a doorway to help with this stretch. In either of the above stretches, stand in a doorway and place your hands on the upper, horizontal doorframe. Be sure to keep your spine straight as you carefully lean in to apply the stretch.

ANTERIOR DELTOID

ORIGIN. Lateral one-third of the clavicle

INSERTION. Deltoid tuberosity, at the lateral midshaft of the humerus (converges there with middle and posterior parts of the deltoid)

PRIMARY ACTION. Flexes and internally rotates the humerus

INNERVATION. Axillary nerve (C5, C6)

STRETCH. To stretch the anterior deltoid of your left arm, extend your arm and hand behind you with your forearm supinated (Fig. 4.17). Next, flex your elbow to about 90 degrees and place your hand on a back of a chair or counter top. Carefully lower your body by flexing your knees, while keeping your body upright and allowing your left elbow to rise up behind you.

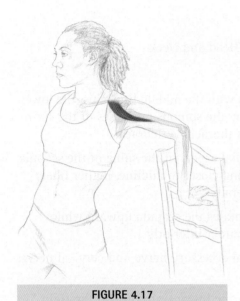

FIGURE 4.17

CORACOBRACHIALIS

ORIGIN. Coracoid process of the scapula

INSERTION. Anterior medial aspect of the humerus, at midshaft

PRIMARY ACTION. Flexes and adducts the humerus

INNERVATION. Musculocutaneous nerve (C5, C6, C7)

STRETCH. To stretch the coracobrachialis of your right arm, abduct your humerus to about 60 degrees, then externally rotate your arm (palm up) (Fig. 4.18). Now extend your arm posteriorly, keeping it abducted roughly 60 degrees.

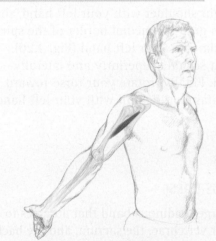

FIGURE 4.18

Shoulder Flexors Acting on the Scapula

Below are stretches for the shoulder flexors acting on the scapula.

SERRATUS ANTERIOR

ORIGIN. Anterior and lateral surfaces of the upper 8 or 9 ribs, generally anterior and inferior to the axilla

INSERTION. Entire medial border of the scapula (passes between the scapula and the rib cage)

PRIMARY ACTION. Upwardly rotates and protracts the scapula. Aids in elevating the arm overhead, particularly at higher angles.

INNERVATION. Long thoracic nerve (C5–C7)

STRETCH. To stretch the serratus anterior of your left shoulder, first fully flex your left elbow allowing the humerus (upper arm) to stay against your left side (Fig. 4.19). Place your left hand, forearm, and anterior shoulder against a wall or doorframe and then carefully apply pressure against your hand, forearm, and shoulder by turning your chest and shoulders toward the right.

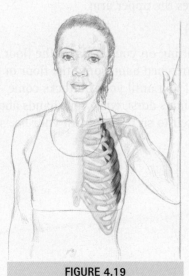

FIGURE 4.19

UPPER TRAPEZIUS

See the stretch for the upper trapezius under Head and Neck.

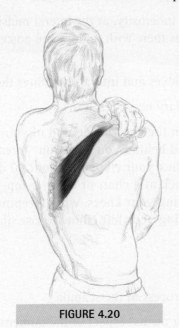

FIGURE 4.20

LOWER TRAPEZIUS

ORIGIN. Continuous with the middle trapezius, the lower trapezius arises from the spinous processes of the sixth through the twelfth thoracic vertebrae.

INSERTION. The medial aspect of the spine of the scapula, lower fibers attaching closer to midline, higher fibers attaching more laterally

PRIMARY ACTION. Rotates the scapula upward while pulling its medial border inferiorly

INNERVATION. Spinal accessory nerve and cervical nerves 3 and 4

STRETCH. To stretch the lower trapezius on the right, reach over your right shoulder with your left hand, so that you are able to grab the medial border of the spine of your right scapula with your left hand (Fig. 4.20). Now pull your right scapula superiorly and laterally with your left hand. Finally, rotate your torso toward the left, while maintaining the pull with your left hand.

Shoulder Extensors

Below are stretches for the shoulder extensors.

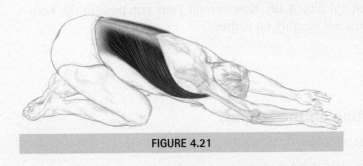

FIGURE 4.21

LATISSIMUS DORSI

ORIGIN. Large tendinous band that attaches to the lumbar vertebrae, the sacrum, and the back of the pelvis

INSERTION. Intertubercular groove on the anterior aspect of the proximal humerus

PRIMARY ACTION. Extends, adducts, and internally rotates the upper arm

INNERVATION. Thoracodorsal nerve (C6, C7, C8)

STRETCH. Assume a position in which you are sitting on your heels on the floor (Fig. 4.21). Now bend over and place both outstretched hands onto the floor in front of you. Reach both hands farther out in front of you until your buttocks come off of your heels. Now to stretch the right latissimus dorsi, walk your hands about 10 inches toward the left. Carefully allow yourself to sit back toward your heels while maintaining the position of your hands.

TERES MAJOR

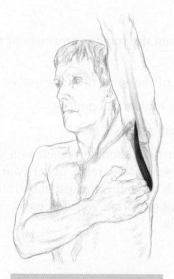

FIGURE 4.22

ORIGIN. Posterior lateral aspect of inferior angle of the scapula

INSERTION. Crest of lesser tubercle of the humerus (anterior aspect of the humerus, below the neck, roughly one-fourth of the way down)

PRIMARY ACTION. Adducts, internally rotates, and extends the humerus

INNERVATION. Lower subscapular nerve (C5, C6, C7)

STRETCH. To stretch your left teres major, maximally abduct and flex your left arm. Now maximally and externally rotate your left shoulder (Fig. 4.22). Using your right hand, reach across your chest and place your fingers on the lateral border of your left scapula. Finally, press the inferior border of your left scapula posteriorly while actively attempting to flex your upper arm behind(posteriorly) the plane of your head.

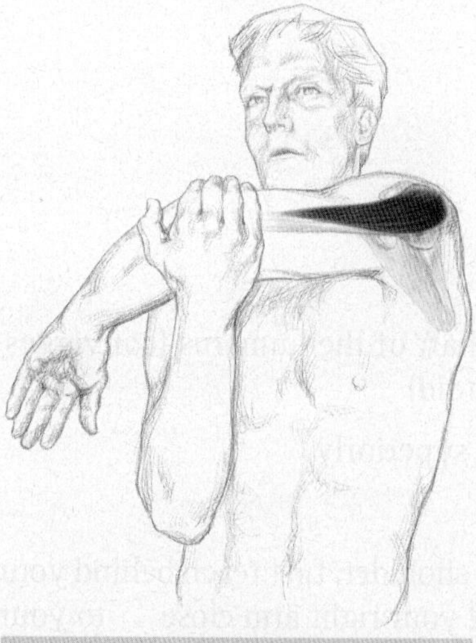

POSTERIOR DELTOID

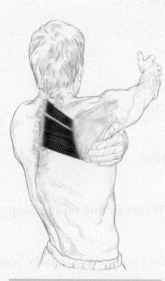

ORIGIN. Most of the spine of the scapula

INSERTION. Deltoid tuberosity, where it converges with both the anterior and middle deltoids

PRIMARY ACTION. Extends and externally rotates the humerus with arm adducted or flexed. Horizontally abducts when arm is elevated.

INNERVATION. Axillary nerve (C5, C6)

STRETCH. To stretch your left posterior deltoid, use your right hand to pull your left elbow high across your chest, allowing your elbow to unlock and your left hand to hang down (Fig. 4.23).

FIGURE 4.23

Shoulder Extensors Acting on the Scapula

Below are stretches for the shoulder extensors acting on the scapula.

RHOMBOID MAJOR AND MINOR

ORIGIN. Rhomboid minor from spinous processes of the seventh cervical and first thoracic vertebrae, rhomboid major from the spinous processes of the second though fifth thoracic vertebrae

INSERTION. Medial border of the scapula with the minor inserting at the level of the spine of the scapula, and the major inserting just inferior to it from the scapular spine down to the inferior angle

PRIMARY ACTION. Adducts the scapula toward midline and rotates it inferiorly

INNERVATION. Dorsal scapular nerve (C4, C5)

STRETCH. To stretch the rhomboids on your right shoulder, reach across your chest and under your right armpit with your left hand (Fig. 4.24). Protract your right shoulder as far as possible and place your left hand across your right scapula. Pull your right scapula superiorly and anteriorly while reaching across toward your left side with your right hand.

FIGURE 4.24

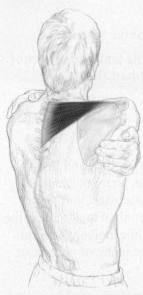

FIGURE 4.25

MIDDLE TRAPEZIUS

ORIGIN. Continuous with the upper trapezius, from the spinous processes of the first through the fifth thoracic vertebrae

INSERTION. The acromion and the lateral aspect of the spine of the scapula

PRIMARY ACTION. Adducts the scapula, pulling it toward the midline

INNERVATION. Spinal accessory nerve and cervical nerves 3 and 4

STRETCH. To stretch the middle trapezius of your right shoulder, reach with your right hand and rest it on the left shoulder (Fig. 4.25). Now reach under your right axilla and place your left hand on the back of your right scapula. Protract your right shoulder while assisting with a strong pull from your left hand, attempting to further protract your right scapula.

Shoulder Abductors

Below are stretches for the shoulder abductors.

MIDDLE DELTOID

ORIGIN. Acromion process of scapula

INSERTION. Deltoid tuberosity, at the lateral midshaft of the humerus (converges there with anterior and posterior parts of the deltoid)

PRIMARY ACTION. Abducts arm laterally and then superiorly

INNERVATION. Axillary nerve (C5, C6)

STRETCH. To stretch the middle deltoid of your right shoulder, first reach behind your back with your right arm (Fig. 4.26). Now, keeping your right arm close   to your body, use your left hand to adduct it (pull it across to the left).

SUPRASPINATUS

See the stretch for the supraspinatus under Rotator Cuff.

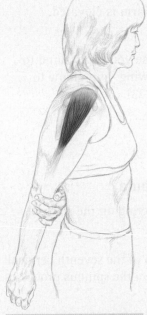

FIGURE 4.26

Shoulder Abductors Acting on the Scapula

Below are stretches for the shoulder abductors acting on the scapula.

UPPER TRAPEZIUS

See the upper trapezius stretch under Head and Neck.

LOWER TRAPEZIUS

See the lower trapezius stretch under Shoulder Flexors Acting on the Scapula.

SERRATUS ANTERIOR

See the stretch for the serratus anterior under Shoulder Flexors Acting on the Scapula.

LEVATOR SCAPULA

See the stretch for the levator scapula under Head and Neck.

Shoulder Adductors

Below are stretches for the shoulder adductors.

LATISSIMUS DORSI

See the stretch for the latissimus dorsi under Shoulder Extensors.

PECTORALIS MAJOR

See the stretch for pectoralis major under Shoulder Flexors.

TERES MAJOR

See the stretch for teres major under Shoulder Extensors.

Shoulder Adductors Acting on the Scapula

Below are stretches for the shoulder adductors acting on the scapula.

RHOMBOIDS MAJOR AND MINOR

See the stretch for rhomboids major and minor under Shoulder Extensors Acting on the Scapula.

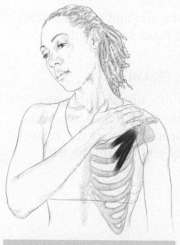

FIGURE 4.27

PECTORALIS MINOR

ORIGIN. Ribs three through five

INSERTION. Coracoid process of the scapula (just medial to the head of the humerus)

PRIMARY ACTION. Depresses and protracts your scapula

INNERVATION. Medial pectoral nerve (C8, T1)

STRETCH. To stretch the pectoralis minor on your left, place your right hand on the left side of your chest so that your middle finger lies over the coracoid process of your left shoulder (Fig. 4.27). Now, guide your left shoulder superiorly and posteriorly with the palm of your right hand, using both the force of your right hand, and the active contraction of the retractors and elevators of your left scapula. You may assist this motion with the elevators of your right scapula.

Rotator Cuff

Below are stretches for the rotator cuff.

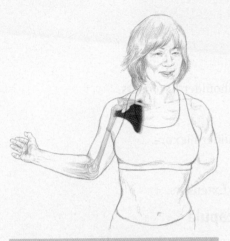

FIGURE 4.28

SUBSCAPULARIS

ORIGIN. Entire anterior surface of the scapula

INSERTION. Lesser tubercle of the humerus

PRIMARY ACTION. Internally rotates the humerus with the arm at the side and is a primary stabilizer of the glenohumeral joint

INNERVATION. Upper and lower subscapular nerves (C5, C6, C7)

STRETCH. To stretch your right subscapularis, bend your right elbow to 90 degrees and externally rotate your right humerus (Fig. 4.28). Keeping your right elbow at your side, place your right hand, palm facing anteriorly, against a doorway or other stationary object. Carefully turn your body toward the left, taking care to maintain the position of your right humerus

SUPRASPINATUS

ORIGIN. Supraspinous fossa

INSERTION. Superior aspect of the greater tubercle of the humerus

PRIMARY ACTION. Assists in abducting the arm and helps stabilize the head of the humerus in the glenoid fossa during motion occurring at the shoulder

INNERVATION. Suprascapular nerve (C4, C5, C6)

STRETCH. To stretch the supraspinatus of your right shoulder, reach behind your back with your right hand (Fig. 4.29). Using your left hand, grasp your right forearm and externally rotate it. Now pull your right arm posteriorly and toward the left, adducting it.

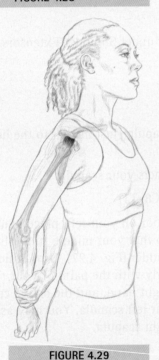

FIGURE 4.29

INFRASPINATUS AND TERES MINOR

ORIGIN. Posterior surface of the scapula, below the scapular spine

INSERTION. The posterior aspect of the head of the humerus along the greater tubercle, with the infraspinatus inserting just superior to the teres minor

PRIMARY ACTION. Externally rotates the humerus and helps stabilize the head of the humerus in the glenoid fossa

INNERVATION. Infraspinatus from subscapular nerve (C5, C6), and teres minor from axillary nerve (C5, C6)

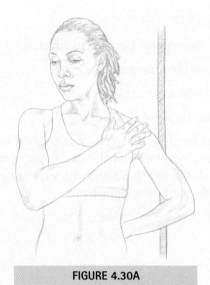

FIGURE 4.30A

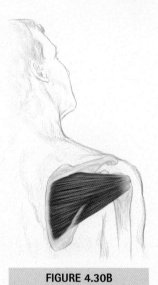

FIGURE 4.30B

STRETCH. To stretch your left infraspinatus and teres minor, stand with your left hand behind your lower back, elbow bent to 90 degrees, and the fingers of your right hand on the anterior aspect of the head of the left humerus (Fig. 4.30). Slowly back into a doorway so that your elbow is being pressed forward by the door jam. Be sure to stabilize the head of your left humerus with the pressure from your right hand.

ELBOW

Below are stretches for specific muscles of the elbow.

Elbow Flexors

Below are stretches for the elbow flexors.

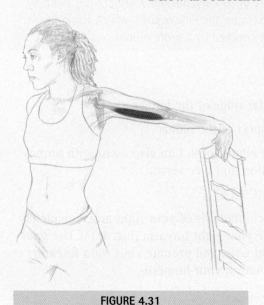

FIGURE 4.31

BICEPS BRACHII

ORIGIN. Long head from the supraglenoid tubercle of the scapula, short head from the coracoid process of the scapula

INSERTION. The bicipital tuberosity of the radius (bony prominence on the medial side of the radius, roughly one inch distal your elbow)

PRIMARY ACTION. Flexes elbow, supinates forearm, and, to a lesser degree, assists in flexing the humerus

INNERVATION. Musculocutaneous nerve (C5, C6)

STRETCH. To stretch the long head of the biceps of your right arm, first extend your right elbow completely (Fig. 4.31). Internally rotate your extended arm and then extend it to end range. From this position, place the palm of your left hand on the back of a chair. Keeping body upright, carefully lower your body by bending at the knees while keeping your right hand stationary on the wall.

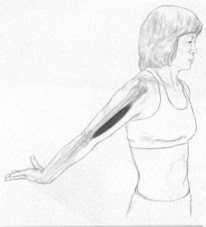

FIGURE 4.32

SHORT HEAD OF BICEPS BRACHII

ORIGIN. Coracoid process of the scapula (see biceps brachii)

INSERTION. Medial midshaft of the humerus

PRIMARY ACTION. Flexes and adducts the humerus

INNERVATION. Musculocutaneous nerve (C5, C6)

STRETCH. To stretch the short head of the biceps brachii, first extend your right elbow, then internally rotate and slightly abduct your right outstretched arm (Fig. 4.32). Reach posteriorly, superiorly, and slightly away from your body with your right hand.

BRACHIALIS

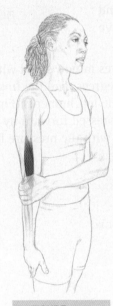

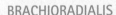

FIGURE 4.33

ORIGIN. Anterior surface of distal one-half of humerus

INSERTION. Coronoid process and tuberosity of the ulna (proximal, anterior surface of the ulna)

PRIMARY ACTION. Flexes the elbow

INNERVATION. Musculocutaneous nerve (C5, C6)

STRETCH. To stretch the brachialis of your right arm, allow your right arm to extend by your side, palm toward hip (Fig. 4.33). Place your left hand on the back of your right elbow and slowly pull your right elbow into extension.

> ⚠ **CAUTION!** The elbow has a bony block at its end of extension. Be sure that the resistance you are getting with this stretch is muscular. It should feel rubbery or springy, not bony. Otherwise, you may be placing unnecessary stress on the elbow joint, which could result in injury. If in doubt, get it checked by a professional.

BRACHIORADIALIS

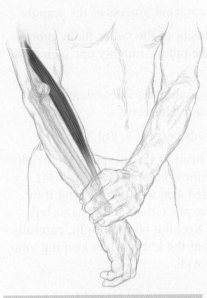

FIGURE 4.34

ORIGIN. Lateral supracondylar ridge of the humerus

INSERTION. Distal, lateral aspect of the radius

PRIMARY ACTION. Flexes the elbow joint. Can also assist with pronation from a supinated position and vice versa.

INNERVATION. Radial nerve (C5, C6)

STRETCH. To stretch the brachioradialis of your right arm, completely extend and internally rotate your right forearm (Fig. 4.34). Use your left hand to grasp your right wrist and pronate your right forearm while actively externally rotating your humerus.

Elbow Extensors

Below are stretches for the elbow extensors.

TRICEPS BRACHII: LONG HEAD

ORIGIN. Infraglenoid tubercle

INSERTION. Joins with the lateral and medial heads and inserts into the olecranon process of the ulna

PRIMARY ACTION. Extends the elbow, and helps extend and adduct the shoulder

INNERVATION. Radial nerve (C6, C7, C8)

STRETCH. To stretch the triceps of your right shoulder, reach overhead with your right hand (Fig. 4.35). Maximally flex your right elbow so that you are essentially reaching to attempt to scratch your right shoulder blade. Now with your left hand, grasp your right elbow and pull it posteriorly and toward the left.

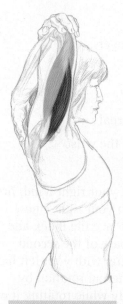

FIGURE 4.35

TRICEPS BRACHII: LATERAL AND MIDDLE HEADS

ORIGIN. Lateral head from the upper third of the posterior and lateral humerus. Medial head from lower two-thirds of the posterior medial surface of the humerus.

INSERTION. Joins with the long head and inserts into the olecranon process of the ulna

PRIMARY ACTION. Extends the elbow

INNERVATION. Radial nerve (C6, C7, C8)

STRETCH. To stretch the lateral and middle heads of the triceps of your left arm, first flex your left elbow as much as possible (Fig. 4.36A). Next, grasp your left forearm just proximal to your wrist with your right hand. Apply pressure to your forearm, pushing it toward your shoulder and flexing your elbow.

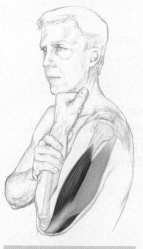

FIGURE 4.36A

ANCONEUS

ORIGIN. Lateral epicondyle of the humerus

INSERTION. Lateral aspect of the olecranon process of the ulna

PRIMARY ACTION. Helps extend the elbow

INNERVATION. Radial nerve (C7, C8, T1)

STRETCH. See stretch above for the lateral and middle heads of the triceps brachii (Fig. 4.36B).

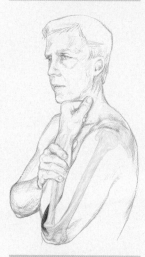

FIGURE 4.36B

WRIST AND HAND

Below are stretches for specific muscles of wrist and hand.

Flexors of the Wrist, Hand, and Fingers

Below are stretches for the flexors of the wrist, hand, and fingers.

FLEXOR CARPI RADIALIS

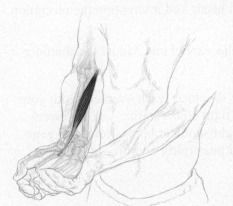

ORIGIN. Medial epicondyle of the humerus

INSERTION. Palmar base of the second metacarpal

PRIMARY ACTION. Flexes and radially deviates the wrist

INNERVATION. Median nerve (C6, C7)

STRETCH. To stretch the flexor carpi radialis of your right hand, first reach your right hand out in front of you with your right elbow extended (Fig. 4.37). Now extend your wrist. Place the index and forefinger of your left hand over the palmar base of the second metacarpal of your right hand. Using a firm grip with your left hand, stretch your right wrist into extension and external rotation by pulling your right hand back toward your body while rotating it out.

FIGURE 4.37

PALMARIS LONGUS

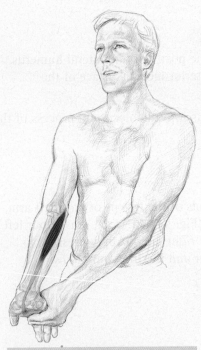

ORIGIN. Medial epicondyle of the humerus

INSERTION. Palmar aponeurosis and flexor retinaculum

INNERVATION. Median nerve (C7, C8)

PRIMARY ACTION. Flexes the wrist

STRETCH. To stretch the palmaris longus of your left hand, first extend your left elbow and wrist in front of you (Fig. 4.38). Now using the fingers of your left hand across the palm of your right, stretch the wrist carefully further back into extension.

FIGURE 4.38

FLEXOR DIGITORUM PROFUNDUS

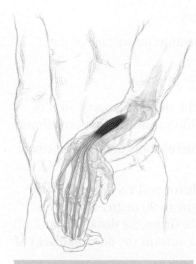

FIGURE 4.39

ORIGIN. Proximal, medial two-thirds of the anterior surface of the ulna

INSERTION. Palmar surface of the distal phalanx of fingers 2–5

PRIMARY ACTION. Flexes the distal interphalangeal joint in fingers 2–5 and assists with flexion of the proximal interphalangeal joints and the wrist. Along with flexor digitorum superficialis, it is responsible for forceful grip.

INNERVATION. Medial part via ulnar nerve (C8, T1), lateral part via median nerve (C8, T1)

STRETCH. To stretch the flexor digitorum profundus of your left hand, place the palm of your right hand over the distal phalanx of fingers 2–5 of your left hand (your left elbow may be slightly flexed) (Fig. 4.39). Use this contact to press the distal phalanx of fingers 2–5 back into extension, continuing until the fingers and the wrist have reached full extension.

FLEXOR DIGITORUM SUPERFICIALIS

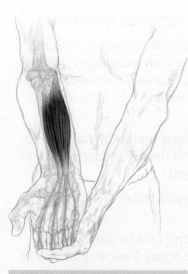

FIGURE 4.40

ORIGIN. Two heads: one from the medial epicondyle of the humerus and the proximal ulna; the other from the proximal half of the radius

INSERTION. Middle phalanx of fingers 2–5

PRIMARY ACTION. Flexes the proximal interphalangeal joint of each finger. Along with the flexor digitorum profundus, it is necessary for forceful grip.

INNERVATION. Median nerve (C7, C8, T1)

STRETCH. To stretch the flexor digitorum superficialis of your right hand, first extend your right elbow and wrist, turning the palm up (Fig. 4.40). Next, place the index finger of your left hand across the middle phalanges of the second through fifth fingers of your right hand. Carefully pull your right wrist and fingers back toward you with your left hand.

FLEXOR CARPI ULNARIS

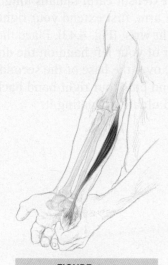

FIGURE 4.41

ORIGIN. Medial epicondyle of the humerus

INSERTION. Pisiform bone of the hand

PRIMARY ACTION. Flexes and ulnar deviates the hand

INNERVATION. Ulnar nerve (C7, C8)

STRETCH. To stretch the flexor carpi ulnaris of your right arm, first actively extend your right elbow, then actively extend and radially deviate your wrist and hand (Fig. 4.41), then use your left hand to apply pressure to the palm of your right hand, guiding it further into extension and radial deviation.

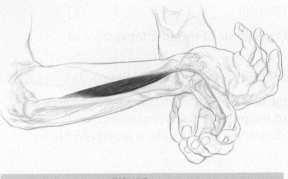

FIGURE 4.42

FLEXOR POLLICUS LONGUS

ORIGIN. Middle half of the anterior surface of the radius

INSERTION. Distal phalanx of thumb

PRIMARY ACTION. Flexes the interphalangeal joint of the thumb, and is critical in grasp with opposed thumb

INNERVATION. Anterior interosseous branch of median nerve (C8, T1)

STRETCH. To stretch the flexor pollicis longus of your right hand, flex your elbow to 90 degrees, palm up (Fig. 4.42). Now actively extend your wrist and thumb. Grasp the distal phalanx of your right thumb with your left hand, and pull it back toward the dorsum (back) of your forearm.

Extensors and Abductors of the Wrist, Hand, and Fingers

Below are stretches for the extensors and abductors of the wrist, hand, and fingers.

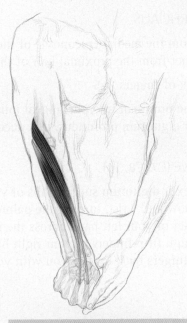

FIGURE 4.43

EXTENSOR CARPI RADIALIS LONGUS AND BREVIS

ORIGIN. Lateral epicondyle of the humerus, with the longus originating slightly more proximally, and the brevis originating from the common extensor tendon with the extensor digitorum and the extensor digiti minimi

INSERTION. The longus inserts into the dorsal base of the second metacarpal, and the brevis inserts into the base of the third metacarpal.

PRIMARY ACTION. Extends and radially deviates the hand

INNERVATION. Extensor carpi radialis longus from radial nerve (C6, C7), and brevis from deep branch of radial nerve (C7, C8)

STRETCH. To stretch the extensor carpi radialis longus and brevis of your right arm, first extend your right elbow and flex your right wrist (Fig. 4.43). Place the index and middle finger of your left hand on the dorsum of your right hand, over the base of the second and third metacarpals and pull your right hand back toward you, flexing and ulnarly deviating it.

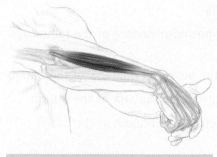

FIGURE 4.44

EXTENSOR DIGITORUM AND EXTENSOR DIGITI MINIMI

ORIGIN. Lateral epicondyle of the humerus (common extensor tendon)

INSERTION. Middle and distal phalanges of fingers 2–5

PRIMARY ACTION. Extends the fingers, mainly at the metacarpal-phalangeal joint of each finger 2–5, with extensor digiti minimi extending the fifth finger alone

INNERVATION. Posterior interosseous branch of the radial nerve (C7, C8)

STRETCH. To stretch the extensor digitorum and extensor digiti minimi of your right hand, first extend your right elbow and make a tight fist (Fig. 4.44). Use your left hand to carefully apply pressure to flex your right wrist.

EXTENSOR CARPI ULNARIS

ORIGIN. Lateral epicondyle of the humerus, and proximal half of the posterior ulna

INSERTION. Dorsomedial aspect of base of the fifth metacarpal

PRIMARY ACTION. Extends and ulnarly deviates the hand

INNERVATION. Posterior interosseous branch of the radial nerve (C7, C8)

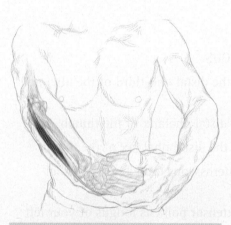

FIGURE 4.45

STRETCH. To stretch the extensor carpi ulnaris of your right hand, first extend your right elbow, palm down (Fig. 4.45). Next, flex your right wrist and, using the fingers of your left hand, gently pull your right hand (not fingers) back toward you, while externally rotating, or rolling out, your hand.

ABDUCTOR POLLICUS LONGUS

ORIGIN. Posterior middle third of both radius and ulna

INSERTION. Ventral (palmar) base of first metacarpal

PRIMARY ACTION. Abducts the thumb

INNERVATION. Posterior interosseous branch of the radial nerve (C7, C8)

STRETCH. To stretch the abductor pollicus longus of your right hand, extend and ulnarly deviate your right wrist (Fig. 4.46). Carefully adduct and extend your right thumb back behind the plane of your hand with the fingers of your left hand.

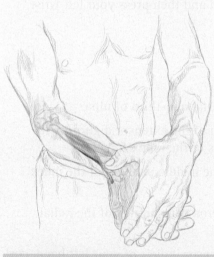

FIGURE 4.46

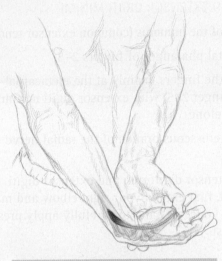

FIGURE 4.47

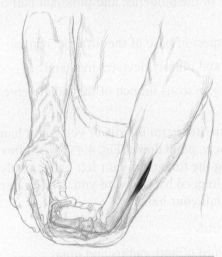

FIGURE 4.48

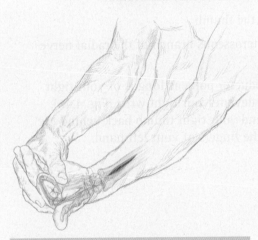

FIGURE 4.49

EXTENSOR POLLICUS BREVIS

ORIGIN. Distal one-third of posterior surface of the radius and interosseous membrane

INSERTION. Dorsal base of the proximal phalanx of the thumb

PRIMARY ACTION. Extends proximal phalanx of the thumb

INNERVATION. Posterior interosseous branch of the radial nerve (C7, C8)

STRETCH. Gently press proximal phalanx of thumb into the palm and then slightly flex and ulnarly deviate the wrist (Fig. 4.47).

EXTENSOR POLLICUS LONGUS

ORIGIN. Dorsal surface of the distal one-third of the ulna and interosseous membrane

INSERTION. Dorsal base of distal phalanx of the thumb

PRIMARY ACTION. Extends the distal phalanx of the thumb

INNERVATION. Posterior interosseous branch of the radial nerve (C7, C8)

STRETCH. To stretch the extensor pollicus longus of your left hand, carefully flex all the joints of your left thumb, curling it into your palm (Fig. 4.48). Using your right hand, carefully hold your left thumb flexed and then press your left wrist into ulnar deviation.

EXTENSOR INDICIS

ORIGIN. Dorsal surface of distal one-third of ulna

INSERTION. Joins the tendon of the extensor digitorum to middle and distal phalanges of the index finger

PRIMARY ACTION. Extends the middle phalanx of the index finger

INNERVATION. Posterior interosseous branch of the radial nerve (C7, C8)

STRETCH. To stretch the extensor indicis of your left hand, curl your index finger into your palm (Fig. 4.49). With the help of your right hand, keep your right index finger tightly flexed and then carefully flex and radially deviate your left wrist.

Pronators and Supinators of the Forearm

Below are stretches for the pronators and supinators of the forearm.

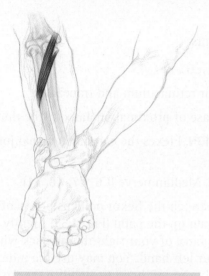

FIGURE 4.50

PRONATOR TERES

ORIGIN. Two heads: humeral head from the medial epicondyle of the humerus, just superior to the common flexor tendon; ulnar head from the coronoid process of the ulna

INSERTION. Lateral aspect of midshaft of the radius

PRIMARY ACTION. Pronates the forearm and hand

INNERVATION. Median nerve (C6, C7)

STRETCH. To stretch the pronator teres of your right arm, extend your right elbow and supinate your forearm and hand (Fig. 4.50). Grasp your right forearm with your left hand, palm up, so that the fingers of your left hand hook over and grasp the radius of your right forearm. Using this grasp, assist your right forearm into more supination while not allowing your upper arm to externally rotate.

PRONATOR QUADRATUS

ORIGIN. Distal one-quarter of anterior ulna

INSERTION. Distal one-quarter of anterior radius

PRIMARY ACTION. Pronates the forearm

INNERVATION. Anterior interosseous branch of the median nerve (C6, C7)

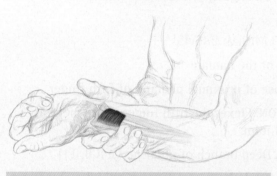

FIGURE 4.51

STRETCH. To stretch the pronator quadratus of your left hand, bend your left elbow and supinate your forearm so that your palm is right in front of your chest (Fig. 4.51). Grasp your left wrist with your right hand, palm up. Using the fingers of your right hand, supinate your left forearm.

SUPINATOR

ORIGIN. Lateral epicondyle of humerus and posterolateral aspect of the ulna

INSERTION. Proximal one-third of radius on lateral anterior and posterior surfaces

PRIMARY ACTION. Supinates the forearm

INNERVATION. Deep branch of radial nerve (C5, C6)

STRETCH. To stretch the supinator of your right forearm, flex your right elbow to about 30 degrees and pronate your forearm (Fig. 4.52). Grasp your right forearm with your left hand. Be sure to grasp your right forearm *proximal* to your radio-carpal (wrist) joint to avoid unnecessarily stressing it. Using a firm grip with your left hand, carefully pronate your right forearm further.

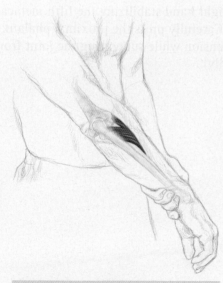

FIGURE 4.52

INTRINSIC HAND MUSCLES

Below are stretches for intrinsic hand muscles.

Finger Flexors

Below are stretches for the finger flexors.

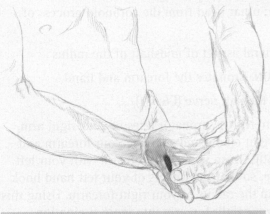

FIGURE 4.53

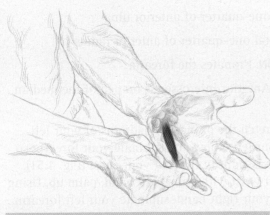

FIGURE 4.54

FLEXOR POLLICUS BREVIS

ORIGIN. Flexor retinaculum and trapezium

INSERTION. Base of proximal phalanx of the thumb

PRIMARY ACTION. Flexes the carpometacarpal joint of the thumb

INNERVATION. Median nerve (C6, C7, C8, T1)

STRETCH. To stretch the flexor pollicus brevis of your right hand, first open up the palm (Fig. 4.53). Gently press the proximal phalanx of your right thumb back with the thumb of your left hand. You may use the index and middle fingers of your left hand to stabilize the first metacarpal while you slightly extend and radially deviate your right thumb.

FLEXOR DIGITI MINIMI BREVIS

ORIGIN. Hook of the hamate

INSERTION. Base of proximal phalanx of fifth finger

PRIMARY ACTION. Flexes the fifth finger at the metacarpophalangeal joint

INNERVATION. Deep branch of ulnar nerve (C8, T1)

STRETCH. To stretch the flexor digiti minimi brevis of your left hand, first open your palm (Fig. 4.54). Next, place the thumb of your right hand against the proximal phalanx of your left little finger, with the index and middle fingers of your right hand stabilizing the fifth metacarpal from behind. Carefully press the proximal phalanx backward into extension while supporting the joint from behind (dorsally).

Finger Adductors and Opposers

Below are stretches for the finger adductors and opposers.

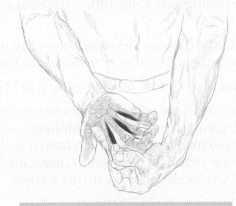

FIGURE 4.55

PALMAR INTEROSSEI (3)

ORIGIN. Anterior, or palmar surfaces of the second, fourth, and fifth metatarsals for the first, second, and third palmar interossei, respectively

INSERTION. Extensor hood and proximal base of second, fourth, and fifth proximal phalanges

PRIMARY ACTION. Adducts each finger toward midline of the hand (i.e., the middle finger)

INNERVATION. Deep branch of ulnar nerve (C8, T1)

STRETCH. To stretch the palmar interossei of your right hand, use your left hand to slowly flex the proximal and distal interphalangeal joints, and then extend and abduct the second, fourth, or fifth finger from its proximal base at the carpo-metacarpal joints (Fig. 4.55).

ADDUCTOR POLLICIS: OBLIQUE AND TRANSVERSE HEADS

ORIGIN. Oblique fibers originate from the capitate and the bases of the second and third metacarpals. The transverse fibers originate from the palmar surface of the third metacarpal.

INSERTION. Base of the proximal phalanx of the thumb

PRIMARY ACTION. Pulls the thumb in toward the middle of the palm

INNERVATION. Deep branch of ulnar nerve (C8, T1)

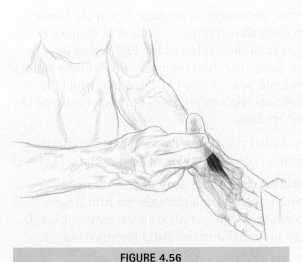

FIGURE 4.56

STRETCH. To stretch the adductor pollicus of the left hand, grasp the base of your left thumb with your right hand and carefully abduct the proximal phalanx of your left thumb diagonally away from your left palm (Fig. 4.56). You may stabilize your left index finger with a stationary surface such as a tabletop.

OPPONENS POLLICIS

ORIGIN. Flexor retinaculum and trapezium

INSERTION. Radial border of first metacarpal

PRIMARY ACTION. Opposes base of the thumb

INNERVATION. Median nerve (C6, C7, C8, T1)

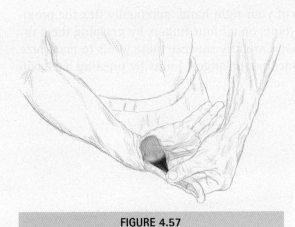

FIGURE 4.57

STRETCH. To stretch the opponens pollicis of your right thumb, grasp the base of your right thumb with your left hand so that the metacarpophalangeal joint is supported between the thumb and the index and middle finger of your left hand (Fig. 4.57). Pressing with your left thumb, extend and externally rotate the base of your right thumb.

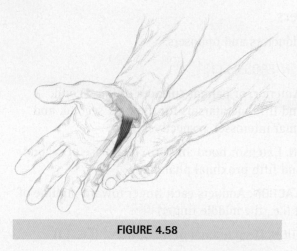

FIGURE 4.58

OPPONENS DIGITI MINIMI

ORIGIN. Hook of hamate

INSERTION. Ulnar aspect of the fifth metacarpal along its length

PRIMARY ACTION. Opposes (flexes and internally rotates) the fifth metacarpal, assisting in "closing" the hand

INNERVATION. Deep branch of ulnar nerve (C8, T1)

STRETCH. To stretch the opponens digiti minimi of your right hand, grasp the base of your fifth finger between the thumb and forefinger of your left hand (Fig. 4.58). While keeping your right hand steady, move the fifth metacarpal into extension and external rotation.

Finger Extensors

Below are stretches for the finger extensors.

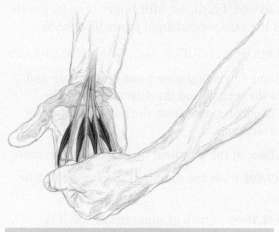

FIGURE 4.59

LUMBRICALES

ORIGIN. From the respective tendons 2–5 of the flexor digitorum profundus (FDP) (i.e., lumbrical number 2 takes origin from the tendon of the FDP which goes to the second digit). The third lumbrical takes origin from both the second and the third FDP tendon, while the fourth lumbrical takes origin from both the third and the fourth FDP tendons.

INSERTION. Radial side of the extensor hood (basically into the base of the palmar side of the proximal phalanx)

PRIMARY ACTION. Flexes the proximal metacarpophalangeal joint on the second through the fifth fingers. Also, through their connection with the extensor hood, extends the proximal and the distal interphalangeal joints.

INNERVATION. Lumbricales 1 and 2: median nerve (C8, T1), and lumbricales 3 and 4: deep branch of ulnar nerve (C8, T1)

STRETCH. To stretch the lumbricales of your right hand, maximally flex the proximal and the distal interphalangeal joints on all four fingers by grasping them in the palm of your left hand (Fig. 4.59). Carefully squeeze these joints to maximize flexion, then gently extend the metacarpophalangeal joints by pressing back with your left hand.

Finger Abductors

Below are stretches for the finger abductors.

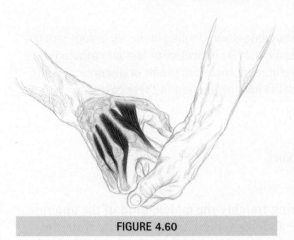

FIGURE 4.60

DORSAL INTEROSSEI (4)

ORIGIN. Proximal one-half of first and second, second and third, third and fourth, and fourth and fifth metacarpals, for the first, second, third, and fourth dorsal interossei, respectively

INSERTION. Extensor hoods and proximal phalanx of fingers 2, 3, and 3 and 4, respectively

PRIMARY ACTION. First dorsal interosseus abducts the second digit, the fourth dorsal interossei abducts the fourth digit. The second and the third dorsal interossei radially deviate, and laterally deviate the second digit, respectively.

INNERVATION. Deep branch of the ulnar nerve (C8, T1)

STRETCH. To stretch the respective abductor, carefully adduct the finger at the metacarpal phalangeal joint with the fingers flexed at the proximal and the distal interphalangeal joints, and extended at the metacarpal phalangeal joints (Fig. 4.60). Deviate the middle finger medially to stretch the second, and laterally to stretch the third.

ABDUCTOR POLLICUS BREVIS

ORIGIN. Flexor retinaculum, trapezium, scaphoid bones

INSERTION. Lateral base of proximal phalanx of the thumb

PRIMARY ACTION. Abducts the thumb

INNERVATION. Recurrent branch of the median nerve (C8, T1)

STRETCH. To stretch the abductor pollicus brevis of your right hand, place the palm of your left hand against the palm of your right so that your left thumb can press against the base of your right (Fig. 4.61). While stabilizing the second metacarpal of your right hand with the grip of your left, use your left thumb to push the base of your right thumb into adduction and extension (back behind the plane of your right hand).

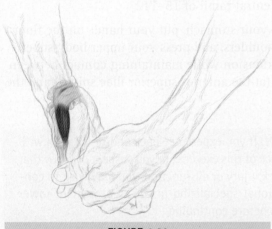

FIGURE 4.61

ABDUCTOR DIGITI MINIMI

ORIGIN. Pisiform and tendon of flexor carpi ulnaris

INSERTION. Base of the proximal phalanx of the fifth digit

PRIMARY ACTION. Abducts the base of the little finger and assists in opposition

INNERVATION. Deep branch of ulnar nerve (C8, T1)

STRETCH. Extend and adduct the proximal phalanx of your little finger by pressing it behind the fourth finger (Fig. 4.62). Continue tilting your wrist into radial deviation.

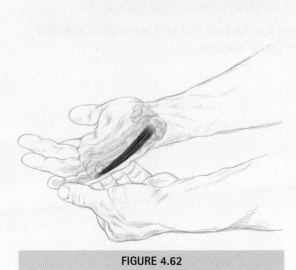

FIGURE 4.62

TRUNK

Below are stretches for specific muscles of the trunk.

> ⚠ **CAUTION!** Severe pain, or pain numbness and tingling in the leg or foot brought on by any movement of the lumbar spine may be indicative of lumbar pathology. The exercise should be modified so as to eliminate these symptoms or discontinued altogether. Further evaluation by a specialist may be prudent in these cases.

Trunk Flexors

Below are stretches for the trunk flexors.

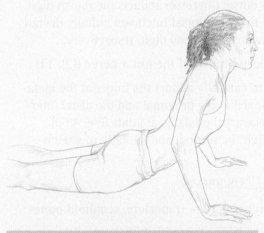

FIGURE 4.63A

RECTUS ABDOMINUS

ORIGIN. Covering roughly the middle third of the anterior surface of the abdomen, these fibers originate from the costal cartilages of the fifth, sixth, and seventh ribs and the xiphoid process

INSERTION. Into the superior ramus of the pubis

PRIMARY ACTION. Flexes the abdomen by pulling the pelvis and the ribcage closer together

INNERVATION. Ventral ramii of T5–T12

STRETCH. Lie on your stomach, put your hands on the floor beneath your shoulders, and press your upper body superiorly and into extension while maintaining contact between your hip bones (at the anterior superior iliac spines) and the floor (Fig. 4.63).

> ⚠ **CAUTION!** If you experience back and/or leg pain with the performance of this exercise, or you suspect or know that you have a back injury or dysfunction, you may wish to consult a professional specializing in the treatment of lower back disorders before continuing.

EXTERNAL AND INTERNAL ABDOMINAL OBLIQUES

See the stretches for the external and internal abdominal obliques under Trunk Rotators.

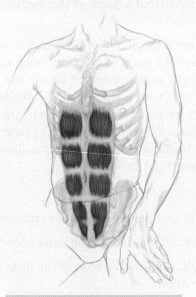

FIGURE 4.63B

Trunk Extensors

Below are stretches for the trunk extensors.

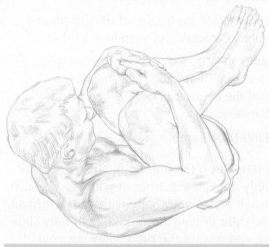

FIGURE 4.64A

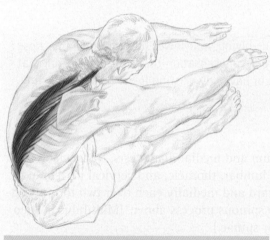

FIGURE 4.64B

ERECTOR SPINAE

ORIGIN. The sacrum, the middle third of the iliac crests, the transverse processes, and the spinous processes of most of the lumbar, thoracic, and cervical vertebrae, and the medial ribs

INSERTION. These individual muscle fibers span multiple segments and are arranged in three roughly parallel columns (spinalis, longissimus, and iliocostalis). According to the particular column, each of the muscle groups spans several segments and inserts into proximal ribs, transverse processes, or spinous processes one or more segments above the origin.

PRIMARY ACTION. When acting bilaterally, extends the spine. When acting unilaterally, extends and side-bends toward the contracting muscle. The erector spinae is very important in maintaining an upright posture.

INNERVATION. Posterior ramii of spinal nerves (T1–T12, L1–L5, S1–3)

STRETCH. Lie on your back and pull both of your knees up to your chest, then carefully pull your head up toward your knees (Fig. 4.64A).

As an alternative, you may sit with both legs extended in front of you while carefully reaching your head down toward your knees (Fig. 4.64B). To emphasize the more laterally positioned components (longissimus and iliocostalis) on the left, lean over toward the right and rotate your torso also toward the right.

> ⚠ **CAUTION!** Be careful doing both of these stretches, particularly if you have lower back or neck problems. In a number of different conditions these positions are contraindicated and may worsen your condition! Please see Chapter 10 (Stretching for Rehabilitation of Injuries).

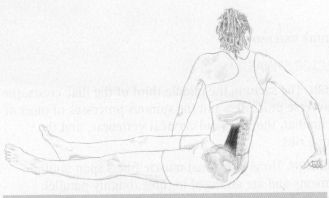

FIGURE 4.65

QUADRATUS LUMBORUM

ORIGIN. Middle third of posterior iliac crests just lateral to the iliocostalis muscle

INSERTION. Inferior border of twelfth rib and transverse processes of vertebrae L1–L4

PRIMARY ACTION. Extends the lumbar spine when acting bilaterally. Side-bends torso toward the contracting side when acting unilaterally.

INNERVATION. Lumbar plexus (T12, L1, L2, L3)

STRETCH. Sit on the floor with your legs comfortably extended in front of you (Fig. 4.65). To stretch your left quadratus lumborum, reach across your body with your left hand, placing your palm on the floor just to the right of your right thigh. Carefully slide your left hand diagonally away, forward, and toward the right, allowing your spine to flex, rotate, and side-bend toward the right. Keep your left buttock on the floor.

> ⚠️ **CAUTION!** As with any exercise involving your lower back, particularly those involving flexion and rotation, be aware of any sensation that is different from that of "stretch." If you experience any pain or have any existing lower back dysfunction, consult a specialist before proceeding.

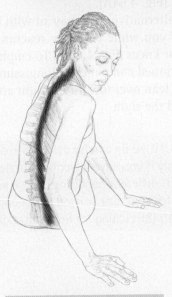

FIGURE 4.66

MULTIFIDUS

ORIGIN. Sacrum and medial iliac crests, transverse processes of lumbar, thoracic, and cervical vertebrae passing upward and medially each over two to four segments to the spinous process above. (Multifidus is deep to the erector spinae.)

INSERTION. Spinous processes of vertebrae two to four segments above the origin

PRIMARY ACTION. Acting bilaterally, extends the lumbar, thoracic, or lower cervical spines. Acting unilaterally, side-bends toward and rotates away the spinal segments above on those below (referenced from the side of the working muscles).

INNERVATION. Posterior ramii of spinal nerves (C1–C8, T1–T12, L1–L5, S1–S4)

STRETCH. To stretch the multifidi on your right side, sit on the floor with your left knee flexed to 90 degrees and your right leg extended (Fig. 4.66). Place both hands on the floor on the right side of your right leg then carefully flex and rotate your spine to the right.

ROTATORES

ORIGIN. Sacrum, transverse processes of lumbar, thoracic, and cervical vertebrae

INSERTION. Spanning only one or two segments and inserting into the lamina above

PRIMARY ACTION. Acting bilaterally, extend the segment above on the segment below. Acting unilaterally, rotate the segment above in the opposite direction. Rotatores work as major stabilizers of the spine.

INNERVATION. Posterior ramii of spinal nerves (C1–C8, T1–T12, L1–L5, S1–S4)

STRETCH. To stretch the rotatores on your left side, first reach your right hand in front of you and place it on your left hip (Fig. 4.67). Reach your left hand behind you and place it on your right hip. With the help of your hands, rotate your head and torso to the left as far as possible. (You may emphasize the area of rotatores as needed, that is, to emphasize the thoracic area, focus the rotation here, while relaxing the cervical and lumbar rotation.) Then flex forward and side-bend toward the right.

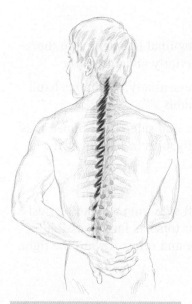

FIGURE 4.67

Trunk Rotators

Below are stretches for the trunk rotators.

EXTERNAL OBLIQUE

ORIGIN. Lower six or seven ribs, with fibers passing at an angle anteriorly and inferiorly toward the iliac crests

INSERTION. Tendinous sheath alongside the rectus abdominus (semilunar line), and along the anterior half of the iliac crest to the pubic tubercle

PRIMARY ACTION. The left side turns the upper body toward the right and vice versa. When working in concert with the internal oblique on the same side, side-bends the trunk to the same side.

INNERVATION. Anterior ramii of T5–T12

STRETCH. To stretch the external oblique on your left side from a standing position, first place your left hand on your lower lumbar area, and your right hand on your right hip for support (Fig. 4.68). Side-bend your torso to the right as far as possible, then rotate your chest and torso toward the left.

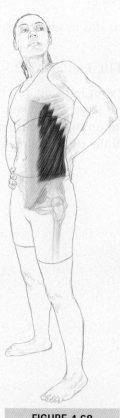

FIGURE 4.68

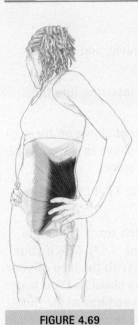

FIGURE 4.69

INTERNAL OBLIQUE

ORIGIN. Middle one-third of iliac crest and lateral inguinal ligament, and thoracolumbar fascia, with fibers running generally superiorly and anteriorly

INSERTION. Lower two or three ribs, the linea alba (essentially, tendinous band from rib cage to pubic bone), and the crest of the pubis

PRIMARY ACTION. Acting unilaterally, rotates, flexes, and side-bends upper body toward the side that is contracting. Acting bilaterally, aids in flexion of the trunk.

INNERVATION. Anterior ramii of T5–T12

STRETCH. To stretch the internal oblique on your left side from a standing position, place your hands on your hips and rotate your torso as far as possible toward the right (Fig. 4.69). Now extend your spine and rotate toward the right.

SERRATUS POSTERIOR INFERIOR

ORIGIN. Lower two thoracic and upper two lumbar vertebrae

INSERTION. Middle third of lower four ribs

PRIMARY ACTION. Depresses and retracts the lower four ribs as an accessory muscle of inspiration

INNERVATION. Posterior ramii of thoracic nerves T9, T10, T11, and T12

STRETCH. To stretch the serratus posterior inferior on your left side, reach your right hand around in front of you and place it on your lower ribs about as far back as you can reach (Fig. 4.70). Place your left hand on top of your right, and use this combination to help rotate your torso toward the right while pulling your ribs superiorly and then anteriorly.

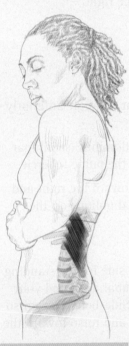

FIGURE 4.70

Trunk Stabilizers

Most muscles can act as stabilizers. The category is used here for transverse abdominus, as this muscle does not precisely qualify as a flexor, extensor, etc.

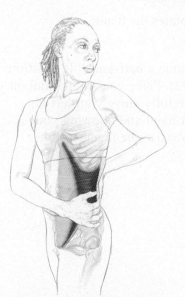

FIGURE 4.71

TRANSVERSE ABDOMINUS

ORIGIN. Subcostal margin, thoracolumbar fascia, along the iliac crests, and the inguinal ligament

INSERTION. Linea alba

INNERVATION. Anterior ramii of T5–T12

PRIMARY ACTION. Helps support the abdomen, aids in respiration, and helps support the spine via increasing intra-abdominal pressure and pulling the thoracolumbar fascia tight

STRETCH. To stretch the transverse abdominus on the left side from a standing position, first place your right hand on your left hip (Fig. 4.71). Next, place your left hand on your lower back and turn toward the left. Now take a deep breath and lean toward the right.

HIP

Below are stretches for specific muscles of the hip.

Hip Flexors

Below are stretches for the hip flexors.

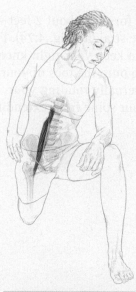

FIGURE 4.72

PSOAS MAJOR AND MINOR

ORIGIN. Anterior-lateral vertebral bodies and transverse processes of the last thoracic and all five lumbar vertebrae (the psoas minor from the twelfth thoracic and first lumbar)

INSERTION. Blending with the iliacus muscle and inserting into the lesser trochanter of the femur. The psoas minor inserts into the arcuate line of the ilium. It has no attachment to the femur.

PRIMARY ACTION. Flexes and externally rotates the femur. If the thigh is fixed, then the psoas muscles can pull the trunk forward while acting bilaterally. When acting unilaterally, side-bends the lumbar spine toward the same side. Tightness can result in hyperextension of the lumbar spine. The psoas minor has no influence on the hip but may affect the lumbar spine through stabilization or side-bending toward the same side.

INNERVATION. Anterior ramii of L1, L2, L3

STRETCH. To stretch the right psoas, assume a half-kneeling position with the right knee on the floor (Fig. 4.72). Carefully move your left hip and knee forward, being conscious of keeping your spine straight by tightening the abdominal muscles. Side-bend your upper body slightly toward the left.

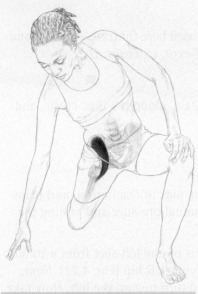

FIGURE 4.73

ILIACUS

ORIGIN. Iliac crest and iliac fossa

INSERTION. Blends with the psoas muscles (see above)

PRIMARY ACTION. Flexes and externally rotates the femur

INNERVATION. Femoral nerve (L2, L3)

STRETCH. To stretch the right iliacus, assume a half-kneeling position with the right knee on the floor (Fig. 4.73). Place your right hand on the floor just opposite your left foot. Carefully move your left hip forward while leaning toward your right hand and allowing your spine to extend slightly (in order to emphasize the iliacus vs. the psoas).

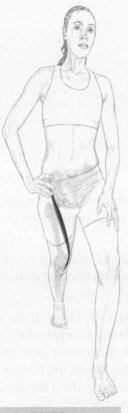

FIGURE 4.74

SARTORIUS

ORIGIN. Anterior superior iliac spine

INSERTION. Superior medial surface of the tibia where it is joined by the tendons of the gracilis and semitendinosus (collectively called the pes anserine tendon)

PRIMARY ACTION. Flexes, abducts, and externally rotates the hip, flexes the knee while internally rotating the tibia on the femur

INNERVATION. Femoral nerve (L2, L3)

STRETCH. To stretch the right sartorius, step forward about 2 feet with your left foot while keeping your right knee straight (Fig. 4.74). Flex your left knee and lunge forward. Be sure to keep your right knee straight while allowing yourself to come up onto the toes of your right foot. Roll your right heel laterally, internally rotating your right leg. Tighten your abdomen to keep your spine from extending.

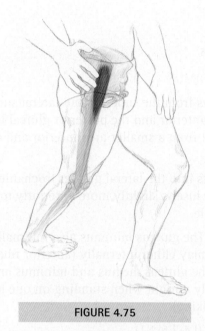

FIGURE 4.75

TENSOR FASCIA LATA

ORIGIN. Anterior end of the crest of the ilia, including the anterior superior iliac spine

INSERTION. Into the iliotibial tract roughly one-third of the way down the lateral thigh. The iliotibial tract is a wide tendon that runs along the lateral side of the thigh, originating at the anterior iliac crest and crossing the knee joint to insert into the lateral tibial condyle.

PRIMARY ACTION. Flexes, abducts, and internally rotates the thigh

INNERVATION. Superior gluteal nerve (L4, L5, S1)

STRETCH. To stretch your right tensor fascia lata from a standing position, step your right foot behind and to the left of your left foot (Fig. 4.75). Internally rotate your right foot and leg. Place your right hand on your right hip and guide it forward and toward the right.

Hip Extensors

Below are stretches for the hip extensors.

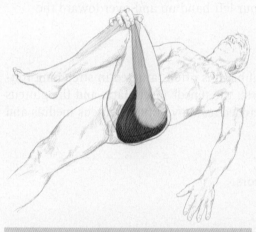

FIGURE 4.76

GLUTEUS MAXIMUS

ORIGIN. Posterior ilium, lateral sacrum, and coccyx

INSERTION. Into the iliotibial band and gluteal tuberosity of the femur

PRIMARY ACTION. Extends and externally rotates the femur

INNERVATION. Inferior gluteal (L4, L5, S1, S2)

STRETCH. To stretch your left gluteus maximus, lie on your back and use your right hand to pull your left knee up to your chest and over toward your right shoulder, thereby flexing and adducting your femur (Fig. 4.76). The origin of this muscle is very large, so you should stretch it in many variants of this position (e.g., on one occasion pull more toward your right shoulder, and the next time pull more toward your right hip).

HAMSTRINGS

The hamstrings help with hip extension, but are primarily knee flexors. See hamstrings in the section on Knee Flexors.

Hip Abductors

Below are stretches for the hip abductors.

GLUTEUS MEDIUS AND GLUTEUS MINIMUS

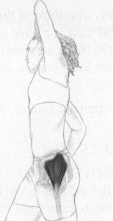

FIGURE 4.77

ORIGIN. The gluteus medius originates from the superior and lateral surface of the ilia below its crest, between the anterior and the posterior gluteal lines. The gluteus minimus arises similarly, but from a smaller area inferior and deep to the gluteus medius.

INSERTION. The gluteus medius inserts into the lateral greater trochanter of the femur, whereas the gluteus minimus inserts slightly more anteriorly to the greater trochanter and the hip capsule.

PRIMARY ACTION. Abducts the thigh. The gluteus minimus also internally rotates, whereas the gluteus medius may either internally (anterior fibers) or externally (posterior fibers) rotate. The gluteus medius and minimus are also critical in holding the rest of the body upright when standing on one leg (e.g., every time you take a step while walking).

INNERVATION. Superior gluteal nerve (L4, L5, S1)

STRETCH. To stretch the left gluteus medius and minimus, lift your left foot and step behind and to the right of your right foot (Fig. 4.77). Then carefully ease your greater trochanter toward the left adducting your left femur. You may accentuate this motion by reaching your left hand up and over toward the right.

ILIOTIBIAL BAND

Note: While not a muscle, the iliotibial band is often targeted in stretching routines. It takes origin from the iliac crest, the tensor fascia lata, and the gluteus maximus. It should be effectively stretched as above under gluteus medius and gluteus minimus.

Hip Adductors

Below are stretches for the hip adductors.

PECTINEUS

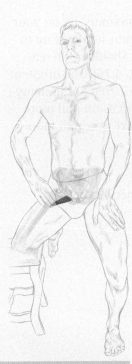

FIGURE 4.78

ORIGIN. Superior pubic ramus just lateral to the origin of the adductor longus, which originates just below and lateral to the easily palpable pubic tubercle

INSERTION. Pectineal line, just inferior to the lesser trochanter of the femur

PRIMARY ACTION. Flexes and adducts the thigh

INNERVATION. Femoral nerve (L2, L3); may also receive branches from the obturator nerve (L2, L3, L4)

STRETCH. To stretch the right pectineus from a standing position, flex your right knee and support it on a chair (Fig. 4.78). Step your left foot forward and toward the left about 12 inches. Place your right hand on your right hip and guide your pelvis inferiorly and toward the left by flexing your left knee.

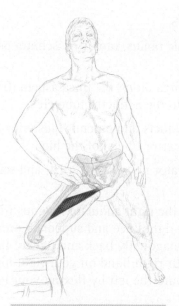

FIGURE 4.79

ADDUCTOR LONGUS

ORIGIN. Just inferior to the pubic tubercle

INSERTION. Middle third of medial aspect of linea aspera (ridge along the posterior femur)

PRIMARY ACTION. Adducts the thigh

INNERVATION. Obturator nerve (L2, L3, L4)

STRETCH. To stretch the right adductor longus from a standing position, bend your right knee and support it on a chair (Fig. 4.79). Step your left foot toward the left about 12–15 inches and back 2–3 inches. Place your right hand on your right hip and guide your pelvis inferiorly and toward the left by flexing your left knee.

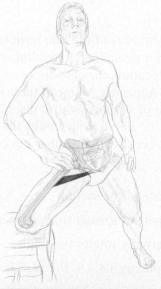

FIGURE 4.80

ADDUCTOR BREVIS

ORIGIN. Body and inferior pubic ramus. Adductor brevis is just deep to the adductor longus.

INSERTION. Pectineal line and upper one-third of linea aspera

PRIMARY ACTION. Adducts the thigh

INNERVATION. Obturator nerve (L2, L3, L4)

STRETCH. To stretch the right adductor longus from a standing position, bend your right knee and support it on a chair (Fig. 4.80). Step your left foot toward the left about 12–15 inches and back 4–5 inches. Place your right hand on your right hip and guide your pelvis down and toward the left by flexing your left knee.

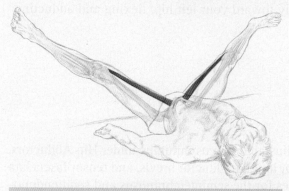

FIGURE 4.81

GRACILIS

ORIGIN. Body and inferior ramus of the pubic bone (slightly medial to the origin of adductor brevis)

INSERTION. Joins with the tendons of the semitendinosus and the sartorius and inserts into the superior medial surface of the tibia

PRIMARY ACTION. Adducts the hip. Also flexes and medially rotates the tibia on the femur.

INNERVATION. Obturator nerve (L2, L3, L4)

STRETCH. Lie on your back with your buttocks against a wall and your legs straight up the wall (i.e., hips flexed to 90 degrees) (Fig. 4.81). Carefully lower both legs into abduction, allowing gravity to perform the stretch.

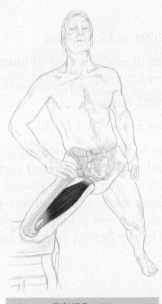

FIGURE 4.82

ADDUCTOR MAGNUS

ORIGIN. Inferior pubic ramus, ramus of ischium posteriorly to the ischial tuberosity

INSERTION. A large area along the linea aspera (from all but the upper one-fourth), to the adductor tubercle

PRIMARY ACTION. Adducts and extends (posterior fibers) or may assist in flexion (anterior fibers) of the hip

INNERVATION. Obturator nerve (L2, L3, L4) and sciatic nerve (L4, L5, S1)

STRETCH. To stretch the right adductor magnus from a standing position, bend your right knee and support it on a chair (Fig. 4.82). Step your left foot diagonally back and toward the left about 15 inches. Place your right hand on your right hip and guide your pelvis back and toward the left by flexing your left knee.

Hip External Rotators

There are actually six small external rotators of the hip: piriformis, obturator internus and externus, inferior and superior gemelli, and quadratus femoris. Because of the complexity of their function and location, they are discussed here as a group. For more detailed information, please see Appendix A. One of these external rotators, the piriformis, is often cited as the cause of various painful disorders of the hip likely because of its proximity with the sciatic nerve, which exits the pelvis just below it. The stretch below for piriformis will also stretch the other hip external rotators.

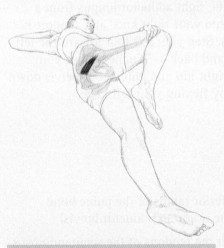

FIGURE 4.83

PIRIFORMIS

ORIGIN. Anterior surface of the sacrum

INSERTION. Medial aspect of greater trochanter of the femur

PRIMARY ACTION. Externally rotates the thigh

INNERVATION. Sacral plexus (L4, L5, S1, S2, S3)

STRETCH. To stretch your right piriformis, lie on your back with your legs extended (Fig. 4.83). Use your left hand to pull your right knee across your body toward your left hip, flexing and adducting your right hip.

Hip Internal Rotators

See the stretches for the gluteus medius and gluteus minimus under Hip Abductors. Also, see the stretches for the adductor longus, adductor brevis, and tensor fascia lata under Hip Adductors. See the stretches for the semimembranosus and semitendonosus under Knee Flexors.

KNEE

Below are stretches for specific muscles of the knee.

Knee Extensors

Knee extensors are often referred to collectively as "quadriceps." Below are stretches for the knee extensors.

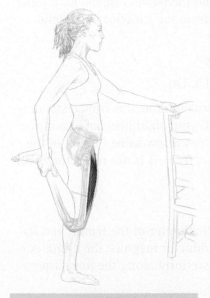

FIGURE 4.84

RECTUS FEMORIS

ORIGIN. Two heads: one originates from the anterior inferior iliac spine; a second originates from the ilium, just superior to the acetabulum

INSERTION. Connects to the patella via the quadriceps tendon, which essentially connects all the quadriceps muscles to the tibia at the tibial tuberosity, via the patella and the patellar ligament

PRIMARY ACTION. Extends the knee and flexes the hip

INNERVATION. Femoral nerve (L2, L3, L4)

STRETCH. To stretch your right rectus femoris from a standing position, first bend your right knee enough to be able to grab your right ankle behind you (Fig. 4.84). Tighten your abdomen to avoid any hyper-extension of your lower back. Now pull your ankle backward until your thigh is vertical or slightly extended (angled back). Finally, pull your ankle up toward your buttock, taking care not to allow your lower back to extend.

> **CAUTION!** It is quite common for this exercise to be performed without attention to stabilizing the pelvis via contracting the abdomen. This results in hyperextension of the lumbar spine and anterior rotation of the pelvis. This may not only be injurious to the lower back but decreases the effectiveness of the stretch on the rectus femoris since it allows the origin of the muscle to move.

VASTUS INTERMEDIUS

ORIGIN. Upper two-thirds of the anterior and lateral aspects of the femur

INSERTION. Connects to the patella via the quadriceps tendon, which then essentially connects all the quadriceps muscles to the tibial tuberosity, via the patella and the patellar ligament

PRIMARY ACTION. Extends the knee

INNERVATION. Femoral nerve (L2, L3, L4)

STRETCH. To stretch your right vastus intermedius from a standing position, use your right hand to pull your right heel back toward your buttock (Fig. 4.85). You may allow slight flexion of the hip in this stretch, so that the rectus femoris is not restricting your stretch of the vastus intermedius.

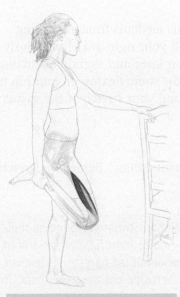

FIGURE 4.85

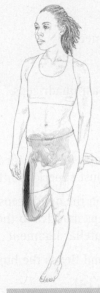

FIGURE 4.86

VASTUS LATERALIS

ORIGIN. The inferior, anterior, and lateral aspect of the greater trochanter, wrapping posteriorly around the femur and descending along the lateral aspect of the distal half of the linea aspera

INSERTION. Connects to the patella via the quadriceps tendon, which then essentially connects all the quadriceps muscles to the tibial tuberosity, via the patella and the patellar ligament. It joins the quadriceps tendon obliquely, from the superior and lateral direction.

PRIMARY ACTION. Extends the knee

INNERVATION. Femoral nerve (L2, L3, L4)

STRETCH. To stretch your right vastus intermedius from a standing position, use your left hand to pull your right heel back toward your left buttock (Fig. 4.86). You may allow some flexion of the hip in this stretch so that the rectus femoris is not restricting your stretch of the vastus lateralis.

VASTUS MEDIALIS

ORIGIN. Just inferior to the lesser trochanter of the femur, and the tendons of adductor longus and adductor magnus; the origin continues wrapping inferiorly and posteriorly along the linea aspera to its inferior end

INSERTION. Connects to the patella via the quadriceps tendon, which then essentially connects all the quadriceps muscles to the tibial tuberosity, via the patella and the patellar ligament. Lower and more medial fibers attach into the medial side of the patella via the medial patellar retinaculum.

INNERVATION. Femoral nerve (L2, L3, L4)

PRIMARY ACTION. Extends the knee; important in stabilizing the patella

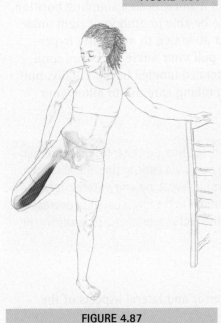

FIGURE 4.87

STRETCH. To stretch your right vastus medialis from a standing position, use your right hand to pull your right ankle posteriorly and away from midline, flexing your knee and slightly abducting your thigh (Fig. 4.87). You may allow some flexion of your hip in this stretch, so that the rectus femoris is not restricting your stretch of the vastus medialis.

Knee Flexors

Knee flexors are often referred to collectively as "hamstrings." Below are stretches for the knee flexors.

> ⚠ **CAUTION!** It is common for people to stretch their hamstrings via rounding their back and shoulders. This is not necessary and can be quite harmful, particularly in those with existing low back pathology. Because the origin of the hamstrings (except the short head of the biceps femoris) is the ischial tuberosity, not the lower back, it is not necessary to flex the spine in order to get an effective stretch in the hamstrings. In addition, few people need additional flexion in their lower back.

BICEPS FEMORIS: SHORT HEAD

ORIGIN. Lower half of the linea aspera

INSERTION. Joins a common tendon with the long head, and inserts into the lateral aspect of the head of the fibula

PRIMARY ACTION. Flexes the knee; may aid in externally rotating the tibia on the femur

INNERVATION. Peroneal branch of sciatic nerve (L5, S1, S2)

STRETCH. To stretch the short head of the biceps femoris on your left from a standing position, place both of your hands on your thigh just above your left knee and carefully press your knee into extension (Fig. 4.88).

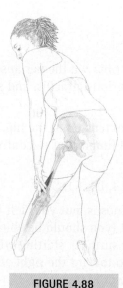

FIGURE 4.88

BICEPS FEMORIS: LONG HEAD

ORIGIN. Ischial tuberosity and distal part of sacrotuberous ligament

INSERTION. Joins a common tendon with the short head, and inserts into the lateral aspect of the head of the fibula

PRIMARY ACTION. Flexes the knee, helps extend the hip, and externally rotates the tibia on the thigh if the knee is unlocked

INNERVATION. Tibial branch of sciatic nerve (L5, S1, S2, S3)

STRETCH. To stretch the long head of your left biceps femoris, put your left heel up on a stool or other object of comfortable height (you should be able to maintain an upright spine; if not, choose a lower surface) (Fig. 4.89A). Be sure your hips are facing forward. Turn your torso slightly toward the left. Without bending forward, extend your lower back (which moves your ischial tuberosity posteriorly). In very flexible individuals, bending forward may be necessary to achieve a stretch; however, this should be accomplished by flexing at the hip of the stance leg, not by flexing the lumbar spine.

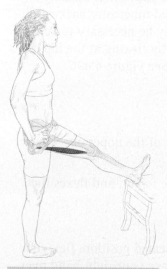

FIGURE 4.89A

SEMIMEMBRANOSUS

ORIGIN. Ischial tuberosity

INSERTION. Posterior medial aspect of tibial condyle

PRIMARY ACTION. Flexes the knee and helps with extension at the hip. Also internally rotates the tibia if the knee is unlocked (important in control of the knee).

INNERVATION. Tibial branch of the sciatic nerve (L4, L5, S1, S2)

STRETCH. Same as the stretch above, except rather than turning your torso slightly toward the left, turn it slightly toward the right. See Figure 4.89B.

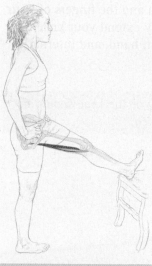

FIGURE 4.89B

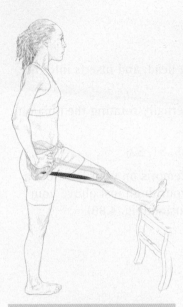

FIGURE 4.89C

SEMITENDINOSUS

ORIGIN. Ischial tuberosity

INSERTION. Anterior medial shaft of the proximal tibia via the pes anserine tendon (common tendon for insertion of the sartorious, gracilis, and semi-tendinosus)

PRIMARY ACTION. Flexes the knee and helps with extension at the hip. Also internally rotates the tibia if the knee is unlocked (important in control of the knee).

INNERVATION. Tibial branch of the sciatic nerve (L4, L5, S1, S2)

STRETCH. As above. To stretch your left semitendinosus, put your left heel up on a stool or any object of comfortable height (you should be able to maintain an upright spine; if not, choose a lower surface), starting with your hips directly facing forward. Turn your torso toward the right about 20–30 degrees, and externally rotate your left lower extremity 15–20 degrees. Without bending forward, extend your lower back by extending your lumbar spine (moving your ischial tuberosity backward). In very flexible individuals, bending forward may be necessary to achieve a stretch; however, this should be accomplished by flexing at the hip of the stance leg, not by flexing the lumbar spine. See Figure 4.89C.

POPLITEUS

ORIGIN. Lateral aspect of lateral femoral condyle

INSERTION. Posterior surface of the medial aspect of the upper one-quarter of the tibia superior to the soleal line

PRIMARY ACTION. Medially rotates the tibia on the femur, and flexes the knee

INNERVATION. Tibial nerve (L4, L5, S1)

STRETCH. To stretch your right popliteus from a seated position, flex your right knee to about 15–20 degrees (Fig. 4.90). Place your right hand over the outside of your lower leg, so that your thumb rests over your tibial tuberosity. Place your left hand on the medial aspect of your right thigh, so that your left thumb is above your right patella and the fingers of your left hand wrap around behind your knee. Carefully extend your knee while externally rotating your tibia with your right hand, and internally rotating your femur with your left hand.

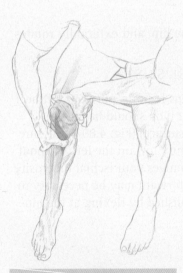

FIGURE 4.90

⚠ **CAUTION!** Those with known or suspected pathology of the knee should be properly screened by a specialist before performing this stretch.

ANKLE AND FOOT

Below are stretches for specific muscles of the ankle and foot.

Ankle Plantarflexors

Below are stretches for the ankle plantarflexors.

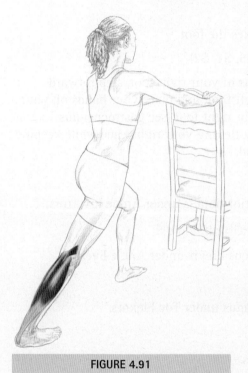

FIGURE 4.91

GASTROCNEMIUS

ORIGIN. Two heads: one originates from the posterior surface of each of the medial and the lateral femoral condyles and the other from the posterior capsule of the knee

INSERTION. Both heads converge in the belly of the muscle which joins the achilles tendon and inserts into the posterior aspect of the calcaneus

PRIMARY ACTION. Plantar flexes the foot and aids in flexion of the knee

INNERVATION. Tibial nerve (S1, S2)

STRETCH. To stretch the gastrocnemius of your right foot, stand 3–4 feet from a chair or wall (Fig. 4.91). Step forward about 1.5 feet with your left foot, and place your hands on the chair or wall in front of you. Supinate your right foot. Slowly move your hips forward, keeping your right knee extended and your right heel on the ground.

Note that most people, particularly over time, lose the integrity and ligamentous support of their arches. This may lead to excessive pronation in stance and gait, which can lead to various maladies including plantar fascitis, metatarsalgias, and patellofemoral pain syndromes. Because the force applied to dorsiflex the foot/ankle also causes pronation and flattening of the arch, it is prudent to supinate, or at least neutralize the arch, to allow its bony structure to support it. This allows a greater percentage of the stretching force to be applied to the gastrocnemius/soleus complex, rather than possibly further destabilizing the arch. Supinate your foot before the stretch by actively pulling the head of the first metatarsal of your first toe toward the heel, while keeping both of these on the ground. This will generally cause a slight external rotation of your tibia.

PLANTARIS

ORIGIN. Distal and lateral part of the supracondylar line, just medial and slightly superior to the origin of the lateral head of the gastrocnemius, and the oblique popliteal ligament

INSERTION. Joins with the achilles tendon and inserts into the posterior aspect of the calcaneus

PRIMARY ACTION. Assists in plantar flexion of the foot

INNERVATION. Tibial nerve (L4, L5, S1, S2)

STRETCH. Same as in gastrocnemius (above). May be emphasized by externally rotating the lower leg 30–45 degrees. See Figure 4.91.

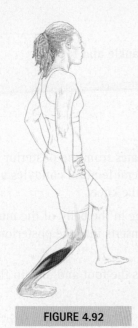

FIGURE 4.92

SOLEUS

ORIGIN. Posterior middle third of the tibia and upper one-fourth of the posterior fibula

INSERTION. Joins with the tendon of the gastrocnemius to form the achilles tendon, and inserts into the posterior aspect of the calcaneus

PRIMARY ACTION. Plantar flexes the foot

INNERVATION. Tibial nerve (L5, S1, S2)

STRETCH. To stretch the soleus of your right foot, step forward about 15 inches with your left foot, and place your hands on your hips (Fig. 4.92). Supinate your right foot (see gastrocnemius above). Slowly sink down by flexing your right knee while keeping your right heel on the ground.

POSTERIOR TIBIALIS

See the stretch for the posterior tibialis under Ankle Invertors.

PERONEUS LONGUS AND PERONEUS BREVIS

See stretches for peroneus longus and peroneus brevis under Ankle Evertors.

FLEXOR DIGITORUM LONGUS

See the stretches for the flexor digitorum longus under Toe Flexors.

Ankle Dorsiflexors

Below are stretches for the ankle dorsiflexors.

TIBIALIS ANTERIOR

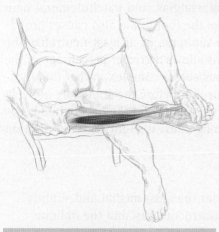

FIGURE 4.93

ORIGIN. Upper two-thirds of the lateral aspect of the tibia and adjacent parts of the interosseous membrane

INSERTION. Crosses over the foot just anterior to the medial malleolus and inserts into the inferior and medial aspect of the medial cuneiform and the base of the first metatarsal

PRIMARY ACTION. Dorsiflexes and inverts the foot

INNERVATION. Deep peroneal nerve (L4, L5, S1)

STRETCH. To stretch the tibialis anterior of your right foot while sitting, cross your right ankle across your left knee (Fig. 4.93). Grasp your right forefoot with your left hand and plantar flex your ankle, while everting (turn plantar surface away from you) and abducting your forefoot.

EXTENSOR DIGITORUM LONGUS

See the stretch for the extensor digitorum longus under Toe Extensors.

Ankle Invertors

Below are stretches for the ankle invertors.

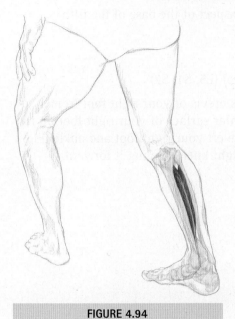

TIBIALIS POSTERIOR

ORIGIN. Posterior aspect of the upper half of the lateral border of the tibia, the interosseus membrane, and the proximal two-thirds of the fibula

INSERTION. Plantar aspect of navicular and all three cuneiforms, the cuboid and the bases of metatarsals 2, 3, and 4

PRIMARY ACTION. Inverts and plantar flexes the foot

INNERVATION. Tibial nerve (L5, S1)

STRETCH. To stretch the tibialis posterior of your right leg, assume a lunge position with your feet roughly 2 feet apart and the right foot slightly rotated inward (Fig. 4.95). Flex your right knee and dorsi-flex your right ankle while guiding your knee anterior-laterally (diagonally toward the right), while keeping your right foot flat on the floor.

TIBIALIS ANTERIOR

See the stretch for the tibialis anterior under Ankle Dorsiflexors.

FIGURE 4.94

Ankle Evertors

Below are stretches for the ankle evertors.

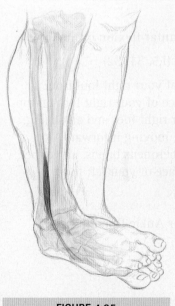

PERONEUS TERTIUS

ORIGIN. Distal third of anterior fibula and adjacent interosseous membrane

INSERTION. Dorsal aspect of the base of the fifth metatarsal

PRIMARY ACTION. Aides in dorsiflexion and eversion

INNERVATION. Deep peroneal nerve (L4, L5, S1)

STRETCH. To stretch the peroneus tertius of your right foot from a standing position, place the plantar surface of your right foot on top of your left foot, and carefully invert your right foot and ankle (Fig. 4.94).

FIGURE 4.95

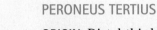

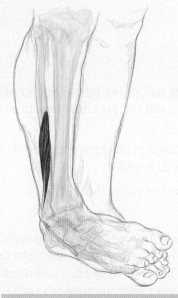

FIGURE 4.96

PERONEUS BREVIS

ORIGIN. Lower two-thirds of the lateral aspect of the fibula

INSERTION. Superior and lateral aspect of the base of the fifth metatarsal

PRIMARY ACTION. Everts the foot

INNERVATION. Superficial peroneal (L5, S1, S2)

STRETCH. To stretch the peroneus brevis of your right foot from a standing position, place the plantar surface of your right foot on top of your left foot and carefully invert your right foot and ankle (Fig. 4.96). Now carefully flex your right knee, moving it forward.

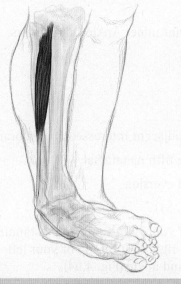

FIGURE 4.97

PERONEUS LONGUS

ORIGIN. Head and upper two-thirds of the lateral aspect of the fibula

INSERTION. Dropping down the lateral aspect of the leg and passing behind the lateral malleolus, crossing under the foot, and inserting into the plantar and lateral aspects of the first metatarsal and the medial cuneiform

PRIMARY ACTION. Everts and assists in plantar flexion of the foot

INNERVATION. Superficial peroneal nerve (L5, S1, S2)

STRETCH. To stretch the peroneus longus of your right foot from a standing position, place the plantar surface of your right foot on top of your left foot and carefully invert your right foot and ankle (Fig. 4.97). Now carefully flex your right knee, moving it forward. To emphasize the peroneus longus over the peroneus brevis, move the right forefoot further over the dorsal surface of your left foot.

PERONEUS TERTIUS

See the stretch for peroneus tertius under Ankle Dorsiflexors.

Toe Flexors

Below are stretches for the toe flexors.

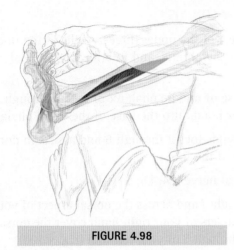

FIGURE 4.98

FLEXOR DIGITORUM LONGUS

ORIGIN. Middle half of posterior aspect of the tibia

INSERTION. Passes posterior and inferior to the medial maleolus, then beneath the foot where it splits into four tendons that insert into the bases of the distal phalanges of toes 2–5

PRIMARY ACTION. Flexes toes 2 through 5 and aids in plantar flexion and inversion of the foot

INNERVATION. Tibial nerve (S2, S3)

STRETCH. To stretch the flexor digitorum longus of your right foot from a seated position, cross your right foot over your left knee (Fig. 4.98). Use your right hand to pull toes 2 through 5 into complete extension and then your ankle into complete dorsiflexion.

FLEXOR DIGITORUM BREVIS

See the stretch for the flexor digitorum brevis under Intrinsic Foot Muscles.

FLEXOR HALLICUS LONGUS

ORIGIN. Distal two-thirds of the posterior aspect of the fibula

INSERTION. Passes posterior and inferior to the medial maleolus and inserts into the plantar surface of the distal phalanx of the great toe

PRIMARY ACTION. Flexes the great toe and assist in plantar flexion and inversion of the foot

INNERVATION. Tibial nerve (L5, S1, S2)

STRETCH. To stretch the flexor hallicus longus of your right foot, sit with your right foot across your left knee (Fig. 4.99). Use your right hand to extend the great toe while dorsiflexing and everting the foot and ankle.

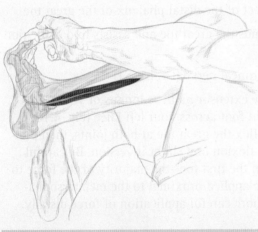

FIGURE 4.99

Toe Extensors

Below are stretches for the toe extensors.

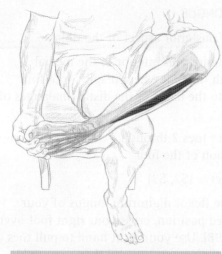

FIGURE 4.100

EXTENSOR DIGITORUM LONGUS

ORIGIN. Anterior aspect of the upper three-fourths of the fibula, adjacent interosseous membrane, and inferior lateral tibial condyle

INSERTION. Dorsal base of middle phalanx of toes 2 through 5, and through extensor hood, into the base of the distal phalanx

PRIMARY ACTION. Extends toes 2 through 5 and assists in dorsiflexion and eversion of the foot

INNERVATION. Peroneal nerve (L4, L5, S1)

STRETCH. Place your right hand across the dorsal aspect of your left foot so that the fingers of your right hand cover the dorsal aspect of the toes 2 through 5 of your left foot (Fig. 4.100). Carefully plantar flex your toes back toward you, continuing with plantar flexion of your foot and ankle.

EXTENSOR HALLICUS LONGUS

ORIGIN. Middle half of anterior and medial aspect of the fibula, and adjacent interosseous membrane

INSERTION. Dorsal aspect of the distal phalanx of the great toe

PRIMARY ACTION. Extends the great toe and assists in dorsiflexion of the foot

INNERVATION. Deep peroneal nerve (L4, L5, S1)

STRETCH. To stretch the extensor hallicus longus of your right foot, sit with your right foot across your left knee (Fig. 4.101). Use your left hand to flex the great toe at both joints, then pull your foot into plantar flexion and slight inversion. Be careful not to pull too hard on the first toe—the majority of the force to flex the foot should be applied proximal to the metatarsophalangeal joint, with a more careful application of force distally.

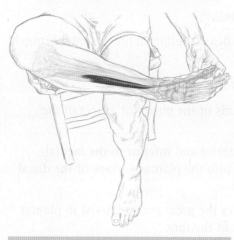

FIGURE 4.101

INTRINSIC FOOT MUSCLES

Below are stretches for intrinsic foot muscles.

Toe Flexors

Below are stretches for the toe flexors.

FLEXOR DIGITORUM BREVIS

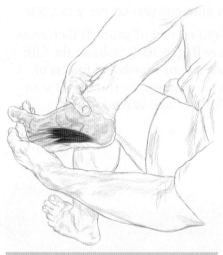

FIGURE 4.102

ORIGIN. Anterior aspect of the tuberosity of the calcaneus and the plantar aponeurosis (plantar fascia)

INSERTION. Plantar surface of the middle phalanges of toes 2 through 5

PRIMARY ACTION. Flexes the proximal interphalangeal joints of toes 2 through 5

INNERVATION. Medial plantar nerve (S2, S3)

STRETCH. To stretch the flexor digitorum brevis of your right foot, sit with your right foot across your left knee (Fig. 4.102). Support your right ankle in a neutral to plantar flexed position with your right hand, and use the palm and fingers of your left hand to push toes 2 through 5 into complete extension.

FLEXOR HALLICUS BREVIS

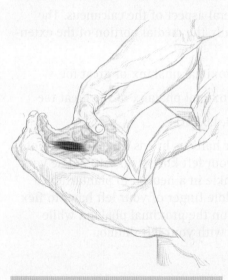

FIGURE 4.103

ORIGIN. Plantar aspect of the distal cuboid and lateral cuneiform

INSERTION. Plantar aspect of the base of the proximal phalanx of the great toe

PRIMARY ACTION. Flexes the proximal phalanx of the big toe

INNERVATION. Medial plantar nerve (S2, S3)

STRETCH. To stretch the flexor hallicus brevis of your right foot, sit with your right foot across your left knee (Fig. 4.103). Support your right ankle in a neutral to plantar flexed position with your right hand. Use the palm of your left hand to push the proximal phalanx of your great toe into complete extension, while preventing ankle dorsiflexion with your right hand.

QUADRATUS PLANTAE

ORIGIN. Two heads: one originates from the medial border of the calcaneus and the long plantar ligament; the other originates from the lateral border of the calcaneus and the long plantar ligament

INSERTION. Posterior lateral surface of the tendon of flexor digitorum longus

PRIMARY ACTION. Assists in flexing the second through the fifth digits via modifying the line of pull of the flexor digitorum longus

INNERVATION. Lateral plantar nerve (S2, S3)

STRETCH. See the stretch for flexor digitorum longus under Toe Flexors.

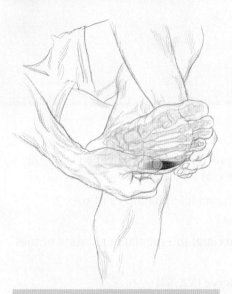

FIGURE 4.104

FLEXOR DIGITI MINIMI BREVIS

ORIGIN. Plantar surface of the base of the fifth metatarsal

INSERTION. Plantar base of proximal phalanx of the fifth toe

PRIMARY ACTION. Flexes the metatarsophalangeal joint of the fifth toe

INNERVATION. Superficial branch of lateral plantar nerve (S2, S3)

STRETCH. To stretch the flexor digiti minimi of your left foot, cross your left foot over your right knee (Fig. 4.104). Stabilize the fifth metatarsal of your left foot between your thumb and fingers of your right hand. Using your left hand, grasp the fifth toe of your left foot at its base, and pull it dorsally into extension.

Toe Extensors

Below are stretches for the toe extensors.

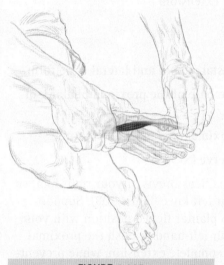

FIGURE 4.105

EXTENSOR HALLICUS BREVIS

ORIGIN. Distal, superior, and lateral aspect of the calcaneus. The extensor hallicus brevis is actually the medial portion of the extensor digitorum brevis.

INSERTION. Dorsal base of the proximal phalanx of great toe

PRIMARY ACTION. Extends the proximal phalanx of the great toe

INNERVATION. Deep peroneal (L4, L5, S1)

STRETCH. To stretch the extensor hallicus brevis of your right foot, sit with your right foot across your left knee (Fig. 4.105). Use your right hand to hold your right ankle in a neutral to plantarflexed position. Use the index and middle finger of your left hand to flex the great toe by pressing down on the proximal phalanx while stabilizing your first metatarsal with your left thumb.

EXTENSOR DIGITORUM BREVIS

ORIGIN. Superior aspect of lateral calcaneus

INSERTION. Joins the tendons of the extensor digitorum longus to toes 2 through 4, which insert into the base of the middle phalanges and through lateral slips into the base of the distal phalanges

PRIMARY ACTION. Extends all joints of toes 2 through 4

INNERVATION. Deep peroneal nerve (L4, L5, S1)

STRETCH. Sit with your right ankle across your left knee (Fig. 4.106). Use your right hand to stabilize your right ankle in a neutral position as you use your left hand to curl toes 2 to 4 of your right foot into full flexion.

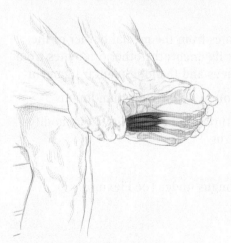

FIGURE 4.106

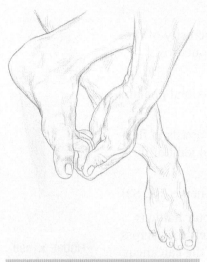

FIGURE 4.107A

LUMBRICALS

ORIGIN. From the tendons of the flexor digitorum longus at a level roughly midshaft of the respective metatarsal 2–5

INSERTION. Medial side of the proximal phalanx and the "extensor hood" of toes 2–5, respectively

PRIMARY ACTION. Assist in flexion of the metatarsophalangeal joints, and via their connection into the extensor hood, assist in extension of the middle and the distal interphalangeal joints 2–5

INNERVATION. Lumbrical I: Medial plantar nerve (S2, S3). Lumbricales II–IV: Lateral plantar nerve (S2, S3).

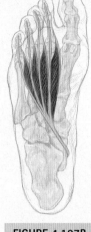

FIGURE 4.107B

STRETCH. To stretch the lumbricals of your left foot, first cross your left foot over your right knee (Fig. 4.107). Using your left hand to flex the interphalangeal joints of your second through your fifth toes, and carefully extend the metatarsophalangeal joints.

Toe Abductors

Please note that abduction and adduction of the individual toes of the foot are defined relative to a midline which is defined as the second metatarsal; abduction being movement in a lateral direction from the second metatarsal, and adduction being movement in a medial direction from the second metatarsal. This is an accepted convention and we are merely reminding the reader of it here.

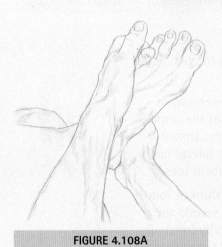

FIGURE 4.108A

ABDUCTOR DIGITI MINIMI

ORIGIN. Medial and lateral processes of the tuberosity of the calcaneus and the plantar aponeurosis (plantar fascia)

INSERTION. Lateral base of the proximal phalanx of the fifth toe

PRIMARY ACTION. Abducts the fifth toe

INNERVATION. Lateral plantar nerve (S2, S3)

STRETCH. To stretch the abductor digiti minimi of your left foot, place your left foot across your right knee (Fig. 4.108). Use your right hand to firmly grasp and stabilize your left calcaneus. Use your left hand to adduct the entire forefoot while slightly adducting and extending the fifth toe.

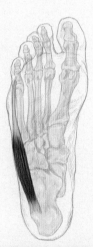

FIGURE 4.108B

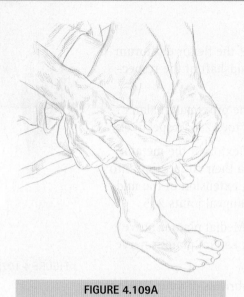

FIGURE 4.109A

ABDUCTOR HALLICUS

ORIGIN. Medial process of tuberosity of the calcaneus and the plantar aponeurosis (plantar fascia)

INSERTION. Medial base of proximal phalanx of the great toe

PRIMARY ACTION. Abducts and assists in flexion of the metatarsophalangeal joint of the great toe

INNERVATION. Medial plantar nerve (S2, S3)

STRETCH. To stretch the abductor hallicus of your left foot, place your left foot across your right knee and stabilize the calcaneus of your left foot with firm pressure from the heel of your right hand (Fig. 4.109). Grasp the proximal phalanx of your great toe and abduct and slightly extend it. Because this muscle's origin is the calcaneus, it is necessary to allow abduction of the entire forefoot on the hindfoot in addition to abducting the great toe.

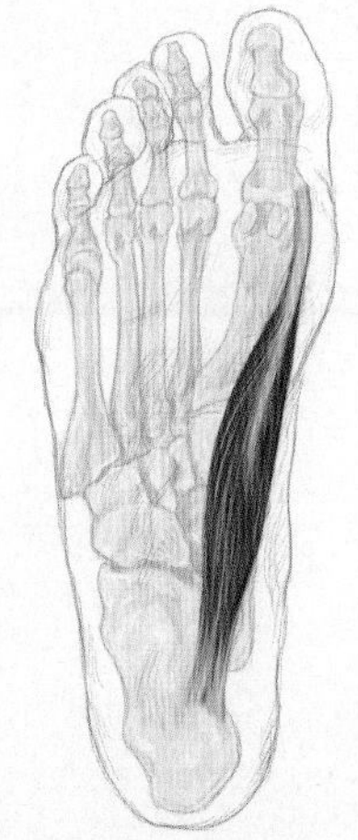

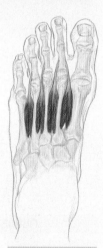

FIGURE 4.109B

> ⚠ **CAUTION!** As the nature of the weightbearing foot is to pronate and lengthen over time, it is unlikely that the abductor hallicus will need significant stretching. It may be stretched for brief periods (10 seconds or less) to relieve cramping, but a thorough evaluation should be performed by a professional knowledgeable in foot and ankle mechanics before undergoing any aggressive stretching of the abductor hallicus.

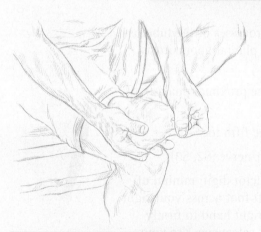

FIGURE 4.110A

DORSAL INTEROSSEI (4)

ORIGIN. Roughly midshaft of the two adjacent metatarsals 1–5

INSERTION. The first dorsal interosseous inserts into the medial base of the proximal phalanx of the second toe. Dorsal interossei 2–4 insert into the lateral bases of the second through the fourth toes.

PRIMARY ACTION. Abduct the third or fourth toe laterally, and deviate the second toe either medially (first) or laterally (second). Each may assist in flexion at the metatarsophalangeal joints.

FIGURE 4.110B

INNERVATION. Lateral plantar nerve (S2, S3)

STRETCH. To stretch the dorsal interossei of the left foot, cross your left foot over your right knee and, with your left hand, grasp the toe to be adducted at the proximal phalanx, about midshaft with your left hand (Fig. 4.110). With your right hand, stabilize the metatarsal of the toe to be stretched and the metatarsal that is just lateral. Carefully adduct and extend the digit. In the case of the first dorsal interosseus, first deviate the proximal second phalange laterally, then extend.

Toe Adductors

Below are stretches for the toe adductors.

ADDUCTOR HALLICUS: TRANSVERSE AND OBLIQUE HEADS

ORIGIN. Oblique head from the bases of the second, third, and fourth metatarsals, and the transverse head from the plantar metatarsophalangeal ligaments (connect the metatarsal heads of the first through the fifth metatarsals) of the third, fourth, and fifth metatarsals

INSERTION. Lateral side of the base of the proximal phalanx of the great toe

PRIMARY ACTION. Adducts and assists in flexion of the great toe

INNERVATION. Deep branch of lateral plantar nerve (S2, S3)

STRETCH. To stretch the adductor hallicus of your right foot, place your right foot over your left knee and stabilize your first metatarsal between the thumb and fingers of your right hand (Fig. 4.111). Carefully abduct and extend the great toe of your right foot with your left hand by pulling it away from the other toes, and dorsally.

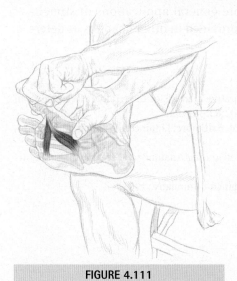

FIGURE 4.111

CAUTION! Many people have a condition in which the great toe deviates laterally or out toward the lesser toes. This is often accompanied by an enlarged metatarsophalangeal joint, which may be stiff and possibly painful. Because this restriction may be ligamentous, capsular, or even bony, attempting to stretch the great toe into abduction may be difficult or injurious. Professional consultation is wise if this restriction is severe or painful.

PLANTAR INTEROSSEI (3)

ORIGIN. Medial surface and base of third–fifth metatarsals

INSERTION. Medial base of proximal phalange of same digit

PRIMARY ACTION. Deviates the respective digit toward the great toe (adducts), and may assist in flexion at the metatarsophalangeal joint

INNERVATION. Lateral plantar nerve (S2, S3)

STRETCH. To stretch the plantar interossei of your left foot, cross your left foot over your right knee (Fig. 4.112). Grasp the metatarsal of the toe to be stretched with your right hand. With your left hand, grasp the proximal phalanx and carefully deviate it laterally (abduct) while extending it slightly.

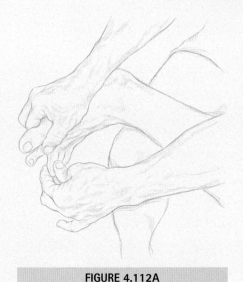

FIGURE 4.112A

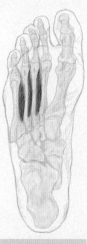

FIGURE 4.112B

SUMMARY   This chapter has been designed for use by the practitioner who wishes to apply specific stretches to areas of carefully diagnosed need. The use of these stretches should be reserved for this purpose and more general applications of stretching should be addressed by the information provided in other chapters as determined by the table of contents.

REFERENCES

1. Fredericson M, White JJ, MacMahon JM, et al. Quantitative analysis of the relative effectiveness of 3 iliotibial band stretches. Arch Phys Med Rehabil 2002;83:589–92.
2. Agur AM, Dalley AF. Grant's Atlas of Anatomy. 11th Ed. Baltimore: Lippincott Williams and Wilkins, 2005.
3. Clay JH, Pounds DM. Basic Clinical Massage Therapy: Integrating Anatomy and Treatment. Baltimore: Lippincott Williams and Wilkins, 2003.
4. Pratt NE. Clinical Musculoskeletal Anatomy. J. B. Lippincott Company, 1991.

Stretches for Major Muscle Groups

This chapter identifies stretches for many of the body's most important muscle groups. These muscle groups enable us to produce the majority of our voluntary movement, making our daily activities, as well as our participation in exercise and athletic endeavors, possible. You may find the chapter most useful as a reference to help you develop flexibility programs based on unique movement needs.

The chapter addresses different muscle groups according to the motion produced by their contraction. For example, there is a stretch for the muscle group that produces flexion at the shoulder, and another for the muscle group that produces external rotation at the shoulder. This method of organization should allow for the design of a flexibility program tailored to the individual's functional needs. You need to determine only the movement patterns fundamental to the desired activity in order to be able to choose the stretches that should be most beneficial. If you are unsure about particular range of motion (ROM) needs, it may be helpful to perform a full range-of-motion assessment as described in Chapter 3.

Each stretch in this chapter is described in detail, with an accompanying figure illustrating the stretch technique. Included in the description of each stretch is a list of all of the individual muscles that make up the group being stretched. Stretches for each of these individual muscles are provided in the previous chapter, which details the origin, action, insertion, and innervation of each muscle listed.

For ease of navigation, the stretches in this chapter are arranged by body region, from head to toe. For each joint, the primary functional movements are identified such as elbow flexion and extension. The muscles involved in producing that particular motion are then listed, followed by the description of a stretch designed to enhance that motion. Please notice that to stretch the muscles that produce extension, the direction of the stretch will generally be into flexion; this is why, for example, the stretch for neck extension involves motion in the direction of cervical *flexion*.

For clarity, most of the stretches are described for either the right or the left side of the body. Obviously, you'll need to reverse all of the references to "left" or "right" to stretch the muscle on the side opposite the one described. Each stretch should be held for 30 seconds. As with the stretches for individual muscles, significant pain in the muscle, pain in the joint, and/or significant limitation in either the muscle or joint is cause for more detailed evaluation. Consultation with a physician or other specialist may be advisable before proceeding.

UPPER BODY

The stretches in this section are designed to increase flexibility throughout the upper body including the neck, shoulders, and upper extremities.

Neck

Below are stretches for the neck.

EXTENSION

MUSCLES INVOLVED. Extensors include the obliquus capitus superior, rectus capitus superior major, rectus capitus superior minor, obliquus capitus inferior, semispinalis capitus, splenius cervicus, longissimus capitus, and levator scapulae.

POSITION. Standing or sitting

STRETCH. Starting with the superior segments, slowly flex your cervical spine so that your chin moves toward your chest (Fig. 5.1). Maintain your chest and shoulders in a static position.

RESULT. You should feel a stretch in the back of your neck.

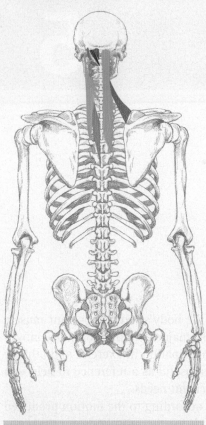

FIGURE 5.1A

obliquus capitis superior
rectus capitis posterior major
rectus capitis posterior minor
obliquus capitis inferior
semispinalis capitis
splenius cervicis
longissimus capitis
levator scapulae

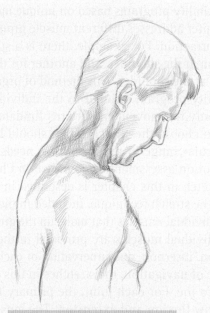

FIGURE 5.1B

longus capitis
longus colli
sternohyoid
omohyoid
platysma

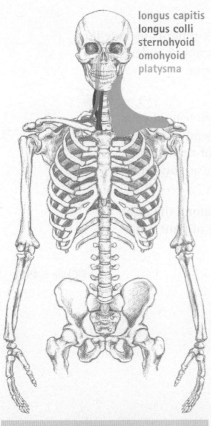

FIGURE 5.2A

FLEXION

MUSCLES INVOLVED. Cervical flexors include the longus capitus, longus coli sternohyoid, omohyoid, and platysma.

POSITION. Standing or sitting

STRETCH. Place both hands behind your neck so that your fingers are just below your occiput and along the upper vertebrae on both sides (Fig. 5.2). Carefully look back and up, extending your cervical spine while supporting your head and neck with your hands.

RESULT. You should feel a stretch along the front of your neck down to your clavicles.

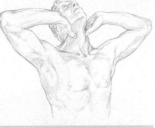

FIGURE 5.2B

> **CAUTION!** While this is normal movement for the cervical spine, extension deserves great caution particularly in older adults and is contraindicated in individuals with a history of cervical injury or dysfunction. If any discomfort or pain is experienced, consult a physician to rule out serious pathologies before continuing. This is especially true if the pain is severe, if there is also associated or isolated dizziness, or nausea, or if there are symptoms referred into the arms or hands.

SIDE-BENDING

MUSCLES INVOLVED. Side-benders include the upper trapezius, anterior, middle, and posterior scalenes, sternocleidomastoid, and splenius capitus.

POSITION. Standing or sitting

STRETCH. Take your right hand and reach over the top of your head, placing it palm down on your head so that your middle two fingers touch your left ear (Fig. 5.3). Carefully, pull your head directly toward the right side, being careful not to let your head move forward or back. Repeat to the left.

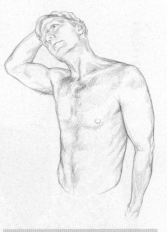

FIGURE 5.3B

RESULT. You should feel a stretch in the left side of your neck and across the top of your left shoulder.

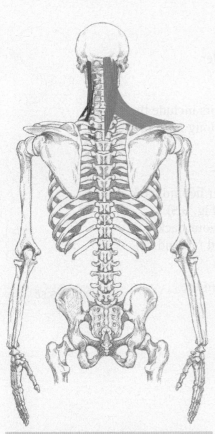

FIGURE 5.3A

upper trapezius
anterior, middle and posterior scalenes
sternocleidomastoid
splenius capitis

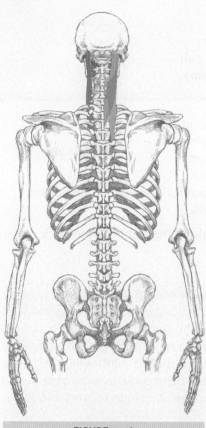

FIGURE 5.4A

ROTATION

MUSCLES INVOLVED. Head and neck rotators include the sternocleidomastoid, longissimus capitus, splenius capitus, and obliquus capitus inferior.

POSITION. Standing or sitting

STRETCH. Use your left hand to reach behind your back and pull your right forearm gently inferiorly and toward the left, depressing your right shoulder (Fig. 5.4). Carefully turn your head toward the left. Repeat toward the right.

RESULT. You should feel a stretch along the right side of your neck and into the top of your right shoulder.

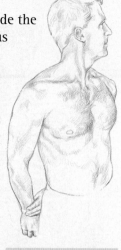

FIGURE 5.4B

sternocleidomastoid
longissimus capitis
splenius capitis
obliquus capitis inferior

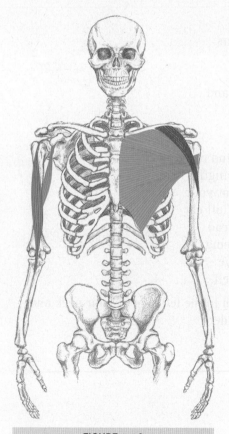

FIGURE 5.5A

Shoulder

Below are stretches for the shoulder.

FLEXION

MUSCLES INVOLVED. Shoulder flexors include the pectoralis major, anterior deltoid, long head of biceps brachii, and coracobrachialis.

POSITION. Standing

STRETCH. Lock your hands together behind back with elbows only slightly flexed (Fig. 5.5). Lift interlocked hands up behind your back, extending your shoulders. No need to bend your back forward!

RESULT. You should feel a stretch in the anterior aspect of both shoulders.

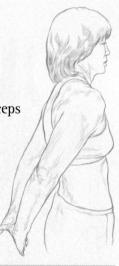

FIGURE 5.5B

pectoralis major
anterior deltoid
long head of biceps brachii
coracobrachialis

EXTENSION

MUSCLES INVOLVED. Shoulder extensors include the latissimus dorsi, teres major, posterior deltoid, long head of the triceps brachii; they also include rhomboid major and minor through their action on the scapula.

POSITION. Standing in front of a chair

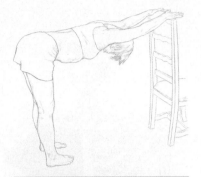

FIGURE 5.6B

STRETCH. Place both hands on the back of a chair or object of similar height (Fig. 5.6). Then carefully bend at the waist until arms are straightened overhead with a roughly 90-degree angle at the waist. Be careful to keep your lower back straight, allowing the forward bend to come from flexion at the hips.

RESULT. You should feel a stretching sensation in the axillary area of both shoulders.

latissimus dorsi
teres major
posterior deltoid
long head of the triceps brachii
rhomboid minor
rhomboid major

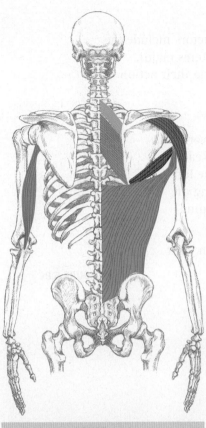

FIGURE 5.6A

ABDUCTION

MUSCLES INVOLVED. Shoulder abductors include the middle deltoid, supraspinatus, and upper trapezius through its action in superiorly rotating the scapula (a necessary and integral motion in abducting the shoulder).

POSITION. Standing

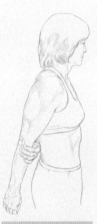

FIGURE 5.7B

STRETCH. Reach your right hand behind your back (Fig. 5.7). Grasp your right forearm with your left hand. Adduct your right arm by carefully pulling it toward the left until a gentle stretch is felt at the right shoulder. Then slowly lean your head toward the left, increasing the stretch at both your right shoulder and your upper trapezius. Repeat toward the right.

RESULT. You should feel a stretch along the lateral aspect of your right shoulder and upper trapezius.

middle deltoid
supraspinatus
upper trapezius

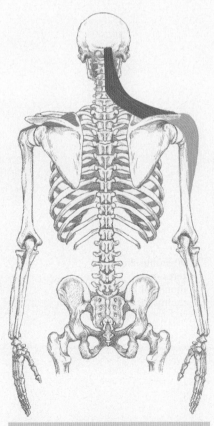

FIGURE 5.7A

ADDUCTION

MUSCLES INVOLVED. Shoulder adductors include the pectoralis major, latissimus dorsi, teres major, and rhomboids major and minor via their action on the scapula.

POSITION. Standing

STRETCH. Extend your right arm overhead, palm facing to the left (Fig. 5.8). Reach your entire arm directly toward the left and continue with left side-bending of your torso. Repeat to the right leading with your left hand.

RESULT. You should feel a stretch in your right axillary area.

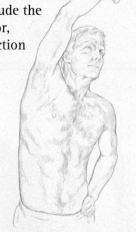

FIGURE 5.8C

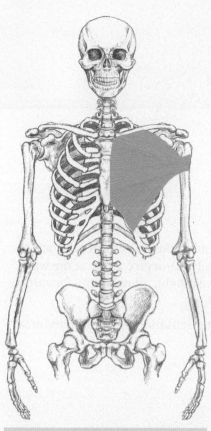

FIGURE 5.8A

pectoralis major

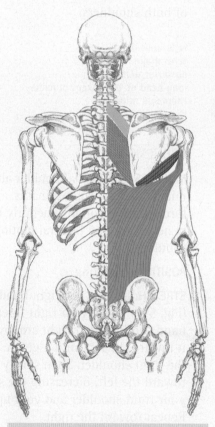

FIGURE 5.8B

latissimus dorsi
teres major
rhomboid major
rhomboid minor

HORIZONTAL ADDUCTION

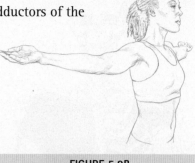

MUSCLES INVOLVED. Horizontal adductors of the shoulder include the anterior deltoid, sternal portion of pectoralis major, and cora-cobrachialis.

POSITION. Standing

STRETCH. Abduct arms to shoulder level with palms facing upward (Fig. 5.9).

FIGURE 5.9B

Horizontally abduct both shoulders, keeping them at shoulder level. You may use a doorway to help assist with this movement. Ideally, both sides can be stretched simultaneously (as the tension from one side stabilizes the origin on the other side); however, this is not necessary, and effective stretches can be performed unilaterally.

RESULT. You should feel a stretch in the anterior aspect of your chest and shoulders.

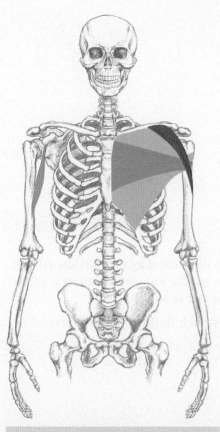

FIGURE 5.9A

anterior deltoid
sternal pectoralis major
coracobrachialis

HORIZONTAL ABDUCTION

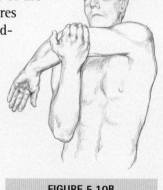

MUSCLES INVOLVED. Horizontal abductors of the shoulder include the posterior deltoid, teres minor, infraspinatus, and upper and mid-dle trapezius and rhomboid major and minor via their attachment to the scapula.

POSITION. Standing

STRETCH. To stretch your left shoulder horizontal abductors, grasp the posterior aspect of your left elbow with your right hand (Fig. 5.10). Horizontally adduct your left shoulder by pulling

FIGURE 5.10B

your left elbow horizontally across toward your right shoulder just beneath the chin. Repeat with the right.

RESULT. You should feel a stretch in the posterior aspect of your left shoulder and scapula.

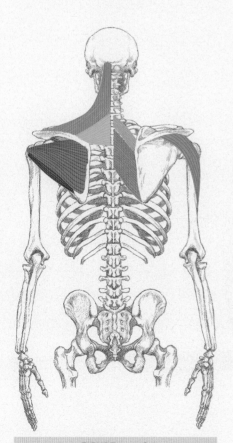

FIGURE 5.10A

posterior deltoid
teres minor
infraspinatus
upper trapezius
middle trapezius
rhomboid major
rhomboid minor

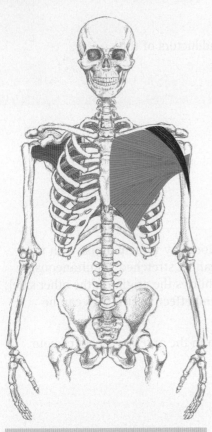

FIGURE 5.11A

pectoralis major
anterior deltoid
subscapularis

INTERNAL ROTATION

MUSCLES INVOLVED. Internal rotators of the shoulder include the subscapularis, latissimus dorsi, pectoralis major, teres major, and anterior deltoid.

POSITION. Standing in a doorway, right arm at your side, elbow flexed to 90 degrees, and palm facing forward against the doorframe

STRETCH. To stretch your right shoulder internal rotators, keep your right elbow at your side and right hand against the doorframe, then carefully turn your body toward the left until you feel a gentle stretch (Fig. 5.11). Repeat for your left shoulder.

RESULT. You should feel a gentle stretch in the anterior aspect of your right shoulder.

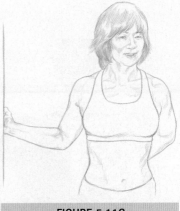

FIGURE 5.11C

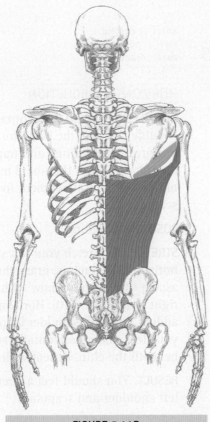

FIGURE 5.11B

latissimus dorsi
teres major

posterior deltoid
teres minor
infraspinatus

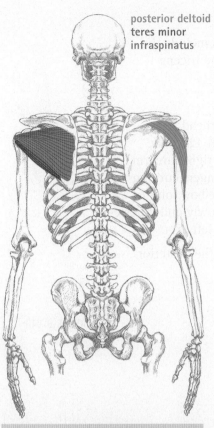

FIGURE 5.12A

EXTERNAL ROTATION

MUSCLES INVOLVED. External rotators of the shoulder include the infraspinatus, teres minor, and posterior deltoid.

POSITION. Standing

STRETCH. Internally rotate your left shoulder by placing your left hand behind your back with the palm facing posteriorly (Fig. 5.12). Place the palm of your right hand over the anterior aspect of your left shoulder. Back into a doorway with the posterior surface of the left elbow against the door jam. While maintaining firm support of the anterior shoulder with the left palm and hand (do not let the shoulder push forward), carefully move your entire body backward, forcing the elbow forward, until an easy stretch is felt in your left shoulder. Repeat on the opposite side to stretch your right shoulder.

RESULT. You should feel a gentle stretch in the posterior aspect of your left shoulder.

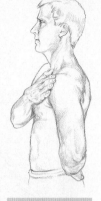

FIGURE 5.12B

> **⚠ CAUTION!** Individuals with shoulder pain, dysfunction, or suspected pathology should consult their physician before performing this exercise.

Elbow

Below are stretches for the elbow.

FLEXION

MUSCLES INVOLVED. Elbow flexors include the long and short heads of the biceps brachii, brachialis, and brachioradialis.

POSITION. Standing

STRETCH. Clasp your hands together behind your lower back, extend your elbows completely, and then externally rotate your arms so that your palms are facing your buttocks (Fig. 5.13). Now extend both shoulders by lifting the hands up and away from your buttocks.

RESULT. You should feel a stretch across your anterior upper arms and shoulders.

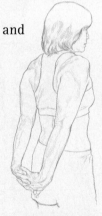

FIGURE 5.13B

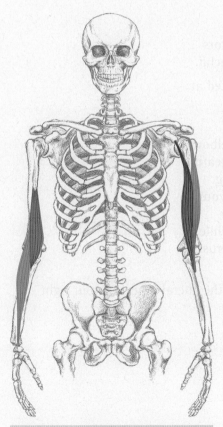

FIGURE 5.13A

long head biceps brachii
short head biceps brachii
brachialis
brachioradialis

EXTENSION

MUSCLES INVOLVED. Elbow extensors include the long, medial, and middle heads of the triceps brachii and the anconeus.

POSITION. Standing

STRETCH. Extend your right arm overhead and flex your elbow maximally (Fig. 5.14). Place the palm of your left hand against your right forearm just distal to the elbow, with your fingers curving over your right elbow. Squeeze your elbow joint to keep it maximally flexed, and then slowly pull it posteriorly and medially. Repeat with the left arm.

RESULT. You should feel a stretch in the posterior aspect of your right upper arm.

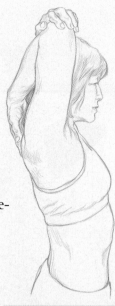

FIGURE 5.14B

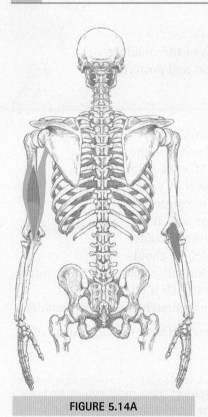

long head triceps brachii
medial head triceps brachii
lateral head triceps brachii
anconeus

FIGURE 5.14A

SUPINATION

MUSCLES INVOLVED. Forearm supinators include the supinator and biceps brachii.

POSITION. Standing with arms relaxed at sides

STRETCH. To stretch the supinators of your right arm, flex your right elbow slightly, and pronate your right forearm so that the palm is facing down (Fig. 5.15). Using your left hand, grasp your right forearm just proximal to your wrist. Pronate your right forearm while externally rotating your right humerus. Repeat with the left forearm.

RESULT. You should feel a stretch in the lateral aspect of your right forearm.

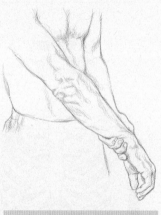

FIGURE 5.15B

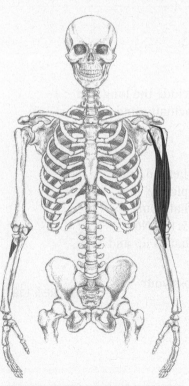

FIGURE 5.15A

biceps brachii
supinator

PRONATION

MUSCLES INVOLVED. Forearm pronators include the pronator teres and pronator quadratus.

POSITION. Standing

STRETCH. To stretch the pronators of your right forearm, extend your right elbow and supinate your right hand (Fig. 5.16). With your left hand, grasp your right forearm just proximal to the wrist. Using your left hand, rotate your right wrist externally, further supinating your right forearm. Be sure to keep your upper arm from externally rotating as well—this may require an active contraction of the shoulder internal rotators. Repeat with the left forearm.

RESULT. You should feel a stretch along the anterior aspect of your forearm.

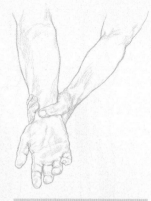

FIGURE 5.16B

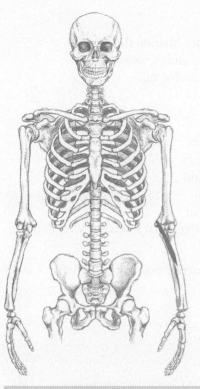

FIGURE 5.16A

pronator teres
pronator quadratus

Wrist and Hand

Below are stretches for the wrist and hand.

EXTENSION

MUSCLES INVOLVED. Wrist and hand extensors include the extensor carpi radialis, extensor digitorum, extensor indicis, extensor digiti minimi, extensor carpi radialis, extensor pollicus longus, and extensor pollicus brevis.

POSITION. Sitting or standing

STRETCH. To stretch the extensors of your left arm and hand, extend your left arm out in front of you with your elbow extended, forearm pronated (Fig. 5.17). Flex your left wrist and then attempt to flex fingers 2–5 into a fist. Repeat on the right arm.

RESULT. You should feel a stretch on the posterior aspect of your left forearm.

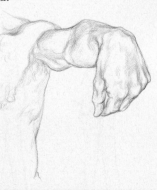

FIGURE 5.17C

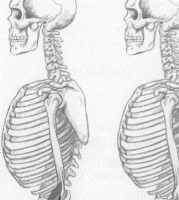
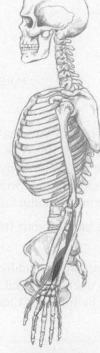

FIGURE 5.17A   FIGURE 5.17B

extensor carpi radialis   extensor digiti minimi
extensor digitorum   extensor carpi radialis
extensor indicis   extensor pollicus longus
                          extensor pollicus brevis

FLEXION

MUSCLES INVOLVED. Wrist and hand flexors include the flexor carpi radialis, flexor digitorum profundus, flexor digitorum superficialis, palmaris longus, flexor pollicis longus, and flexor carpi ulnaris.

POSITION. Sitting or standing

STRETCH. To stretch the flexors of your left wrist and hand, extend your left arm out in front of you with your elbow extended and palm supinated (Fig. 5.18). Use your right hand to extend the fingers and the wrist of your left hand by carefully pulling the fingers back toward you. Repeat with the right.

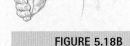

FIGURE 5.18B

RESULT. You should feel a stretch in the anterior aspect of your left forearm.

Fingers

Below are stretches for the fingers.

FLEXION AND ADDUCTION

MUSCLES INVOLVED. Intrinsic hand muscles include the lumbricales, interossei (plantar adductors, dorsal abductors), flexor pollicus brevis, abductor pollicus brevis, abductor pollicus longus, flexor digiti minimi, opponens pollicis, and opponens digiti minimi.

POSITION. Sitting or standing with upper arms at sides, elbows flexed, palms together

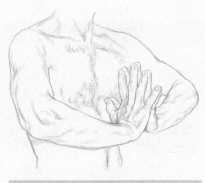

FIGURE 5.19B

STRETCH. Place your hands together in front of you, matching your palms and fingers as if you are about to pray (Fig. 5.19). With elbows flexed and wrists and fingers extended, elevate both elbows by flexing both shoulders, while lowering both hands extending the wrists. Keep palms together and fingers matched. Now maximally abduct all fingers.

RESULT. You should feel a stretch in the base of your fingers and across the palm of both hands.

NOTE. This stretch is very general and attempts to address the intrinsic muscles that serve to close, rather than open, the hand. Detailed stretches of the individual muscles can be found in Chapter 4.

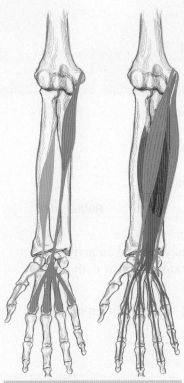

FIGURE 5.18A

flexor carpi radialis
flexor digitorum profundus
flexor digitorum superficialis
palmaris longus
flexor pollicus longus
flexor carpi ulnaris

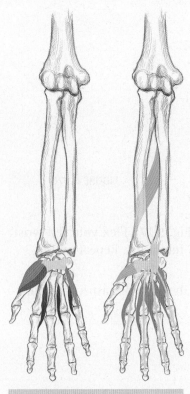

FIGURE 5.19A

lumbricales
interossei
flexor pollicis brevis
abductor pollicis brevis
abductor pollicis longus
flexor digiti minimi brevis
opponens pollicis
opponens digiti minimi

TRUNK

The stretches in this section are designed to increase flexibility of the trunk including the thoracic and lumbar spines, abdomen, and torso areas.

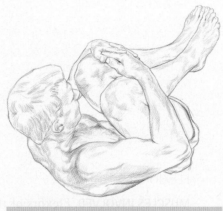

FIGURE 5.20B

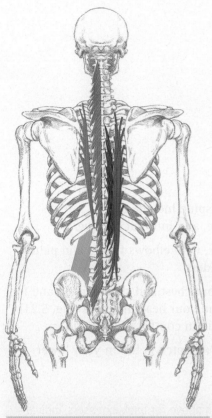

FIGURE 5.20A

multifidi
spinalis thoracis
longissimus thoracis
iliocostalis thoracis
quadratus lumborum

EXTENSION

MUSCLES INVOLVED. Extensors of the spine include the multifidi, spinalis thoracis, longissimus thoracis, iliocostalis thoracis, quadratus lumborum, and erector spinae.

POSITION. Lying on the floor, supine

STRETCH. Bring both of your knees up to your chest flexing both hips (Fig. 5.20). Using your arms and hands, pull both of your knees closer to your chest. Continue pulling until your buttocks are off of the floor, flexing your mid and lower spine. You may carefully flex your cervical and upper thoracic spine by pulling your head up toward your knees.

RESULT. You should feel a stretch in your lower back and hips, and along the posterior aspect of your neck, shoulders, and upper back if you have flexed your cervical and thoracic spines as well.

> ⚠ **CAUTION!** Individuals who have significant or unexplained back pain or have been diagnosed with any significant back dysfunction should consult their physician before doing this exercise. Flexing the lumbar spine should always be undertaken with caution, as many of the maladies associated with the lower back have been either caused or may be exacerbated by excessive flexion. Additionally, many people have excessive flexion in their lumbar spine to begin with and applying a stretching force may not only be unnecessary, but dangerous.

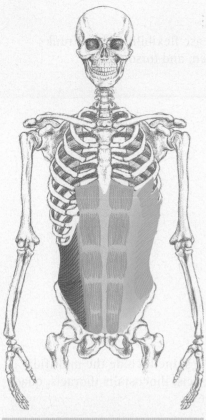

FIGURE 5.21A

rectus abdominus
external oblique
internal oblique

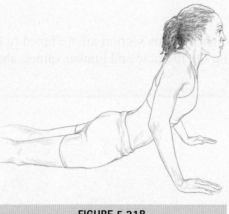

FIGURE 5.21B

FLEXION

MUSCLES INVOLVED. Flexors of the spine include the rectus abdominus, external oblique, and internal oblique.

POSITION. Lying on the floor, prone, with elbows flexed and palms on the floor just beneath the shoulders

STRETCH. Slowly attempt to press your chest and shoulders up and forward while taking care not to extend your head and neck (Fig. 5.21). Your hip bones (ASIS) should remain in contact with the floor.

RESULT. Continue to press up until a stretch is felt in your lower abdominal area.

> **⚠ CAUTION!** As with the stretch above for back extensors, individuals should not do this exercise if it is painful, especially if they have a diagnosed spondylolisthesis. Again, be careful not to hyperextend the cervical spine.

SIDE-BENDING

MUSCLES INVOLVED. Side-benders of the spine include the internal oblique, external oblique, iliocostalis lumborum, multifidis, and quadratus lumborum.

POSITION. Lying on the floor on your left side

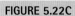

STRETCH. To stretch the side-benders on your left side, side-bend your torso toward the right by pressing up with your left arm and hand (Fig. 5.22). Be sure to bend directly sideways, staying in the frontal plane. Repeat on the right side.

RESULT. You should feel a stretch in the left side of your torso, from above the hip to the rib cage.

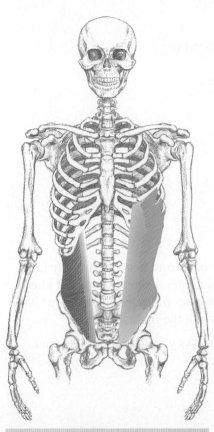

FIGURE 5.22A

external oblique
internal oblique

FIGURE 5.22C

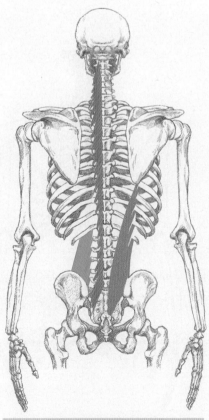

FIGURE 5.22B

multifidi
quadratus lumborum
iliocostalis lumborum

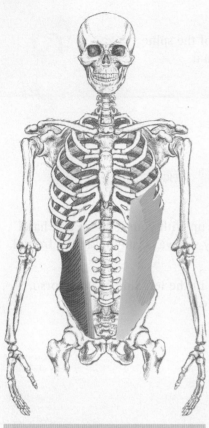

FIGURE 5.23A

ROTATION

MUSCLES INVOLVED. Rotators of the spine include the internal and external oblique, rotatores, semispinalis, and multifidis.

POSITION. Sitting on the floor with both legs extended

STRETCH. Straighten your spine and then step your left foot over and place it on the right side of your right knee (Fig. 5.23). Now rotate your upper body and head toward the left, placing your right elbow against the lateral side of your left knee. Continue turning to the left by applying pressure against your left knee with your right elbow. Repeat on the opposite side.

RESULT. You should feel a stretch across your upper, middle, and lower back and torso.

external oblique
internal oblique

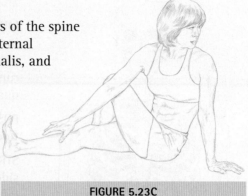

FIGURE 5.23C

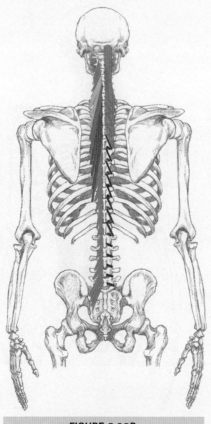

FIGURE 5.23B

multifidi
rotatores
semispinalis thoracsis
semispinalis capitis
semispinalis cervicis

LOWER BODY

The stretches in this section are designed to increase flexibility throughout the lower body, from the hip to the knee, ankle, and foot.

Hip

Below are stretches for the hip.

FLEXION

MUSCLES INVOLVED. Hip flexors include the psoas major and minor, iliacus, rectus femoris, sartorius, and tensor fascia lata.

POSITION. Standing

STRETCH. To stretch the hip flexors on your right side, first step forward about 2 feet with your left foot (Fig. 5.24). While keeping your torso and hips facing forward, move your upper body and hips anteriorly over your left foot by flexing your left knee and allowing a relaxed flexion in your right knee and ankle. You may allow your right heel to come off of the floor. Contract your abdominals to keep your lower back from extending. Repeat on your left side.

FIGURE 5.24B

RESULT. As you continue to move forward, maintaining your stomach tight and your back straight, you should feel a stretch in the anterior aspect of your right hip and upper thigh.

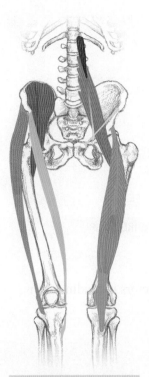

FIGURE 5.24A

psoas major
psoas minor
iliacus
rectus femoris
sartorius
tensor fascia lata

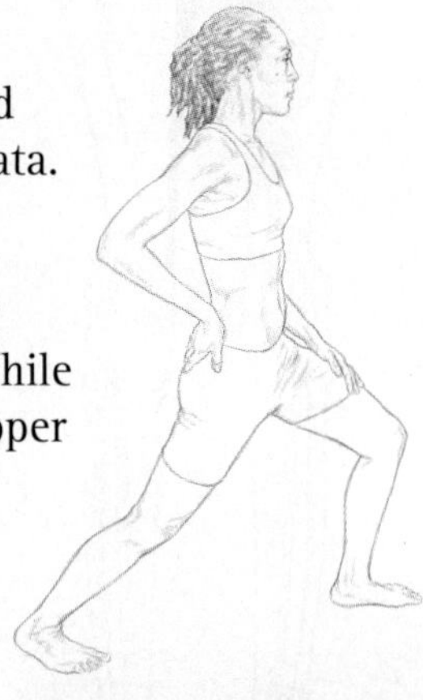

EXTENSION

MUSCLES INVOLVED. Hip extensors include the gluteus maximus and hamstrings: the semimembranosus, semitendinosus, and long head of biceps femoris. (The short head of biceps femoris does not cross the hip joint.)

POSITION. Lying supine

STRETCH. To stretch the hip extensors on your left side, grasp your left knee with your right hand (Fig. 5.25). Using your right arm and hand, pull your left knee up and across your torso toward your right shoulder, flexing and adducting your left hip. While keeping your knee in this position, actively extend your left knee to add stretch to the hamstrings, which also extend the hip. Repeat on the opposite side.

FIGURE 5.25B

RESULT. You should feel a stretch in the left lateral hip and gluteal area.

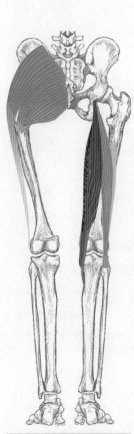

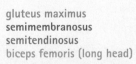

FIGURE 5.25A

gluteus maximus
semimembranosus
semitendinosus
biceps femoris (long head)

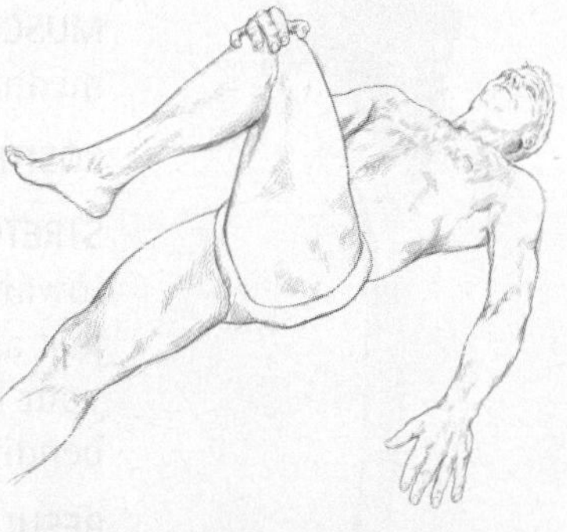

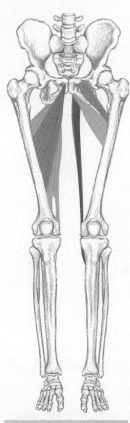

ADDUCTION

MUSCLES INVOLVED. Hip adductors include the adductor magnus, adductor longus, adductor brevis, pectineus, and gracilis.

POSITION. Lying on the floor with knees extended and legs abducted

STRETCH. Using the abductors of your hips, abduct your legs to their end range (Fig. 5.26). You may assist this stretch by placing the medial borders of your feet against a wall. As you achieve a stretching sensation you can scoot your feet slightly farther apart on the wall.

RESULT. You should feel a stretching sensation in your adductors extending from your pubic area to your medial thigh and knee.

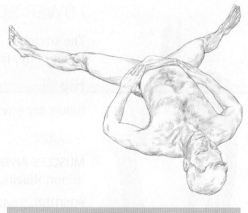

FIGURE 5.26B

adductor magnus
adductor longus
adductor brevis
pectineus
gracilis

FIGURE 5.26A

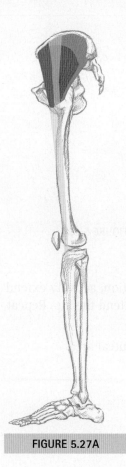

FIGURE 5.27A

ABDUCTION

MUSCLES INVOLVED. Abductors of the hip include the gluteus medius, gluteus minimus, and tensor fascia lata.

POSITION. Standing

STRETCH. To stretch your left hip abductors, step forward and toward the left with your right foot so that your right foot rests just ahead and to the left of your left foot (Fig. 5.27). Using your left hand, reach overhead and toward the right. Continue bending toward the right with your upper body.

RESULT. You should feel a stretch over the left greater trochanter. Note: Some individuals have difficulty feeling a stretch in the hip abductors. Adjusting the greater trochanter anteriorly or posteriorly by rotating the pelvis in the transverse plane may help to achieve the best stretch. Palpating the IT band will assure that it is under tension and being stretched. Repeat in the opposite direction to stretch the right side.

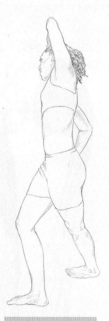

FIGURE 5.27B

gluteus medius
gluteus minimus
tensor fascia lata

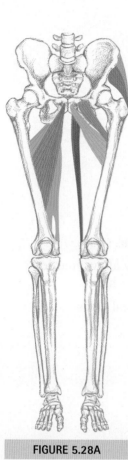

FIGURE 5.28A

gluteus medius
adductor magnus
adductor longus
adductor brevis
pectineus
gracilis

INTERNAL ROTATION

MUSCLES INVOLVED. Internal rotators of the hip include the anterior fibers of the gluteus medius, hip adductors, and medial hamstrings (semimembranosus and semitendinosus).

POSITION. Lying supine, with the left knee flexed to 90 degrees

STRETCH. To stretch the internal rotators of your left hip, place the ankle of your left leg on top of and across the right thigh making sure that the lateral lower left leg is lying on top of the right femur (Fig. 5.28). Now, place your left hand on your left knee and carefully press it toward the floor, taking care not to let your hips twist. Repeat on the right.

RESULT. You should feel a stretch in the groin area on the left.

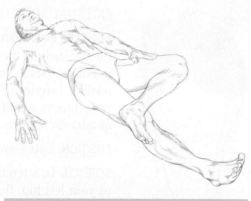

FIGURE 5.28C

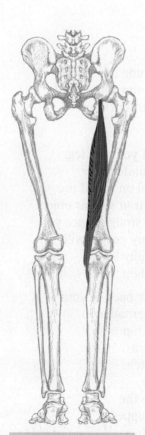

FIGURE 5.28B

semimembranosus
semitendinosus

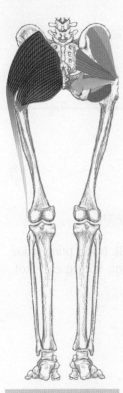

FIGURE 5.29A

piriformis
gluteus maximus
gluteus medius
inferior gemelli
superior gemelli
obturator internus
obturator externus
quadratus femoris

EXTERNAL ROTATION

MUSCLES INVOLVED. External rotators of the hip include the piriformis, gluteus maximus, posterior fibers of gluteus medius, inferior and superior gemelli, obturator internus and externus, and quadratus femoris.

POSITION. Lying on the floor, supine

STRETCH. To stretch the external rotators of your left hip, flex your left hip to just above 90 degrees (Fig. 5.29). Next, adduct your left hip by pulling your left knee over toward the right by pulling with your right hand. You may allow your left hip/buttock to come slightly off of the floor. Repeat for the right hip.

RESULT. You should feel a stretch in the left lateral hip and gluteal areas.

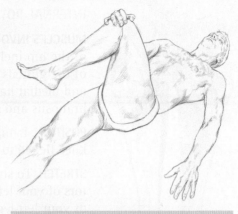

FIGURE 5.29B

Knee

Below are stretches for the knee.

FLEXION

MUSCLES INVOLVED. Knee flexors include the semimembranosus, semitendinosus, long and short heads of biceps femoris, popliteus, and gastrocnemius.

POSITION. Standing

STRETCH. To stretch the knee flexors of your left leg, stand facing a chair so that you can comfortably straighten your leg and place your heel on top of the chair (Fig. 5.30A and B). Choose a chair or similar object that will allow you to keep your spine straight once you have lifted your leg onto it. (Note: many people will have to choose a lower surface.) Carefully lean forward while keeping your spine straight.

RESULT. You should feel a stretch in the back of your thigh and knee. Note: An excellent alternative to this exercise is to lie supine with your hip flexed beyond 90 degrees and knee comfortably stretched. To perform the stretch, extend your knee with the help of one hand while stabilizing your thigh with the other. (You may use a belt or strap wrapped around your lower leg if you have difficulty reaching it.) See Fig. 5.30C.

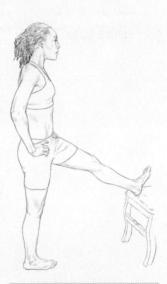

FIGURE 5.30B

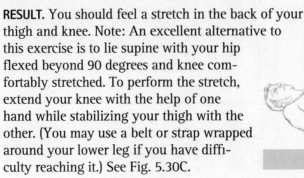

FIGURE 5.30C

FIGURE 5.30A

semimembranosus
semitendinosus
biceps femoris
popliteus
gastrocnemius

EXTENSION

MUSCLES INVOLVED. Knee extensors include the rectus femoris, vastus intermedius, vastus lateralis, and vastus medialis.

POSITION. Standing on your left leg, holding onto a chair or other object with your left hand for support

STRETCH. To stretch the extensors of the right knee, flex your right knee and grab your right shin just proximal to the ankle with your right hand (Fig. 5.31). Tighten your abdominals and concentrate on not allowing your back to arch (extend). Now pull your right ankle posteriorly, and then superiorly toward your buttock. Repeat for the left knee.

RESULT. You should feel a stretch in the middle of your right thigh.

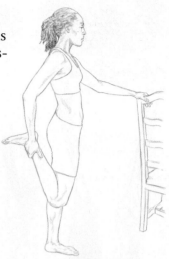

FIGURE 5.31B

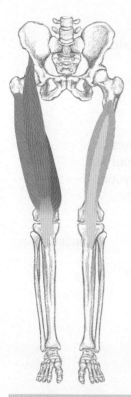

rectus femoris
vastus intermedius
vastus lateralis
vastus medialis

FIGURE 5.31A

Ankle and Foot

Below are stretches for the ankle and foot.

EXTENSION (DORSIFLEXION)

MUSCLES INVOLVED. Extensors of the ankle and foot include the anterior tibialis, extensor digitorum longus, extensor digitorum brevis, extensor hallicus longus, extensor hallicus brevis, and peroneus tertius.

POSITION. Standing

STRETCH. To stretch the extensors of the right ankle, foot, and toes, flex the right knee and plantarflex the foot and toes (Fig. 5.32). Place the dorsum of your right foot and toes on the floor about 18 inches behind you. Slowly bend your left knee, applying a gentle stretch to your right ankle, foot, and toes, bending them further into plantarflexion. Repeat on the left.

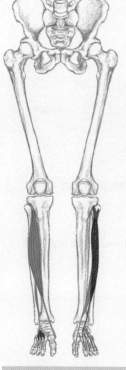

FIGURE 5.32B

RESULT. You should feel a stretch along the dorsal surface of the right foot and toes.

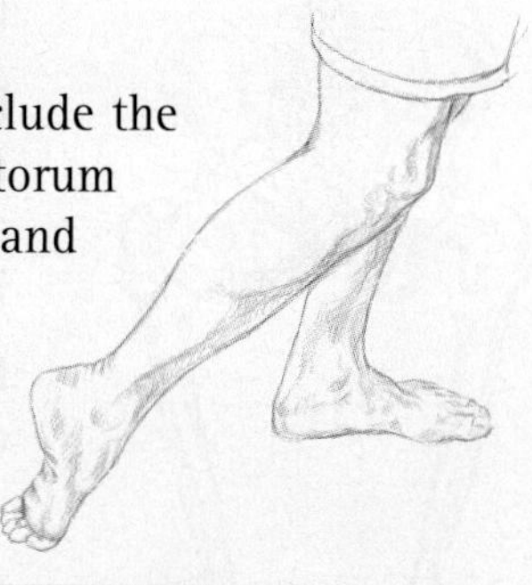

tibialis anterior
extensor digitorum longus
extensor digitorum brevis
extensor hallucis longus
extensor hallicus brevis
peroneus tertius

FIGURE 5.32A

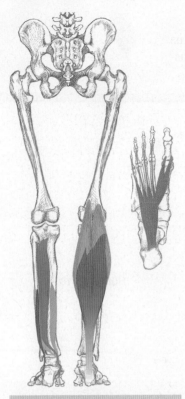

FLEXION (PLANTARFLEXION)

MUSCLES INVOLVED. Flexors of the ankle and foot include the gastrocnemius, soleus, peroneus brevis, posterior tibialis, flexor digitorum longus, flexor digitorum brevis, flexor hallicus longus, and flexor hallicus brevis.

POSITION. Standing

STRETCH. To stretch the flexors of the ankle, foot, and toes of your right leg, step forward about 18 inches with your left foot (Fig. 5.33A and B). Flex both knees while keeping your right heel on the ground. Maintain a neutral to high right arch (this may require a slight external rotation of your right tibia). You may move slightly forward over your left foot. Repeat to stretch the left ankle, foot, and toes.

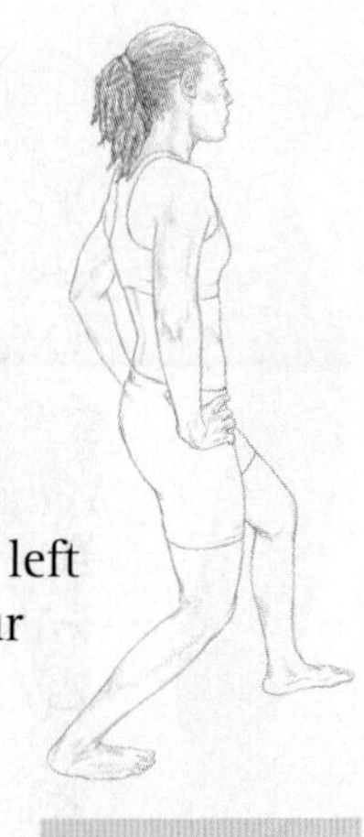

RESULT. You should feel a stretch in the posterior lower right leg. Note: To emphasize the gastrocnemius, which crosses both the ankle and the knee joints, step forward as above with your left foot, but in this case, keep the right knee extended while moving forward over your left foot (Fig. 5.33C). You may use your outstretched hands on a chair in front of you to support your forward lean.

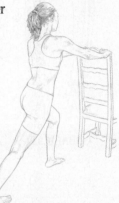

FIGURE 5.33B

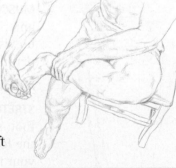

FIGURE 5.33C

FIGURE 5.33A

gastrocnemius	flexor digitorum longus
soleus	flexor digitorum brevis
peroneus brevis	flexor hallucis longus
tibialis posterior	flexor hallucis brevis

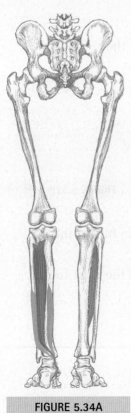

INVERSION

MUSCLES INVOLVED. Invertors of the ankle and foot include the tibialis posterior, tibialis anterior, flexor digitorum longus, and flexor hallicus longus.

POSITION. Seated with your left ankle supported across your right knee

STRETCH. To stretch the invertors of the left foot, use your right hand to dorsiflex the toes of your left foot, and then continue to push your left forefoot into dorsiflexion and eversion (sole of the foot away from you) (Fig. 5.34). Repeat for the right foot.

RESULT. You should feel a stretch along medial aspect of your lower left leg and foot.

FIGURE 5.34B

tibialis posterior
tibialis anterior
flexor digitorum longus
flexor hallucis longus

FIGURE 5.34A

EVERSION

MUSCLES INVOLVED. Evertors of the ankle and foot include the peroneus longus, brevis, and tertius, and the extensor digitorum longus.

POSITION. Standing

STRETCH. To stretch the evertors of your right foot step on top of your left foot with your right. Now carefully allow your right foot to roll over onto its outside edge (Fig. 5.35). Now, carefully bend your right knee, moving it forward.

RESULT. You should feel a stretch along the lateral aspect of your lower right leg and foot.

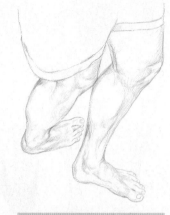

FIGURE 5.35B

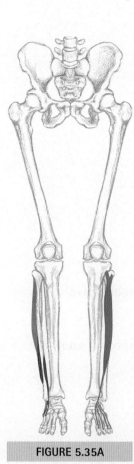

peroneus longus
peroneus brevis
peroneus tertius
extensor digitorum longus

FIGURE 5.35A

Toes

Below are stretches for the toes.

EXTENSION

MUSCLES INVOLVED. Toe extensors include the extensor digitorum longus, extensor digitorum brevis, extensor hallicus longus, extensor hallicus brevis, and extensor digiti minimi.

POSITION. Seated with left ankle crossed over your right knee

STRETCH. To stretch the extensors of your left foot and toes, place your right hand over the dorsal surface of the toes of your left foot (Fig. 5.36). Carefully flex all 5 toes toward you. Repeat for the right foot.

RESULT. You should feel a stretch evenly across the dorsal surface of your foot and toes.

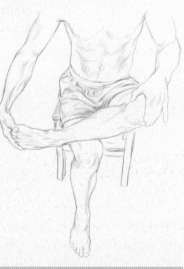

FIGURE 5.36B

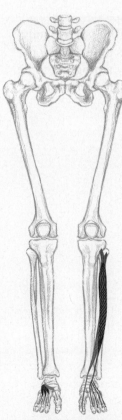

extensor digitorum longus
extensor digitorum brevis
extensor hallucis longus
extensor hallicus brevis

FIGURE 5.36A

FLEXION

MUSCLES INVOLVED. Toe flexors include the flexor digitorum longus, flexor digitorum brevis, flexor hallicus longus, flexor hallicus brevis, and flexor digiti minimi brevis.

POSITION. Seated with your left ankle crossed over the right knee

STRETCH. To stretch the toe flexors of your left foot, grasp the toes of your left foot with the fingers and palm of your right hand (Fig. 5.37). Extend all 5 toes and dorsiflex your ankle by pushing the toes toward the shin and allowing the ankle to dorsiflex. Repeat for your right foot.

RESULT. You should feel a stretch along the plantar aspect of your foot and toes.

flexor digitorum longus
flexor digitorum brevis
flexor hallucis longus
flexor hallucis brevis
flexor digiti minimi brevis

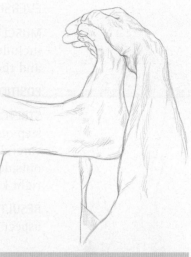

FIGURE 5.37B

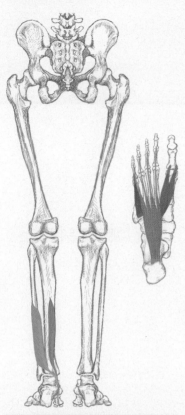

FIGURE 5.37A

SUMMARY

This chapter presents stretches for some of the major muscle groups of the body. The stretches are organized by body region and by movements produced by the contraction of muscles in these groups. It is designed to allow a program to be developed for the individual based on the individual's unique movement needs.

Stretching Programs for the Whole Body

This chapter contains three basic stretching programs, each designed to address all of the major muscle groups of the body from head to toe. These programs are designed to take roughly 10, 20, or 30 minutes to complete. For each stretch, we identify the region involved, the motion affected, the starting position, and the method. We also have provided a figure illustrating proper technique.

Because the chapter is addressed to individuals who may lack understanding of anatomical terminology, the description of each stretch uses words in everyday speech (e.g., *front* rather than *anterior* and *neck* rather than *cervical region*). However, common movement terms such as *flexion* and *extension* are used. For a review of these terms, see Chapter 2.

As this chapter is designed to give the individual safe guidelines, we have included only those stretches that address normal movement patterns, not stretches that require professional supervision. For instance, in the section on the cervical vertebrae, we have left out many possible stretches involving cervical extension, or extension with rotation, because these may cause injury in individuals with cervical dysfunction. Individuals with pain or discomfort in the cervical spine may have injury involving the cervical discs, which may be aggravated by cervical flexion, particularly if combined with rotation. They may also have injury or dysfunction leading to excessive stress on the cervical facet joints or ligaments, which may be aggravated by cervical extension, again particularly with rotation. Cervical extension and rotation also may cause restriction of blood flow through the vertebral artery, which may be dangerous in some individuals. Although these movements are benign in healthy, asymptomatic individuals, avoidance of these movements seems prudent. Stretches to improve cervical extension via stretching anterior tissues are included in the more detailed Chapters 4 and 5 of this book. Indeed, if you need more specific stretches for any body region, please see Chapters 4 and 5.

Table 6.1 lists the three different stretching programs, which are designed to provide a thorough, head-to-toe stretching program in 10, 20, or 30 minutes. The details of each program, including illustrations of each stretch, follows below.

10-MINUTE PROGRAM

This program includes stretches for all of the major muscle groups and functional movements. Although not as thorough as the longer programs, it is an effective stretching program for the entire body that can be performed in a short period of time.

TABLE 6.1 10-, 20-, AND 30-MINUTE STRETCHING PROGRAMS

10-minute Flexibility Program	20-minute Flexibility Program	30-minute Flexibility Program
(1) Front of Neck, Chest, and Abdomen: Extension	(1) Neck and Shoulders: Flexion	(1) Neck and Shoulders: Side-bending with Rotation
(2) Neck, Upper and Middle Back, and Torso: Side-bending	(2) Neck and Back: Flexion	(2) Neck and Shoulders: Flexion with Rotation
(3) Neck, Upper and Middle Back, and Torso: Rotation	(3) Front of Neck, Chest, and Abdomen: Extension	(3) Neck and Shoulders: Flexion
(4) Hip, Shoulders, Back, and Upper Arm: Hip Adduction, Shoulder Abduction, and Back Side-bending	(4) Neck, Upper and Middle Back, and Torso: Side-bending	(4) Neck and Back: Flexion
(5) Back of Shoulders and Upper and Middle Back: Horizontal Adduction	(5) Neck, Upper and Middle Back, and Torso: Rotation	(5) Front of Neck, Chest, and Abdomen: Extension
(6) Front of Chest and Shoulders: Horizontal Abduction	(6) Hip, Shoulders, Back, and Upper Arm: Hip Adduction, Shoulder Abduction, and Back Side-bending	(6) Neck, Upper and Middle Back, and Torso: Side-bending
(7) Hip Adductors (Groin): Abduction	(7) Back of Shoulders and Upper and Middle Back: Horizontal Adduction	(7) Neck, Upper and Middle Back, and Torso: Rotation
(8) Hip, Quadriceps, Ankle, and Foot: Hip Extension, Knee Flexion, and Ankle Plantar Flexion	(8) Chest and Front of Shoulders: Shoulder Horizontal Abduction	(8) Neck, Upper, Middle, and Lower Back, and Torso: Rotation
(9) Hips and Calves: Hip Extension and Ankle Dorsiflexion	(9) Front of Chest and Shoulders: Horizontal Abduction	(9) Middle and Lower Back and Hips: Flexion
	(10) Front of Shoulders: Extension	(10) Shoulders and Middle and Lower Back: Shoulder Flexion and Middle and Lower Back Flexion (and Side-bending)
	(11) Lats (Shoulders): Flexion	(11) Torso and Middle and Lower Back: Rotation
	(12) Elbow: Flexion	(12) Torso, Abdominals, and Middle and Lower Back: Extension
	(13) Wrist, Forearm, and Fingers: Flexion	(13) Hip, Shoulders, Back, and Upper Arm: Hip Adduction, Shoulder Abduction, and Back Side-bending
	(14) Wrist, Forearm, and Fingers: Extension	(14) Back of Shoulders and Upper and Middle Back: Horizontal Adduction
	(15) Glutes: Hip Flexion, Adduction, and Internal Rotation	(15) Chest and Front of Shoulders: Shoulder Horizontal Abduction
	(16) Hip Flexors: Extension	(16) Front of Chest and Shoulders: Horizontal Abduction
	(17) Hip Adductors: Hip Abduction	(17) Front of Shoulders: Extension
	(18) Hip Adductors (Groin): Abduction	(18) Lats (Shoulders): Flexion
	(19) Hamstrings: Standing	(19) Elbow: Flexion
	(20) Hip, Quadriceps, Ankle, and Foot: Hip Extension, Knee Flexion, and Ankle Plantarflexion	(20) Wrist, Forearm, and Fingers: Flexion
	(21) Hips and Calves: Hip Extension and Ankle Dorsiflexion	(21) Wrist, Forearm, and Fingers: Extension
	(22) Feet and Toes: Flexion	(22) Glutes: Hip Flexion, Adduction, and Internal Rotation
	(23) Feet and Toes: Extension	(23) Hip Flexors: Extension
		(24) Hip Adductors: Hip Abduction
		(25) Hip Adductors (Groin): Abduction
		(26) Hamstrings: Lying Supine
		(27) Hamstrings: Standing
		(28) Knee and Front of Thigh: Hip Extension and Knee Flexion
		(29) Hip, Quadriceps, Ankle, and Foot: Hip Extension, Knee Flexion, and Ankle Plantarflexion
		(30) Hips and Calves: Hip Extension and Ankle Dorsiflexion
		(31) Outside of Lower Leg: Ankle Inversion and Dorsiflexion
		(32) Feet and Toes: Flexion
		(33) Feet and Toes: Extension

Hold each stretch for 30 seconds at an intensity sufficient to elicit a feel of strong stretch in the target muscles. You should not feel sharp pain in the target muscles or in related muscles or joints; pain may be a sign of injury or dysfunction for which professional evaluation is necessary. Repeat the program at least 3–4 times a week.

Upper Body

Below are stretches for the upper body in the 10-minute program.

FRONT OF NECK, CHEST, AND ABDOMEN

MOTION AFFECTED. Extension of the neck, upper, middle, and lower back

POSITION. Standing with hands on hips

STRETCH. Carefully extend your neck (DO NOT HYPEREXTEND! Any feeling of discomfort in the back of the neck should be avoided.) by lifting your head up and back, following with your upper, then middle, then lower back (Fig. 6.1). Attempt to "unload" your spine by applying a moderate downward pressure on your hips with your hands. Try to achieve a balanced stretch, distributing the backward curve along the entire spine as evenly as possible.

RESULT. You should feel a stretch along the front of your neck, chest, and abdomen.

> ⚠ **CAUTION!** Pain in your lower back may be a sign of lower back injury or dysfunction. Either modify this exercise to eliminate this symptom or omit it. Pain may also signal that you need to seek medical advice. Similar precautions are in order if you feel pain in the neck or upper back.

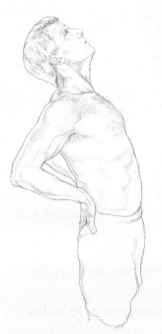

FIGURE 6.1

NECK, UPPER AND MIDDLE BACK, AND TORSO: SIDE-BENDING

MOTION AFFECTED. Side-bending

POSITION. Standing, hands at sides

STRETCH. Lean head to left, and then slowly slide your left hand down the outside of your left leg (Fig. 6.2). Try to bend directly to the side without moving backward or forward. Repeat to the right.

RESULT. You should feel a stretch along the right side of your neck and shoulder, continuing down the right side of your torso to your hip.

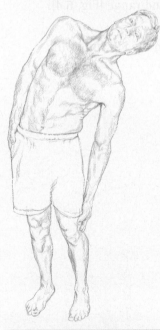

FIGURE 6.2

10-min program

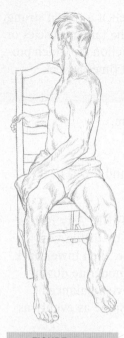

FIGURE 6.3A

NECK, UPPER AND MIDDLE BACK, AND TORSO: ROTATION

MOTION AFFECTED. Rotation

POSITION. Sitting

STRETCH. Turn your head, then your shoulders, and then your entire back maximally toward the right (Fig. 6.3A). You may use your arms to help you rotate. Repeat toward the left.

This stretch may also be performed from a standing position (Fig. 6.3B).

RESULT. You should feel a stretch in your neck and your upper and middle back.

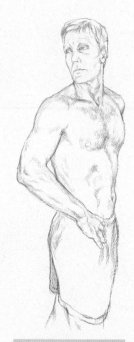

FIGURE 6.3B

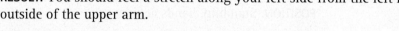

HIPS, SHOULDERS, BACK, AND UPPER ARM

MOTION AFFECTED. Hip adduction, spine and torso side-bending, and shoulder abduction

POSITION. Standing in a lunge position with your right foot roughly 18 inches ahead of your left

STRETCH. Lift your left hand overhead and move it in an arc directly toward the right, eventually taking the ribs, torso, and hip along to end range (Fig. 6.4). Repeat to the left.

RESULT. You should feel a stretch along your left side from the left hip to the outside of the upper arm.

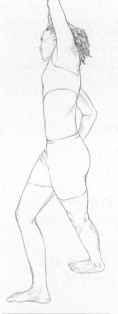

FIGURE 6.4

BACK OF SHOULDERS AND UPPER AND MIDDLE BACK

MOTION AFFECTED. Horizontal adduction (upper arms and shoulder blades forward in horizontal plane)

POSITION. Standing with your right arm reaching across the front of your torso to your left shoulder

STRETCH. Using your left hand, pull your right elbow toward your left shoulder (Fig. 6.5). Continue by twisting your torso toward the left. Repeat in the opposite direction.

RESULT. You should feel a stretch in the back of your right shoulder and across your upper and middle back.

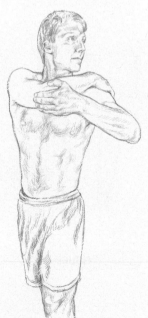

FIGURE 6.5

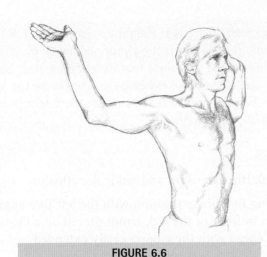

FIGURE 6.6

FRONT OF CHEST AND SHOULDERS

MOTION AFFECTED. Horizontal abduction of shoulders

POSITION. Standing with arms straight out to the side, and elbows bent 90 degrees

STRETCH. Move your elbows back, while also moving your hands backward (you are externally rotating your shoulders) (Fig. 6.6). Keep your posture erect, and avoid allowing your head to project forward.

RESULT. You should feel a stretch in the front of your chest and shoulders.

Lower Body

Below are stretches for the lower body in the 10-minute program.

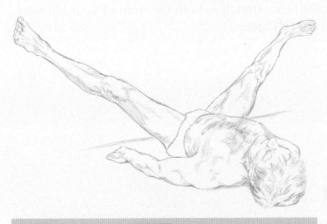

FIGURE 6.7

HIP ADDUCTORS (GROIN)

MOTION AFFECTED. Hip abduction

POSITION. Lying supine perpendicular to a wall, with legs extended straight up the wall, buttocks in contact with the wall. Contract your abdominals to flatten your lower back against the floor. This will stabilize your pelvis and protect your lower back from the strain of your abducting legs.

STRETCH. Relax and allow your legs to fall outward (abduct), sliding down the wall until they reach their end range (Fig. 6.7).

RESULT. You should feel a stretch along your inner thighs, from knee to groin.

HIP, QUADRICEPS, ANKLE, AND FOOT

MOTION AFFECTED. Hip extension, knee flexion, and foot/ankle plantar flexion

POSITION. Standing near a chair or other object for support

STRETCH. Bend your right knee and grab the top of your foot from behind, pulling the entire foot and lower leg toward your buttocks (Fig. 6.8). Be sure to tighten your stomach muscles and keep your back straight. Repeat with the left leg.

RESULT. You should feel a stretch across the top of your foot and ankle, and in the middle of your thigh.

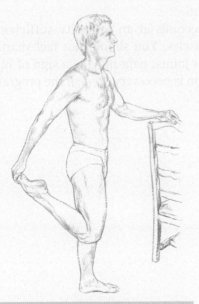

FIGURE 6.8

> **CAUTION!** Carelessly stretching your quads (thigh) can easily result in hyper-extending your lower back. Avoid this by contracting your abdominal muscles and flattening your lower back *before* pulling your right foot back and up. Also, because of the obvious difference in the size of the muscles being stretched in the top of your foot and the front of your thigh, be cautious about applying too much stretch to your foot. If you feel any pain, let up on the stretch.

HIPS AND CALVES

MOTION AFFECTED. Hip extension and ankle dorsiflexion

POSITION. Standing in a lunge position with the left foot approximately 24 inches in front of the left, hands placed on a chair or against the wall ahead with the elbows easily extended

STRETCH. Bend the lead (left) knee and lean forward keeping the right knee straight, allowing the elbows to bend as your body comes closer to the chair or wall (Fig. 6.9). Repeat with the right knee leading.

RESULT. You should feel a stretch in both the front of your hip near the groin and in the calf area.

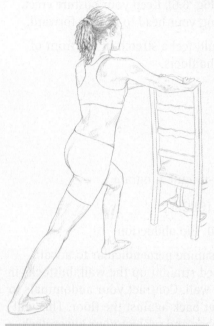

FIGURE 6.9

20-MINUTE PROGRAM

This program enables you to stretch all of the major muscle groups and perform all essential functional movements in roughly 20 minutes. If you have a limited amount of time and no specific flexibility needs, then this is an effective, entry-level stretching program for you.

Hold each stretch for 30 seconds at an intensity sufficient to elicit a feel of strong stretch in the target muscles. You should not feel sharp pain in the target muscles or in related muscles or joints; pain may be a sign of injury of dysfunction for which professional evaluation is necessary. Repeat the program at least 3–4 times a week.

Perform all of the stretches listed in the 10-minute program, then add the following:

Upper Body

Below are stretches for the upper body in the 20-minute program.

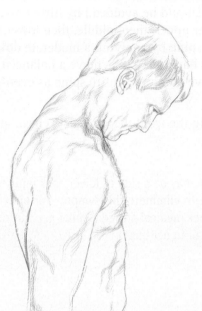

FIGURE 6.10

NECK AND SHOULDERS: FLEXION

MOTION AFFECTED. Neck flexion

POSITION. Standing

STRETCH. Carefully tuck your chin, and then flex your head down toward your chest (Fig. 6.10).

RESULT. You should feel a gentle stretch in the back of your neck and upper shoulders.

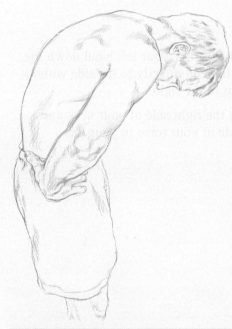

FIGURE 6.11

NECK AND BACK

MOTION AFFECTED. Flexion

POSITION. Standing with hands on hips

STRETCH. Gently tuck your chin, then bend first your head, then your upper back and ribcage down to your hips (Fig. 6.11).

RESULT. You should feel a stretch down along the back of your neck, and farther down into your middle and lower back.

20-min program

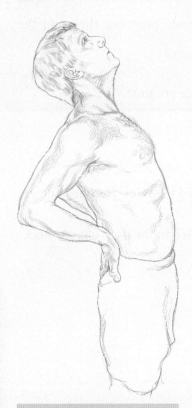

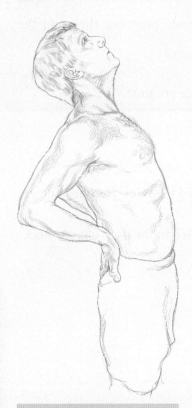

FIGURE 6.12

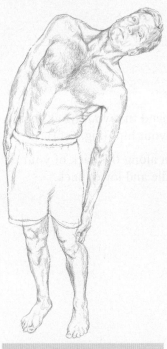

FIGURE 6.13

FRONT OF NECK, CHEST, AND ABDOMEN

MOTION AFFECTED. Extension of the neck, upper, middle, and lower back

POSITION. Standing with hands on hips

STRETCH. Carefully extend your neck (DO NOT HYPEREXTEND! Any feeling of discomfort in the back of the neck should be avoided.) by lifting your head up and back, following with your upper, then middle, then lower back (Fig. 6.12). Attempt to "unload" your spine by applying a moderate downward pressure on your hips with your hands. Try to achieve a balanced stretch, distributing the backward curve along the entire spine as evenly as possible.

RESULT. You should feel a stretch along the front of your neck, chest, and abdomen.

⚠ **CAUTION!** Pain in your lower back may be a sign of lower back injury or dysfunction. Either modify this exercise to eliminate this symptom or omit it. Pain may also signal that you need to seek medical advice. Similar precautions are in order if you feel pain in the neck or upper back.

NECK, UPPER AND MIDDLE BACK, AND TORSO: SIDE–BENDING

MOTION AFFECTED. Side-bending

POSITION. Standing, hands at sides

STRETCH. Lean head to left, and then slowly slide your left hand down the outside of your left leg (Fig. 6.13). Try to bend directly to the side without movement backward or forward. Repeat to the right.

RESULT. You should feel a stretch along the right side of your neck and shoulder, continuing down the right side of your torso to your hip.

NECK, UPPER AND MIDDLE BACK, AND TORSO: ROTATION

MOTION AFFECTED. Rotation

POSITION. Sitting

STRETCH. Turn your head, then your shoulders, and then your entire back maximally toward the right (Fig. 6.14A). You may use your arms to help you rotate. Repeat toward the left.

This stretch may also be performed from a standing position (Fig. 6.14B).

RESULT. You should feel a stretch in your neck and your upper and middle back.

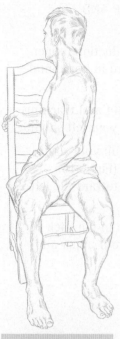

FIGURE 6.14A

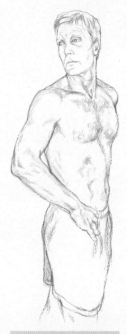

FIGURE 6.14B

HIPS, SHOULDERS, BACK, AND UPPER ARM

MOTION AFFECTED. Hip adduction, spine and torso side-bending, and shoulder abduction

POSITION. Standing in a lunge position with your right foot roughly 18 inches ahead of your left

STRETCH. Lift your left hand overhead and move it in an arc directly toward the right, eventually taking the ribs, torso, and hip along to end range (Fig. 6.15). Repeat to the left.

RESULT. You should feel a stretch along your left side from the left hip to the outside of the upper arm.

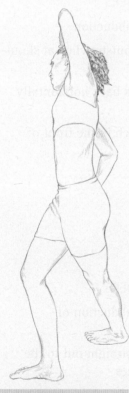

FIGURE 6.15

20-min program

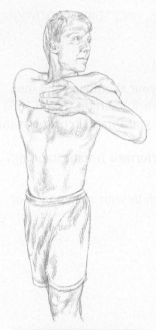

FIGURE 6.16

BACK OF SHOULDERS AND UPPER AND MIDDLE BACK

MOTION AFFECTED. Horizontal adduction (upper arms and shoulder blades forward in horizontal plane)

POSITION. Standing with your right arm reaching across the front of your torso to your left shoulder

STRETCH. Using your left hand, pull your right elbow toward your left shoulder (Fig. 6.16). Continue by twisting your torso toward the left. Repeat in the opposite direction.

RESULT. You should feel a stretch in the back of your right shoulder and across your upper and middle back.

CHEST AND FRONT OF SHOULDERS

MOTION AFFECTED. Horizontal abduction

POSITION. Standing with arms outstretched at shoulder level, palms up

STRETCH. Move arms and hands back horizontally (Fig. 6.17).

RESULT. You should feel a stretch in the front of your chest and shoulders.

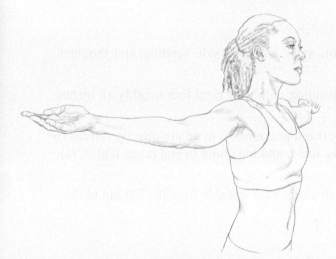

FIGURE 6.17

FRONT OF CHEST AND SHOULDERS

MOTION AFFECTED. Horizontal abduction of shoulders

POSITION. Standing with arms straight out to the side, and elbows bent 90 degrees

STRETCH. Move your elbows back, while also moving your hands backward (you are externally rotating your shoulders) (Fig. 6.18). Keep your posture erect, and avoid allowing your head to project forward.

RESULT. You should feel a stretch in the front of your chest and shoulders.

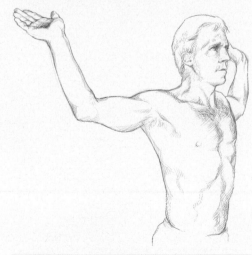

FIGURE 6.18

FRONT OF SHOULDERS

MOTION AFFECTED. Extension

POSITION. Standing with hands clasped behind body, elbows extended

STRETCH. Lift your hands up behind your back as far as possible, keeping your elbows straight and being careful not to bend forward at the waist (Fig. 6.19).

RESULT. You should feel a stretch in the front of your shoulders and upper arms.

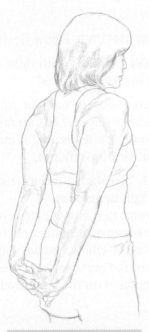

FIGURE 6.19

LATS (SHOULDERS)

MOTION AFFECTED. Flexion

POSITION. Standing within arms' reach of the back of a chair or other object of similar height

STRETCH. Bend over from the waist and reach both arms straight overhead, placing both hands on the back of the chair (Fig. 6.20). Keeping your back straight, bend forward at the waist until a stretch is felt in the area of your armpits.

RESULT. You should feel a stretch in your axillary (armpit) area.

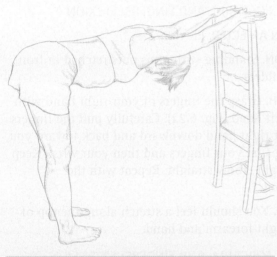

FIGURE 6.20

20-min program

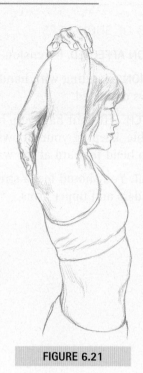

FIGURE 6.21

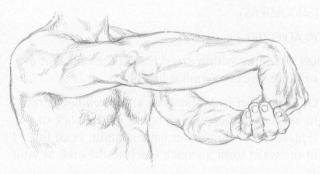

FIGURE 6.22

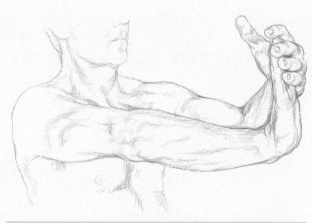

FIGURE 6.23

ELBOW

MOTION AFFECTED. Elbow flexion

POSITION. Standing with right elbow overhead, elbow maximally flexed

STRETCH. Place the palm of your left hand over your right elbow (Fig. 6.21). Carefully push your elbow backwards while keeping it maximally flexed. Repeat with the left arm.

RESULT. You should feel a stretch in the back of your right upper arm.

Notice that elbow extension is not covered here. This is because the earlier stretch for shoulder extension has the elbow extended and will place a stretch on all of the muscles that cross the elbow joint, with the emphasis on the long head of the biceps.

WRIST, FOREARM, AND FINGERS: FLEXION

MOTION AFFECTED. Flexion

POSITION. Standing with arms outstretched in front of shoulders

STRETCH. Grasp the fingers of your right hand with your left hand (Fig. 6.22). Carefully pull the fingers of your right hand downward and back toward you, flexing first your fingers and then your wrist. Keep your right elbow straight. Repeat with the left hand.

RESULT. You should feel a stretch along the top of your right forearm and hand.

WRIST, FOREARM, AND FINGERS: EXTENSION

MOTION AFFECTED. Extension

POSITION. Standing with arms outstretched in front of shoulders

STRETCH. Place the palm of your left hand against the palm and fingers of your right hand (Fig. 6.23). Push the right fingers and then hand backward. Repeat with the left hand.

RESULT. You should feel a stretch along the underside of your forearm, hand, and fingers.

Lower Body

Below are stretches for the lower body in the 20-minute program.

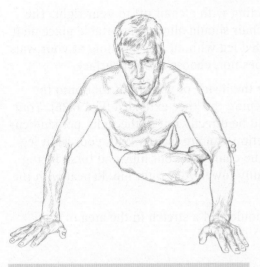

FIGURE 6.24

GLUTES

MOTION AFFECTED. Hip flexion with adduction, and hip external rotation

POSITION. Lying on your stomach (prone)

STRETCH. Lift your chest and shoulders as if doing a pushup (Fig. 6.24). Bring your right knee up and across, in front of you and toward the left, allowing your right knee to bend roughly 100 degrees. If you feel any stress in your right knee increase the amount of bend (flex) in it until these symptoms disappear. Carefully attempt to lie back down onto your right knee, which is now under the left side of your body. Repeat with the left leg.

RESULT. You should feel a stretch in the gluteal area on your right side.

> **⚠ CAUTION!** As soon as you feel a stretch, you have accomplished your goal. Do not continue to lower yourself onto the floor if you feel a stretch early on in this exercise. If you have a ligamentous instability, or are otherwise suspicious of your knee's health, consultation with a professional is recommended before performing this exercise.

HIP FLEXORS

MOTION AFFECTED. Hip extension

POSITION. Standing

STRETCH. Take a large step forward with the left foot, keeping the torso and upper body facing forward (Fig. 6.25). Carefully bend the left knee while moving your body forward over your left foot. Your right leg remains relaxed, with the knee slightly bent. The right heel may come off of the floor. Repeat with the right foot forward.

RESULT. You should feel a stretch in the front of your right thigh/groin.

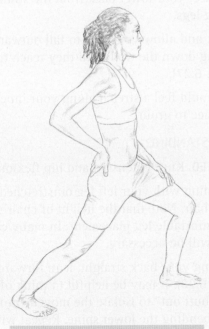

FIGURE 6.25

20-min program

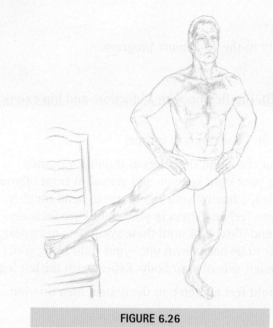

FIGURE 6.26

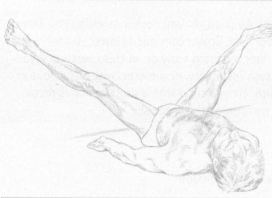

FIGURE 6.27

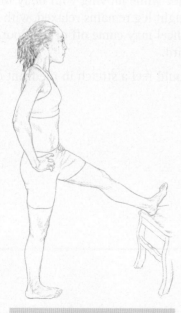

FIGURE 6.28

HIP ADDUCTORS

MOTION AFFECTED. Hip abduction

POSITION. Standing with a chair off to your right. The height of the chair should allow comfortable placement of your extended leg without side-bending at your waist or hips. If it does not, choose a lower surface.

STRETCH. Place the inside of your right foot onto the chair while keeping the knee extended (Fig. 6.26). Your right leg should be directly out to the right, perpendicular to the direction you are facing. With your right leg supported by the chair and your hips and torso facing forward, carefully lower your right hip. Repeat with the left leg.

RESULT. You should feel a stretch in the area of your right groin.

HIP ADDUCTORS (GROIN)

MOTION AFFECTED. Hip abduction

POSITION. Lying supine perpendicular to a wall, with legs extended straight up the wall, buttocks in contact with the wall. Contract your abdominals to flatten your lower back against the floor. This will stabilize your pelvis and protect your lower back from the strain of your abducting legs.

STRETCH. Relax and allow your legs to fall outward (abduct), sliding down the wall until they reach their end range (Fig. 6.27).

RESULT. You should feel a stretch along your inner thighs, from knee to groin.

HAMSTRINGS: STANDING

MOTION AFFECTED. Knee extension and hip flexion

POSITION. Standing with your left leg outstretched and supported on chair. Note that the height of chair should allow for a comfortable leg placement; in many cases, a lower support will be necessary.

STRETCH. Keeping your back straight, lean forward from your hips (Fig. 6.28). It may be helpful to think of "sticking your butt out" to isolate the movement to the hip and avoid bending the lower spine. Repeat with your right leg.

RESULT. You should feel a stretch along the back of your left thigh from the belly of the hamstrings to the back of the knee.

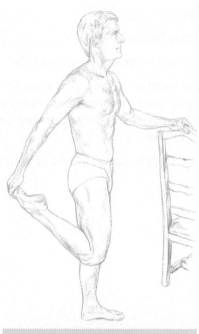

FIGURE 6.29

HIP, QUADRICEPS, ANKLE, AND FOOT

MOTION AFFECTED. Hip extension, knee flexion, and foot/ankle plantar flexion

POSITION. Standing near a chair or other object for support

STRETCH. Bend your right knee and grab the top of your foot from behind, pulling the entire foot and lower leg toward your buttocks (Fig. 6.29). Be sure to tighten your stomach muscles and keep your back straight. Repeat with the left leg.

RESULT. You should feel a stretch across the top of your foot and ankle, and in the middle of your thigh.

> **△ CAUTION!** Carelessly stretching your quads (thigh) can easily result in hyperextending your lower back. Avoid this by contracting your abdominal muscles and flattening your lower back *before* pulling your right foot back and up. In addition, because of the obvious difference in the size of the muscles being stretched in the top of your foot and the front of your thigh, be cautious about applying too much stretch to your foot. If you feel any pain, let up on the stretch.

HIPS AND CALVES

MOTION AFFECTED. Hip extension and ankle dorsiflexion

POSITION. Standing in a lunge position with the left foot approximately 24 inches in front of the left, hands placed on a chair or against the wall ahead with the elbows easily extended

STRETCH. Bend the lead (left) knee, and lean forward keeping the right knee straight. Allow the elbows to bend as your body comes closer to the chair or wall (Fig. 6.30). Repeat with the right knee leading.

RESULT. You should feel a stretch in both the front of your hip near the groin, and in the calf area.

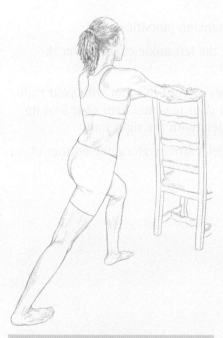

FIGURE 6.30

20-min program

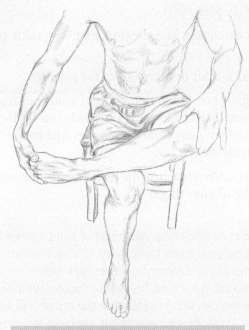

FIGURE 6.31

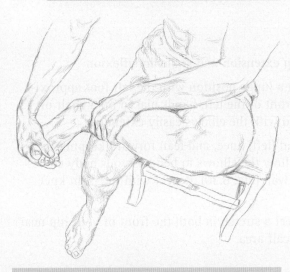

FIGURE 6.32

FEET AND TOES: FLEXION

MOTION AFFECTED. (Plantar) flexion

POSITION. Seated with left ankle crossed over right knee

STRETCH. Place your right hand over the top of your left foot (Fig. 6.31). Gently pull your toes and then your foot back toward your body (you are extending your toes and feet). Repeat with the right foot.

RESULT. You should feel a stretch along the top of your left foot and toes.

FEET AND TOES: EXTENSION

MOTION AFFECTED. Extension (dorsiflexion)

POSITION. Seated with the left ankle crossed over the right knee

STRETCH. Grasp the toes of your left foot with your right hand (Fig. 6.32). Push your toes and then your foot up toward your shin. Repeat with the right foot.

RESULT. You should feel a stretch along the bottom of your foot.

30-MINUTE PROGRAM

This program includes stretches for all of the major muscle groups and functional movements. It can be performed in about 30 minutes. It is designed for people without specific movement needs.

Hold each stretch for 30 seconds at a level of intensity sufficient to elicit a feel of strong stretch in the target muscles. You should not feel sharp pain in the target muscles or in related muscles or joints; pain may be a sign of injury or dysfunction for which professional evaluation is necessary. Repeat the program at least 3–4 times a week.

Perform all of the stretches for the 20-minute program, then add the following.

Upper Body

Below are stretches for the upper body in the 30-minute program.

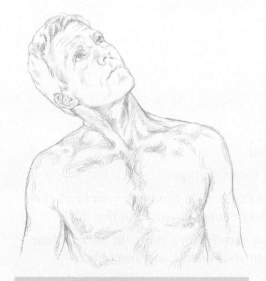

FIGURE 6.33

NECK AND SHOULDERS: SIDE-BENDING WITH ROTATION

MOTION AFFECTED. Side-bending with rotation

POSITION. Standing or sitting

STRETCH. First lean head toward the right, directly sideways (Fig. 6.33). Now turn head toward the left. Repeat in the opposite direction.

RESULT. You should feel a stretch along the left side of your neck into your left shoulder.

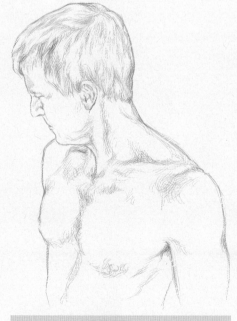

FIGURE 6.34

NECK AND SHOULDERS: FLEXION WITH ROTATION

MOTION AFFECTED. Flexion with rotation

POSITION. Standing or seated

STRETCH. Carefully bend your head and neck forward to its end range, then carefully rotate it toward the right (Fig. 6.34). Repeat to the left.

RESULT. You should feel this in the upper back and neck.

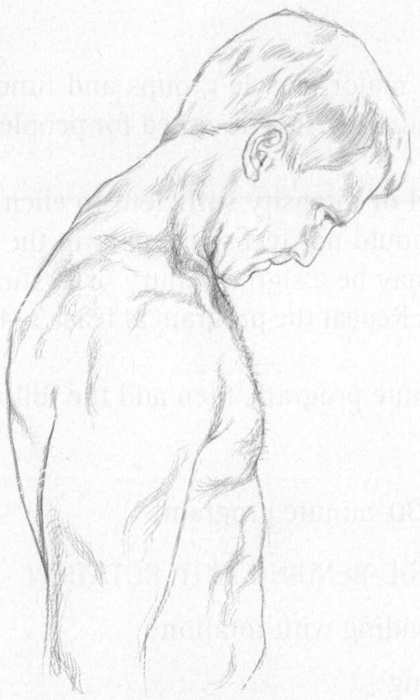

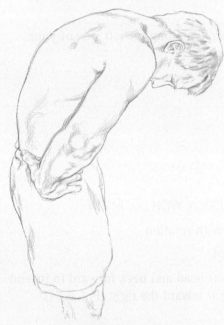

FIGURE 6.35

NECK AND SHOULDERS: FLEXION

MOTION AFFECTED. Neck flexion

POSITION. Standing

STRETCH. Carefully tuck your chin, and then flex your head down toward your chest (Fig. 6.35).

RESULT. You should feel a gentle stretch in the back of your neck and upper shoulders.

NECK AND BACK

MOTION AFFECTED. Flexion

POSITION. Standing with hands on hips

STRETCH. Gently tuck your chin, then bend first your head, then your upper back and ribcage down to your hips (Fig. 6.36).

RESULT. You should feel a stretch down along the back of your neck, and further down to your middle and lower back.

FIGURE 6.36

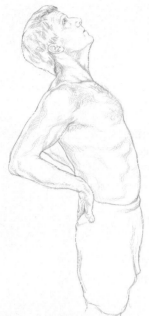
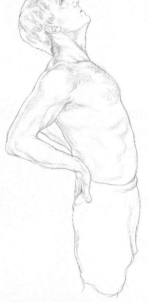

FIGURE 6.37

FRONT OF NECK, CHEST, AND ABDOMEN

MOTION AFFECTED. Extension of the neck, upper, middle, and lower back

POSITION. Standing with hands on hips

STRETCH. Carefully extend your neck (DO NOT HYPEREXTEND! Any feeling of discomfort in the back of the neck should be avoided.) by lifting your head up and back, following with your upper, then middle, then lower back (Fig. 6.37). Attempt to "unload" your spine by applying a moderate downward pressure on your hips with your hands. Try to achieve a balanced stretch, distributing the backward curve along the entire spine as evenly as possible.

RESULT. You should feel a stretch along the front of your neck, chest, and abdomen.

> ⚠ **CAUTION!** Pain in your lower back may be a sign of lower back injury or dysfunction. Either modify this exercise to eliminate this symptom or omit it. Pain may also signal that you need to seek medical advice. Similar precautions are in order if you feel pain in the neck or upper back.

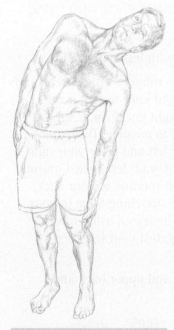

FIGURE 6.38

NECK, UPPER AND MIDDLE BACK, AND TORSO: SIDE-BENDING

MOTION AFFECTED. Side-bending

POSITION. Standing, hands at sides

STRETCH. Lean head to left, and then slowly slide your left hand down the outside of your left leg (Fig. 6.38). Try to bend directly to the side without movement backward or forward. Repeat to the right.

RESULT. You should feel a stretch along the right side of your neck and shoulder, continuing down the right side of your torso into your hip.

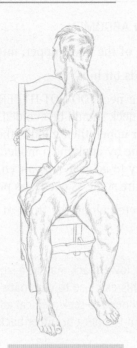

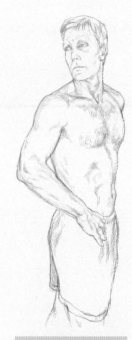

NECK, UPPER AND MIDDLE BACK, AND TORSO: ROTATION

MOTION AFFECTED. Rotation

POSITION. Sitting

STRETCH. Turn your head, then your shoulders, and then your entire back maximally toward the right (Fig. 6.39A). You may use your arms to help you rotate. Repeat toward the left.

This stretch may also be performed from a standing position (Fig. 6.39B).

RESULT. You should feel a stretch in your neck and your upper and middle back.

FIGURE 6.39A

FIGURE 6.39B

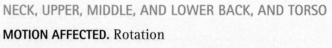

NECK, UPPER, MIDDLE, AND LOWER BACK, AND TORSO

MOTION AFFECTED. Rotation

POSITION. Seated on the floor with legs extended

STRETCH. Bend your left knee to roughly 110 degrees, and step your left foot over your right knee so that it rests on the floor adjacent to your right knee (Fig. 6.40). Straighten your spine as much as possible. Turn your head and shoulders toward the left and place your right elbow against, and to the left of, your left knee. Continue to stretch in the direction of left rotation at your neck, shoulders, and lower back. The stretching force in your middle and lower back can be increased using careful pressure of your right elbow against your left knee. Repeat to the right.

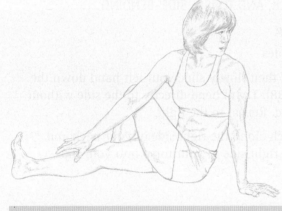
FIGURE 6.40

RESULT. You should feel a stretch along your lower, mid, and upper back and shoulders and to the right side of your neck.

MIDDLE AND LOWER BACK AND HIPS

MOTION AFFECTED. Flexion

POSITION. Lying supine

STRETCH. Using your arms and hands, pull one knee first and then the other knee to your chest (Fig. 6.41). Wrap your arms around your knees and carefully pull them close, while lifting your head and flexing your neck.

RESULT. You should feel a stretch extending from the back of your neck down to your lower back.

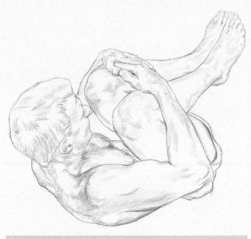
FIGURE 6.41

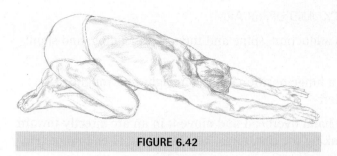

FIGURE 6.42

SHOULDERS AND MIDDLE AND LOWER BACK

MOTION AFFECTED. Shoulder abduction and flexion. Spinal side-bending

POSITION. On the floor, seated back on heels

STRETCH. Place the palms of both hands on the floor in front of you (Fig. 6.42). Slide your hands forward along the floor, following with your chest and shoulders until your arms are outstretched completely and your buttocks have just lifted off of your heels (or have otherwise moved forward from the seated position). Walk your hands slightly further forward and then apply enough downward pressure to fix them in place. Now allow your hips and buttocks to carefully drop backwards while holding your hands in place. To emphasize spinal left side-bending and the right latissimus dorsi muscle, walk both hands about 12 inches to the left before fixing them in place, sitting back, and holding. Repeat to the right.

RESULT. You should feel a stretch in your axilla (armpit area) from the upper chest to upper arms.

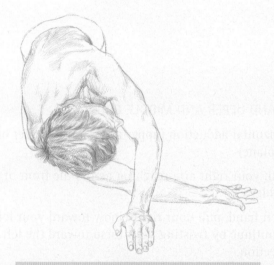

FIGURE 6.43

TORSO AND MIDDLE AND LOWER BACK

MOTION AFFECTED. Rotation

POSITION. On hands and knees, with hands directly below shoulders, and knees directly below hips

STRETCH. Place the back of your right hand on the floor while continuing to support your body weight with your left hand (Fig. 6.43). Slide your right hand toward the left, going underneath your body, beyond your left hand. Continue until you have rotated your entire upper body maximally toward the left. Repeat toward the right, leading with the left hand.

RESULT. You should feel a stretch along the side of your middle and upper back.

TORSO, ABDOMINALS, AND MIDDLE AND LOWER BACK

MOTION AFFECTED. Extension

POSITION. Lying on your stomach (prone)

STRETCH. Place your hands on the floor in front of your chest and shoulders (Fig. 6.44). Press your chest and shoulders up and forward, away from your waist so that your spine forms a gentle curve backward. Be careful not to hyperextend your lower back or neck. Your hip bones should remain in contact with the floor.

RESULT. You should feel a stretch along the front of your hips, abdomen, and chest.

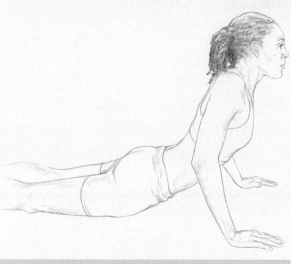

FIGURE 6.44

30-min program

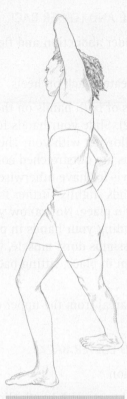

FIGURE 6.45

HIPS, SHOULDERS, BACK, AND UPPER ARM

MOTION AFFECTED. Hip adduction, spine and torso side-bending, and shoulder abduction

POSITION. Standing in a lunge position with your right foot roughly 18 inches ahead of your left

STRETCH. Lift your left hand overhead and move it in an arc directly toward the right, eventually taking the ribs, torso, and hip along to end range (Fig. 6.45). Repeat to the left.

RESULT. You should feel a stretch along your left side from the left hip to the outside of the upper arm.

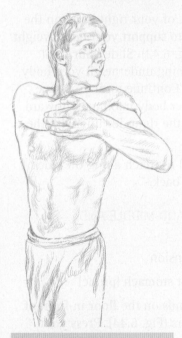

FIGURE 6.46

BACK OF SHOULDERS AND UPPER AND MIDDLE BACK

MOTION AFFECTED. Horizontal adduction (upper arms and shoulder blades forward in horizontal plane)

POSITION. Standing with your right arm reaching across the front of your torso to your left shoulder

STRETCH. Using your left hand, pull your right elbow toward your left shoulder (Fig. 6.46). Continue by twisting your torso toward the left. Repeat in opposite direction.

RESULT. You should feel a stretch in the back of your right shoulder and across your upper and middle back.

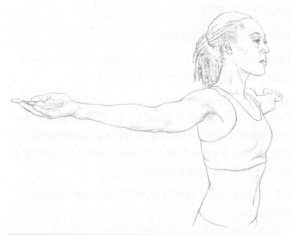

FIGURE 6.47

CHEST AND FRONT OF SHOULDERS

MOTION AFFECTED. Horizontal abduction

POSITION. Standing with arms outstretched at shoulder level, palms up

STRETCH. Move arms and hands back horizontally (Fig. 6.47).

RESULT. You should feel a stretch in the front of your chest and shoulders.

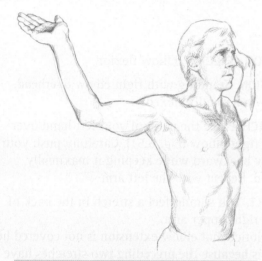

FIGURE 6.48

FRONT OF CHEST AND SHOULDERS

MOTION AFFECTED. Horizontal abduction of shoulders

POSITION. Standing with arms straight out to the side, and elbows bent 90 degrees

STRETCH. Move your elbows back, while also moving your hands backward (you are externally rotating your shoulders) (Fig. 6.48). Keep your posture erect, and avoid allowing your head to project forward.

RESULT. You should feel a stretch in the front of your chest and shoulders.

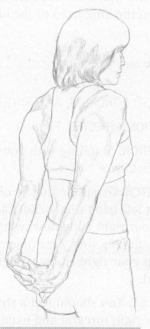

FIGURE 6.49

FRONT OF SHOULDERS

MOTION AFFECTED. Extension

POSITION. Standing with hands clasped behind body, elbows extended

STRETCH. Lift your hands up behind your back as far as possible, keeping your elbows straight and being careful not to bend forward at the waist (Fig. 6.49).

RESULT. You should feel a stretch in the front of your shoulders and upper arms.

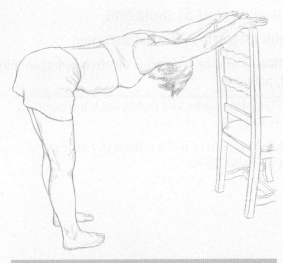

FIGURE 6.50

LATS (SHOULDERS)

MOTION AFFECTED. Flexion

POSITION. Standing within arms' reach of the back of a chair or other object of similar height

STRETCH. Bend over from the waist and reach both arms straight overhead, placing both hands on the back of the chair (Fig. 6.50). Keeping your back straight, bend forward at the waist until a stretch is felt in the area of your armpits.

RESULT. You should feel a stretch in your axillary (armpit) area.

ELBOW

MOTION AFFECTED. Elbow flexion

POSITION. Standing with right elbow overhead, elbow maximally flexed

STRETCH. Place the palm of your left hand over your right elbow (Fig. 6.51). Carefully push your elbow backward while keeping it maximally flexed. Repeat with the left arm.

RESULT. You should feel a stretch in the back of your right upper arm.

Notice that elbow extension is not covered here. This is because the preceding two stretches have the elbow extended and will place a stretch on all of the muscles that cross the elbow joint, with the emphasis on the long head of the biceps.

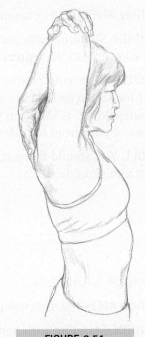

FIGURE 6.51

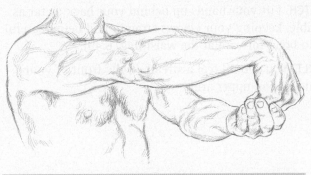

FIGURE 6.52

WRIST, FOREARM, AND FINGERS: FLEXION

MOTION AFFECTED. Flexion

POSITION. Standing with arms outstretched in front of shoulders

STRETCH. Grasp the fingers of your right hand with your left hand (Fig. 6.52). Carefully pull the fingers of your right hand downward and back toward you, flexing first your fingers and then your wrist. Keep your right elbow straight. Repeat with the left hand.

RESULT. You should feel a stretch along the top of your right forearm and hand.

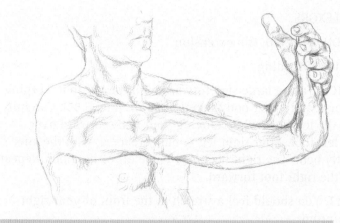

FIGURE 6.53

WRIST, FOREARM, AND FINGERS: EXTENSION

MOTION AFFECTED. Extension

POSITION. Standing with arms outstretched in front of shoulders

STRETCH. Place the palm of your left hand against the fingers of your right hand (Fig. 6.53). Push the right fingers and then your hand backward. Repeat with the left hand.

RESULT. You should feel a stretch along the underside of your forearm, hand, and fingers.

Lower Body

Below are stretches for the lower body in the 30-minute program.

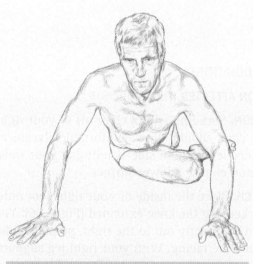

FIGURE 6.54

GLUTES

MOTION AFFECTED. Hip flexion with adduction and hip internal rotation

POSITION. Lying on your stomach (prone)

STRETCH. Lift your chest and shoulders as if doing a pushup (Fig. 6.54). Bring your right knee up and across, in front of you and toward the left, allowing your right knee to bend roughly 100 degrees. If you feel any stress in your right knee increase the amount of bend (flex) in it until these symptoms disappear. Carefully attempt to lie back down onto your right knee, which is now under the left side of your body. Repeat with the left leg.

RESULT. You should feel a stretch in the gluteal area on your right side.

> ⚠ **CAUTION!** As soon as you feel a stretch, you have accomplished your goal. Do not continue to lower yourself onto the floor if you feel a stretch early on in this exercise. If you have a ligamentous instability, or are otherwise suspicious of your knee's health, consultation with a professional is recommended before performing this exercise.

30-min program

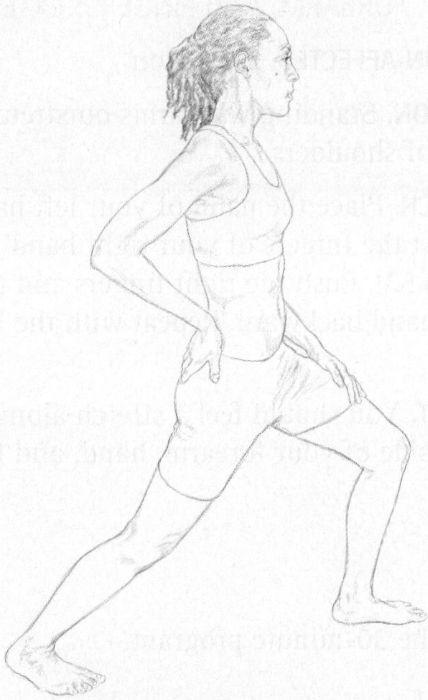

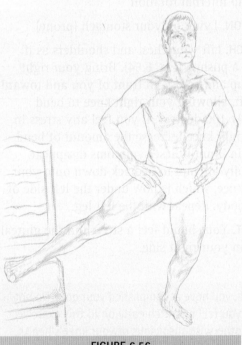

FIGURE 6.55

HIP FLEXORS

MOTION AFFECTED. Hip extension

POSITION. Standing

STRETCH. Take a large step forward with the left foot, keeping the torso and upper body facing forward (Fig. 6.55). Carefully bend the left knee while moving your body forward over your left foot. Your right leg remains relaxed, with the knee slightly bent. The right heel may come off of the floor. Repeat with the right foot forward.

RESULT. You should feel a stretch in the front of your right thigh/groin.

HIP ADDUCTORS

MOTION AFFECTED. Hip abduction

POSITION. Standing with a chair off to your right. The height of the chair should allow comfortable placement of your extended leg without side-bending at your waist or hips. If it does not, choose a lower surface.

STRETCH. Place the inside of your right foot onto the chair while keeping the knee extended (Fig. 6.56). Your right leg should be directly out to the right, perpendicular to the direction you are facing. With your right leg supported by the chair and your hips and torso facing forward, carefully lower your right hip. Repeat with the left leg.

RESULT. You should feel a stretch in the area of your right groin.

FIGURE 6.56

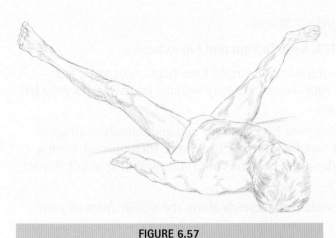

FIGURE 6.57

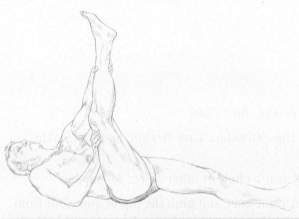

FIGURE 6.58

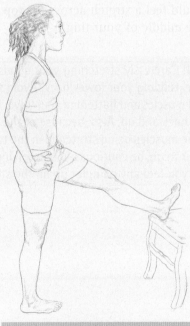

FIGURE 6.59

HIP ADDUCTORS (GROIN)

MOTION AFFECTED. Hip abduction

POSITION. Lying supine perpendicular to a wall, with legs extended straight up the wall, buttocks in contact with the wall. Contract your abdominals to flatten your lower back against the floor. This will stabilize your pelvis and protect your lower back from the strain of your abducting legs.

STRETCH. Relax and allow your legs to fall outward (abduct), sliding down the wall until they reach their end range (Fig. 6.57).

RESULT. You should feel a stretch along your inner thighs, from knee to groin.

HAMSTRINGS: LYING SUPINE

MOTION AFFECTED. Knee extension and hip flexion

POSITION. Lying supine with both legs extended

STRETCH. Lift your right leg straight up and back, relaxing and allowing your right knee to flex (Fig. 6.58). Use your right hand to stabilize your right knee while attempting to straighten your right knee by both actively contracting your quadriceps muscle and pulling back on your right lower leg with your left hand. Repeat with the right knee.

RESULT. You should feel a stretch in the back of your right thigh and behind your right knee.

HAMSTRINGS: STANDING

MOTION AFFECTED. Knee extension and hip flexion

POSITION. Standing with your left leg outstretched and supported on chair. Note that the height of chair should allow for a comfortable leg place-ment; in many cases, a lower support will be necessary.

STRETCH. Keeping your back straight, lean forward from your hips (Fig. 6.59). It may be helpful to think of "sticking your butt out" to isolate the movement to the hip and avoid bending the lower spine. Repeat with your right leg.

RESULT. You should feel a stretch along the back of your left thigh from the belly of the hamstrings to the back of the knee.

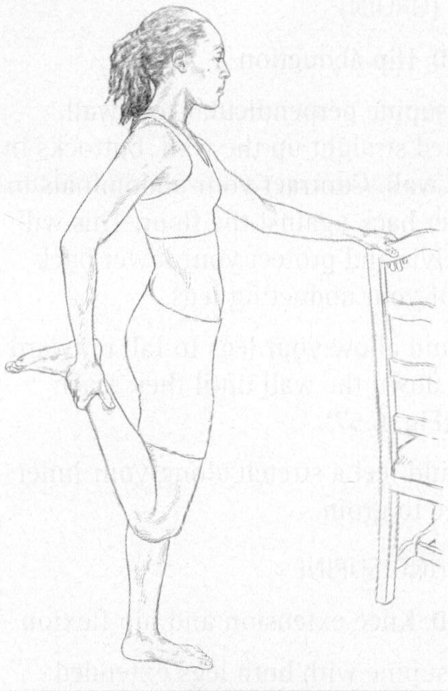

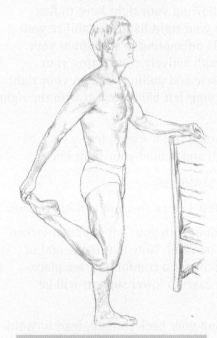

FIGURE 6.60

KNEE AND FRONT OF THIGH

MOTION AFFECTED. Knee flexion and hip extension

POSITION. Standing with your right knee bent, right ankle supported in your right hand. You may support yourself with your left hand if necessary.

STRETCH. Keeping your back straight and abdominals contracted, pull your right foot first directly backward, then upward, until a stretch is felt along the front of your right thigh (Fig. 6.60). Repeat with the left leg.

RESULT. You should feel a stretch along the middle front of your right thigh.

HIP, QUADRICEPS, ANKLE, AND FOOT

MOTION AFFECTED. Hip extension, knee flexion, and foot/ankle plantar flexion

POSITION. Standing near a chair or other object for support

STRETCH. Bend your right knee and grab the top of your foot from behind, pulling the entire foot and lower leg toward your buttocks (Fig. 6.61). Be sure to tighten your stomach muscles and keep your back straight. Repeat with the left leg.

RESULT. You should feel a stretch across the top of your foot and ankle, and in the middle of your thigh.

FIGURE 6.61

> **CAUTION!** Carelessly stretching your quads (thigh) can easily result in hyperextending your lower back. Avoid this by contracting your abdominal muscles and flattening your lower back *before* pulling your right foot back and up. Also, because of the obvious difference in the size of the muscles being stretched in the top of your foot and the front of your thigh, be cautious about applying too much stretch to your foot. If you feel any pain, let up on the stretch.

HIPS AND CALVES

MOTION AFFECTED. Hip extension and ankle dorsiflexion

POSITION. Standing in a lunge position with the left foot approximately 24 inches in front of the left, hands placed on a chair or against the wall ahead with the elbows easily extended

STRETCH. Bend the lead (left) knee, and lean forward keeping the right knee straight, allowing the elbows to bend as your body comes closer to the chair or wall (Fig. 6.62). Repeat with the right knee leading.

RESULT. You should feel a stretch in both the front of your hip near the groin, and in the calf area.

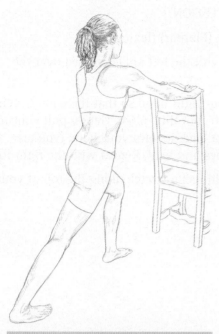

FIGURE 6.62

OUTSIDE OF LOWER LEG

MOTION AFFECTED. Inversion (rolling foot onto outside) and dorsiflexion (flexing foot toward shin)

POSITION. Standing

STRETCH. Step on top of your left foot with your right. Carefully allow your right foot to roll over onto its outside edge. Now, carefully bend your right knee, moving it forward (Fig. 6.63).

RESULT. You should feel a stretch along the outside of your lower right leg just above the ankle.

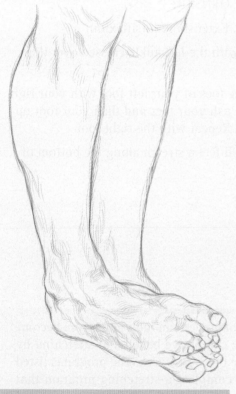

FIGURE 6.63

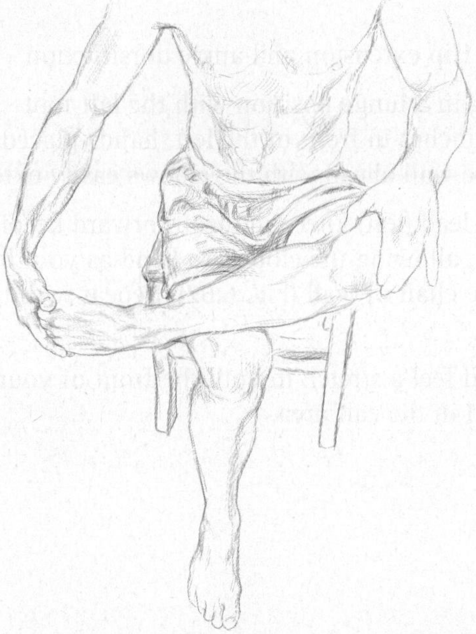

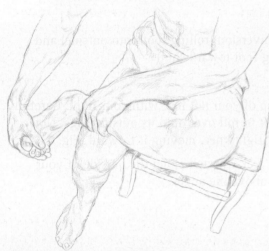

FIGURE 6.64

FEET AND TOES: FLEXION

MOTION AFFECTED. (Plantar) flexion

POSITION. Seated with the left ankle crossed over the right knee

STRETCH. Place your right hand so that the palm covers the top of your left foot (Fig. 6.64). Gently pull your toes and then your foot back toward your body (you are extending your toes and feet). Repeat with the right foot.

RESULT. You should feel a stretch along the top of your left foot and toes.

FEET AND TOES: EXTENSION

MOTION AFFECTED. Extension (dorsiflexion)

POSITION. Seated with the left ankle crossed over the right knee

STRETCH. Grasp the toes of your left foot with your right hand (Fig. 6.65). Push your toes and then your foot up toward your shin. Repeat with the right foot.

RESULT. You should feel a stretch along the bottom of your foot.

FIGURE 6.65

SUMMARY

Having a limited amount of time should not prevent an individual from becoming involved in a flexibility program. One can derive benefits of stretching by investing just a few minutes three or more times per week. The programs listed above should allow for an individual to complete a stretching program that basically addresses the entire body in as little as 10 minutes. The 20-minute and 30-minute programs successively add depth to each of the body areas addressed in the 10-minute program.

30-min program

Improving Posture Through Flexibility

Simply put, *posture* is the interrelationship of body parts. It primarily results from the positioning of one spinal segment in relation to another, but in reality, it is defined by the relative position of each and every joint in the body. Good posture, by definition, minimizes physical stresses to the body by balancing the skeletal system, effectively allowing it to function under reduced loads. Improving posture is therefore likely a worthwhile goal, particularly for those who sit or stand for prolonged periods. This chapter defines "good" posture, and then describes several common postural deviations. We then discuss assessment of posture and identify several interventions to improve it, including education, strengthening, and stretching programs.

GOOD POSTURE

Good posture can be described as an alignment that allows for the most efficient working relationship between various body parts. The spine, for instance, functions most efficiently when it utilizes three balanced curves—the cervical and lumbar lordoses, and the thoracic kyphosis. With the body in anatomical position (see Chapter 2), the lumbar and the cervical curves are concave posteriorly, and the thoracic curve is concave anteriorly. Figure 7.1A shows a lateral view of the spine demonstrating these curves.

Good standing posture, as viewed from a lateral perspective, might be described by a plum line dropping from the ear and passing over the shoulder, hip, knee, and a point just in front of the ankle (see Fig. 7.1A). Head position would be level, the three spinal curves would be present, and the knees would be unlocked with the body weight easily balanced over the middle of the foot. A posterior view might be described as the head sitting straight over level shoulders, with the hips and feet a little less than shoulder width apart (Fig. 7.1B). The spine would follow a plum line dropping from the middle of the back of the head. Good seated posture is discussed in Chapter 8.

POSTURE-FUNCTION RELATIONSHIPS

In their book *Muscle Testing and Function,* Kendall and McCreary provide a definition of posture that emphasizes functional relationships: "In the standard posture, the spine represents the normal curves, and the bones of the lower extremities are in ideal alignment for weight bearing. The neutral position of the pelvis is conducive to good alignment of the abdomen and trunk, and that of the extremities below. The

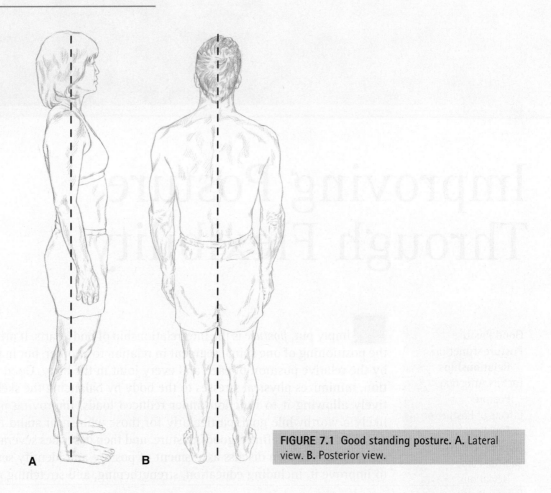

FIGURE 7.1 Good standing posture. A. Lateral view. **B.** Posterior view.

chest and upper back are in a position that favors optimal function of the respiratory organs. The head is erect in a well balanced position that minimizes stress on the neck musculature."[1]

With over 150 significant joints, human bodies were designed to move, and too much time spent in any one position will become uncomfortable. Good body mechanics might be described as the maintenance of optimal joint relationships throughout movement. The fundamental principle behind good body mechanics is the same as that for static posture: loads are supported through a stable spinal position over a balanced base of support. If we can maintain the spinal curves as we move through space, then we can protect the musculoskeletal system while performing our tasks as efficiently as possible. For example, Figure 7.2A shows a basic lift performed while maintaining a "neutral" spine, and Figure 7.2B shows the same lift allowing excessive thoracic and lumbar flexion. The posture in Figure 7.2B places excessive load on the posterior stabilizing structures of the lower lumbar segments, including the intervertebral disc and supporting ligaments. Loading the spine in this position may cause injury to these tissues either immediately with application of a significant load or over time through repetitive stress.

Workplace body mechanics are discussed briefly in Chapter 8, and suggestions for more detailed reading about body mechanics are listed in Appendix A.

Factors Affecting Posture

Posture is a result of a number of factors including, but not limited to, occupation, avocation, lifestyle, health, motivation, and awareness. Though their relative contributions may vary, these factors help determine an individual's posture.

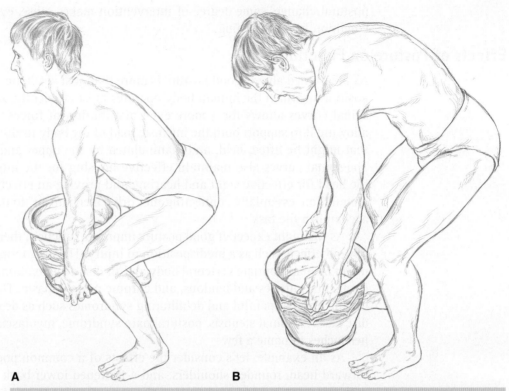

FIGURE 7.2 Lifting. A. A basic lift performed while maintaining a neutral alignment of the spine. **B.** The same lift performed with excessive thoracic and lumbar flexion.

Occupation may be one of the largest factors influencing posture, because for most of us, our choice of occupation dictates how we spend the majority of our waking hours. For example, as an individual sits at his or her desk for several hours each day, gravity exerts a subtle pull that coaxes the head forward, hunches the back, and rounds the shoulders. The effects of occupationally influenced movement patterns and positions on posture are as variable as the occupations themselves. Even activities pursued for just a few hours a week such as gardening, writing, or pottery have characteristic static positions and movement patterns that can influence posture.

Lifestyle may also have a significant influence on posture. Individuals involved in athletic or other movement-related pursuits may be more likely to maintain good posture because of their greater strength, flexibility, and body awareness. This is particularly true for those who participate in endeavors that emphasize body awareness such as yoga, dance, diving, or gymnastics.

An individual's choice of activity, or lack thereof, during non-working hours may also affect posture. Long hours spent hunched over a computer keyboard, or seated in front of a television, may cause the body to permanently assume these positions, especially if that individual makes no effort to counterbalance these positions through awareness or exercise.

An individual's health may also influence his or her posture. Severely debilitating conditions such as hemiplegia, paraplegia, or quadraplegia resulting from stroke or head or spinal cord injury can severely affect posture. Arthritic conditions osteo or rheumatoid arthritis or ankylosing spondylitis, or other maladies such as osteoporosis or scoliosis, may also have dramatic effects on an individual's posture. Interventions such as education, physical medicine, and/or exercise may be helpful in reducing the severity of the postural deficits. Even in the most severe cases of disease-related postural change, some degree of intervention makes sense, even if only to keep the condition from worsening.

Effects of Posture on Function

As mentioned above, good posture is more than just aesthetic: by definition, it is the position in which the human body operates most efficiently. A normal alignment of spinal curves allows for a more even distribution of forces throughout the spine, allowing it to support both the intrinsic load of the body itself and the extrinsic loads that might be lifted, held, and manipulated by the upper and/or lower extremities. The spinal curves also maintain effective housing for the internal organs, position the head for effective sight and hearing, and provide an effective "transmission" for ambulation, essentially connecting the "drive mechanism" to the machinery that may accomplish the task.

As we might expect, if good posture improves function, then "bad" postures might have ill effects such as a predisposition to injury. The long term result of poor posture might be inappropriate vertebral body and/or disc degeneration, lengthening of spinal ligaments, muscles and tendons, and chronic muscle spasm. These changes may hasten the onset of painful and debilitating syndromes such as degenerative joint and or disc disease, spinal stenosis, postural pain syndrome, myofascial pain syndrome, and headaches to name a few.

As an example, let's consider the effects of a common poor standing posture: a forward head, rounded shoulders, and a flattened lower back (Fig. 7.3). Individuals with this posture must hyperextend the cervical spine to bring their head up to view the world. This may lead to chronic overuse and the breakdown of particular cervical spinal segments. The forward position of the head may also cause overuse of the

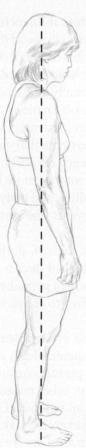

FIGURE 7.3 A common poor standing posture. Notice the forward head, rounded shoulders, and flattened lower back.

posterior muscles and ligaments of the cervical spine and may result in head, neck, or shoulder pain.

The rounded position of the shoulders essentially "lowers the roof" of the shoulder joint. This effectively decreases the amount of space between the head of the humerus and the acromion during any activities that involve shoulder flexion, thereby increasing the likelihood of compression injury to subacromial tissues.

The effects of spinal posture on extremity joint function may be exemplified by a study of shoulder function in erect versus slouched postures. Kebaetse et al showed that slouched posture reduced scapular posterior tilting and the resultant abduction of the humerus by 23 degrees.[2] The slouched position also showed a 16 percent decrease in muscle force generated from a horizontal position. Other researchers also showed changes in scapular mechanics with increased thoracic kyphosis.[3]

Intuitively, we might expect that shortened muscles might be caused by, or result in, postural changes. Borstad et al has shown that shortness of the pectoralis minor causes changes in scapular mechanics and might provide a mechanism for subacromial impingement, or irritation/inflammation of the tissues above the humeral head, trapped below the acromion.[4] Chronically lengthened muscles may cause "stretch weakness," which is defined by Kendall and McCreary as "weakness which results from muscles remaining in an elongated condition, however slight, beyond the neutral physiological rest position, but not beyond the normal range of muscle length."[1] This may be significant enough to affect normal functioning.

It is not hard to imagine the link between poor postures and certain types of headaches, especially with the understanding of the location and basic function of the cervical and sub-occipital musculature. Forward head postures cause hyperextension of the upper cervical joints and increased tone in the cervical, upper thoracic, and even the lumbar musculature. Chronically increased tone in the upper cervical musculature, combined with hyperextension of the joints, plays a likely role in the development of tension headaches. McDonnell et al found that combining postural alignment of cervical, thoracic, lumbar, and scapulothoracic areas with exercise may help in headache relief for some patients.[5]

Perhaps less obvious is the effect of a forward head posture on temporomandibular joint (TMJ) function, which might result in TMJ pain or headaches. A forward head position causes the jaw to move forward from its neutral alignment, resulting in a change in the way the upper and lower jaws articulate, and hence how the upper and lower teeth fit together in bite. In their website, the American Academy of General Dentistry suggests that "this movement puts stress on muscles, joints, and bones and, if left untreated, can create pain and inflammation in muscles and joints when the mouth opens and closes."[6] Dr. Ludwig Leibsohn, DDS, an Academy spokesperson, suggests, "Good posture is important, yet many people don't realize how posture affects their oral health."

The effects of position and posture on the intervertebral discs were first quantified by a classic 1981 study by Nachemson that showed the changes in intradiscal pressures between various positions and postures.[7] Significant increases (40%) in intradiscal pressures, compared with those in standing, were recorded when subjects were sitting unsupported versus reclined positions in which intradiscal pressures decreased 50–80%. More recently, researchers have also measured the changes in intradiscal pressures with somewhat varied results; for example, Wilke et al showed decreased intradiscal pressures in sitting versus standing.[8,9] Other findings were similar to Nachemson's earlier study. What is not in doubt, however, is that intradiscal pressures do change significantly with changes in position (posture).

The effects of poor posture on the function of the lungs and other internal organs are not well documented, but rather, make sense anatomically and physiologically. For example, the lung is designed to function with an erect spine, and hyperflexion of the thoracic spine, as in kyphosis, decreases the effective space in which the lungs can expand and contract. Research does show that altering positions changes respiratory function. Kera et al showed that changes in position (e.g., posture) relate directly to differences in lung volume, and to the demand placed on various respiratory muscles.[10] Even the timing of respiratory muscles may be affected by changes in posture. Abe et al showed significant changes in the timing of the four major abdominal respiratory muscles with changes in posture.[11] Additionally, Yamashita et al showed changes in portal and hepatic arterial flows in response to changing postures.[12] Obviously, more specific research needs to be done to detail the relationships of various postures to specific muscle and organ function, but the fact that muscle and organ function is affected is hard to ignore.

Even the available motion of the spine itself may be affected by the posture present when the spinal movements are taking place.[13] The list of possible postural challenges continues down the spine and through the lower extremities to the feet. (Deviations in seated posture are discussed in Chapter 8.)

ABNORMAL POSTURES

Abnormal postures can be defined as any posture that differ significantly from those we have defined as "good." In reality, most people have some degree of postural abnormality such as a slightly forward head and a slightly longer left leg. In fact, certain deviations from the norm are expected, such as a lower shoulder on the dominant side.

Deviations from the norm become significant when they cause alterations in movement patterns that lead to dysfunction and/or pain. In some cases, individuals will have postural abnormalities that are quite noticeable but result in no symptoms. Conversely, an individual may suffer significant pain and dysfunction from seemingly minor abnormalities that are quite difficult to detect even with a thorough manual examination.

Ultimately, the body's reaction to postural abnormalities varies greatly. Some reactions are fairly obvious and easy to explain, whereas others may seem impossible to understand. For example, it is easy to understand how a 1/4-inch leg length discrepancy might prove completely asymptomatic for a sedentary individual, while proving disastrous for a runner in training for a marathon. It is harder to see why another individual will react with back and neck pain from something as apparently benign as a change in the type of shoes he or she is wearing. Obviously, people vary in both their physiology and reactions to different stresses.

Abnormal postures occur primarily in one of three planes: the sagittal, frontal, or transverse plane (see Chapter 2). Nevertheless, most postural deviations involve all three planes to some degree, because so many of the body's joints affect motion across planes. For example, it is very difficult to side-bend an intact spine without introducing a rotation. Similarly, the knee joint does not only function in the sagittal plane like a hinge, because its axis of rotation changes continually throughout its range, particularly as it nears extension. A quick look at musculature will also reveal why few muscles cause motion in a single plane. Pecs, lats, obliques, hip flexors, and glutes are all oriented diagonally in the body, producing and resisting motion in a multi-planar environment.

The postural deviations described next should be examined in all three planes. With this understanding, you can design stretching programs that will help improve individual's postures. Stretches for each type of postural distortion are identified later in this chapter.

Sagittal Plane Deviations

Probably the most common postural deviations occur in the sagittal plane. Recall that the sagittal plane is that which you would view when looking at someone from the side. From this view, you could easily notice a forward head, rounded shoulders, or excessive or absent cervical, thoracic, or lumbar curves. Additionally, changes in the sagittal plane orientation of the pelvis and hyperextension at the knees would be easily visible.

From a muscular perspective, sagittal plane changes may be the result of inappropriately shortened and/or lengthened muscles. For example, a forward head posture may result from shortened upper cervical extensors, lengthened lower cervical extensors, and shortened cervical flexors. Rounded shoulders may result from shortened anterior chest muscles and lengthened posterior scapular and upper back muscles.

An increased thoracic kyphosis might be caused by lengthened thoracic paraspinal musculature and shortened abdominals. An increased lumbar lordosis might be indicative of shortened hip flexors and lengthened, and/or weak, abdominals. Finally, hyperextended knees may result from shortened calves, the soleus in particular.

Figure 7.4 shows an individual with shortened anterior cervical, pectoral, lumbar paraspinal, hip flexor, and calf muscles. The cervical flexors, scapular retractors, and abdominals are likely *overstretched*. Note the forward head, rounded shoulders, hyperextended lumbar spine, and hyperextended knees.

Frontal Plane Deviations

Changes in the frontal plane are visible from either an anterior or a posterior view, and they reveal such abnormalities as scoliosis, actual or functional leg length discrepancies, hip, knee, or ankle (subtalar) varum or valgum, and excessively pronated feet.

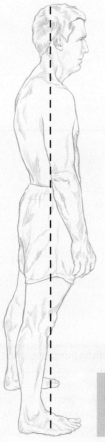

FIGURE 7.4 Sagittal plane distortions. Note the shortened anterior cervical, pectoral, lumbar paraspinal, hip flexor, and calf muscles. The cervical extensors, scapular retractors, and abdominals are likely *overstretched*. Note the forward head, rounded shoulders, hyperextended lumbar spine, and hyperextended knees.

Possible muscular implications at the head and neck include unilateral shortness in the cervical flexors and/or extensors on the same side. Frontal plane distortions of the spine can be caused by unilateral shortness in the paraspinal musculature, as well as in the psoas and/or quadratus lumborum on one side. The spinal posture may be affected from below by the position of the pelvis, which is in turn affected by the muscles attaching the lower extremities to the pelvis. An example of this might be excessive shortness of the adductors on the right side, which might cause a lowering of the left side of the pelvis and a commensurate lumbar scoliosis, concave to the right.

Though more likely to be bony or ligamentous in origin, frontal plane distortions in the knees and feet might be caused or exacerbated by shortness and/or lengthening of the hip abductors or adductors, or the invertors and evertors of the ankle and foot. Deviations below the hips may be either bilateral, such as in bilateral genu valgus, or unilateral. Unilateral changes may occur on opposite sides of the "norm," such as genu valgum, and foot pronation on the right, concurrent with genu varum and foot supination on the left.

Figure 7.5 shows shortness of the cervical musculature on the right, obliques and quadratus lumborum on the left, hip adductors on the left and abductors on the right, and foot evertors on the right. Note the cervical right side-bending, the lumbar left side-bending and higher left iliac crest and proximity of the rib cage to the crest of the ilia on the left versus the right. Also note the hyper-pronated right foot.

Transverse Plane Deviations

Abnormalities in the transverse plane are best viewed from above. Because this is impractical, we advise careful observation of the individual from the front, back, and side to ascertain possible transverse plane abnormalities. These are generally

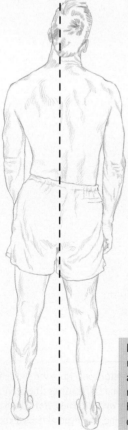

FIGURE 7.5 Frontal plane distortions. Note the shortness of the cervical musculature on the right, the obliques and quadratus lumborum on the left, hip adductors on the left and abductors on the right, and foot evertors on the right. Note the cervical right side-bending, the lumbar left side-bending and higher left iliac crest, and the proximity of the ribcage to the crest of the ilia on the left versus the right. Also note the hyper-pronated right foot.

rotations about a vertical axis. In the cervical spine, a transverse plane imbalance might be seen as a rotation of the head. Short rotator musculature in the spine may be at fault. Postural abnormality in the thoracic spine might be seen as a rib "hump," which usually becomes visible if the subject bends over to touch his or her toes; as the subject does so, one side of the ribcage may appear obviously higher than the other.

Another example of a deviation in the transverse plane is an internally or externally rotated position of the humerus in a relaxed position. In a neutral position, the palm of the hand will generally face the hip on the same side. If the internal rotators of the shoulder are tight, the hand might be facing slightly posteriorly, and if the external rotators are tight, the hand might be turned slightly anteriorly. Similarly at the hips, excessive tightness in the external rotators might cause the knees to point slightly outward. On the other hand, excessive laxity and/or weakness of the external rotators, with or without a commensurate shortness of the internal rotators might cause, or allow, the knees to turn in toward each other. Most likely, however, those showing internally rotated femurs are a victim of a congenital bony abnormality called femoral anteversion, in which the neck of the femur is rotated anteriorly versus the norm. Stretching to change this position would be futile. Even if this internally rotated position could be changed, it would likely destabilize the hip joint by altering the angle of articulation of the head of the femur into the acetabulum.

Figure 7.6 shows an example of transverse plane distortions including shortened cervical right rotators, glenohumeral internal rotators, right hip flexors, trunk left rotators, hip external rotators, and ankle and foot evertors.

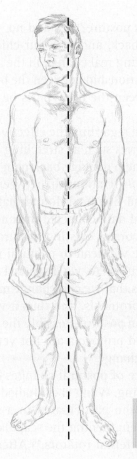

FIGURE 7.6 Transverse plane distortions. Note the shortened cervical right rotators, glenohumeral internal rotators, right hip flexors, trunk left rotators, hip external rotators, and ankle and foot evertors.

ASSESSING POSTURE

Assessing posture should begin with an observation of sitting, standing, and walking postures. It should take place from general to specific, first determining large patterns of deviation and then later identifying the individual components of these deviations.

Initially we can attempt to determine if there are any gross deviations from a normal, healthy "good" posture. These deviations may include points such as an obviously higher hip on one side, a tilted head, or spinal curves that differ significantly from the norm. These observations should be taken from anterior, posterior, and lateral (both left and right) vantage points.

Helpful clues often include the height of the shoulders, the difference in the space between the arm and torso on the left versus the right, and the angles of the legs at the hips, knees and ankles, from each view.

Next, more specific information must be gleaned from the gross observations above. Why is the hip higher on the right? Is there a significant leg length difference or spinal scoliosis? Is there a pelvic torsion or shift? Are there any specific muscular length issues that may be causing or contributing to these deviations? Chapter 3 discusses the assessment of muscle length and joint range of motion (ROM) and identifies stretches for assessed muscular shortness issues. Examples of postural deviations and their possible muscular causes are listed in the following section on "Stretching." These deviations are grouped according to the plane in which the primary restriction is occurring; however, few postural deviations occur only in one plane. A thorough evaluation and treatment program should consider deviations in all three planes.

INTERVENTIONS TO IMPROVE POSTURE

Is it possible to change an individual's posture? Yes and no. Certainly we can sit or stand more erect, hold our shoulders back, and tuck our chin. But can we actually change the structure of our body affecting real change in the actual length of the tissues and the resulting distance and relationship between the bony segments? Can the actual physiological relationship between the body parts be changed? These are is less clear.

The research is, as yet, inconclusive regarding the effectiveness of changing posture with exercise. Long accepted theories such as stretching hamstrings to improve pelvic position and lumbar posture to help manage back pain do not seem to be supported in the literature. Li et al showed *no* relationship between hamstring length and lumbo pelvic posture.[14] Hyrsomallis and Goodman found that "a review of the literature has found a lack of reliable, valid data collected in controlled settings to support the contention that exercise will correct existing postural deviations. Likewise, objective data to indicate that exercise will lead to postural improvement are lacking."[15] What about stretching in particular? As we discussed in Chapter 1, epidemiological and research evidence suggests that we can change muscle lengths and joint positions with appropriate flexibility protocols, and thus it would seem reasonable to conclude that we can effect change in posture. Possibly the research does not confirm this yet because the programs and protocols are not yet well defined, and the research has not yet defined postural change.

There are examples in the literature of postural changes effected with a combination of stretching and strength-training. Wang et al studied 20 asymptomatic subjects with forward shoulder posture who participated in a structured program of stretching the pectoral muscles and strengthening the scapular retractors and elevators and the humeral abductors and external rotators.[16] After 6 weeks at three sessions per week, there was no change in resting scapular position, but there was a significant decrease in the anterior inclination of the thoracic spine (i.e., a decrease in poor thoracic posture). Katzman et al showed a significant decrease in thoracic kyphosis in a group of 24 elderly women who had a significantly increased kyphosis (>50 degrees), with a 12-week stretching and strengthening intervention.[17] Falla et al showed an improved ability in subjects with chronic neck pain, to maintain neutral cervical posture during prolonged sitting, after undergoing a 6-week specific cervical strengthening program.[18] Itoi et al showed improvements in thoracic posture in elderly women who had a significant existing kyphosis, as a result of a 6-week strengthening program.[19] They also showed little change in those with mildly kyphotic postures to begin with.

Though abundant research is lacking, few healthcare or fitness professionals would dispute the value of stretching short muscles and strengthening weak ones in attempting to improve posture. Even in the unlikely event that no "real" change is possible, it makes sense to balance postural imperfections to support optimal function, reduce the likelihood of injury, and reduce the chance of further declines in posture. Three interventions for improving posture include education, strength training, and stretching.

Education

Probably the most dramatic impact that can be made on posture is through education. Understanding the basics of spinal anatomy, function, and care, including good standing, sitting, bending, and lifting mechanics, can help make dramatic changes in "operating" posture. Information about good seated posture and workplace body mechanics is included in Chapter 8. See Appendix A for additional sources of information on good body mechanics.

Strengthening

Strengthening weak muscles is of obvious importance in the enhancement of posture. Weakness may be due to general or specific deconditioning, postural habits, injury, disease, or even activities that strengthen some muscles but leave others hopelessly weak. Weakness may also be due to chronically elongated muscles, as mentioned above (stretch weakness).

Appropriate strengthening programs can help individuals improve their posture by improving the balance of strength from anterior to posterior, or left to right. Strength training can also help overcome a generally deconditioned musculoskeletal system. It may be especially helpful to those with a weak "core," which generally includes abdominals, obliques, spinal stabilizers, pelvic floor, and other muscles that generally effect stability by controlling the pelvis and spine. Strengthening weak core muscles will help maintain more efficient postures, especially under loads such as prolonged sitting, standing, bending, lifting, or athletics.

An effective strengthening program should be based on a thorough evaluation, which will help you identify particular training needs in response to both posture and individual areas of muscular weakness, which may or may not be related. Assess strength training needs in conjunction with an appropriate ROM/flexibility assessment (as described in Chapter 3), because findings in one area can provide valuable information about needs in another area. For example, identification of shortened anterior chest and shoulder muscles suggests not only the need to improve flexibility anteriorly but also to strengthen the antagonistic musculature—the upper back and posterior shoulders in this case. General guidelines for designing strength-training programs are presented in Chapter 10.

Stretching

Stretching may be an essential component of a health and fitness program designed to improve posture. Particularly in cases involving significantly shortened muscle groups, stretching may be the key to allowing more effective postures. Significantly shortened hamstrings are a good example. Sitting keeps the hamstrings in a chronically shortened position. As people spend more and more time sitting, in many cases without the balance of activity calling for a lengthened position, the hamstrings may respond by permanently shortening. This in turn may alter the resting position of the pelvis during sitting, increasing its posterior tilt and making upright sitting even more difficult.

Having identified shortened hamstrings in an individual who spends several hours each day sitting allows for the design of an appropriate program for stretching the hamstrings (see Chapter 5). Consistent stretching may, over time, increase hamstring length and allow improved standing and sitting postures.

This section identifies specific stretches for individuals with common sagittal, frontal, and transverse plane deviations.

STRETCHES FOR SAGITTAL PLANE DEVIATIONS

As mentioned above, common cases of muscular shortening include tightness of the cervical flexors, the shoulder horizontal adductors, the abdominals, the lumbar extensors, the hip flexors, and the ankle plantar flexors. Stretches for these muscle groups can be found in Chapter 5 (Stretches for Major Muscle Groups). These muscle groups should be stretched to improve posture only after having determined which groups are actually tight. See Chapter 3 (Assessing Flexibility).

As an example, consider the individual with a forward head, rounded shoulders, hyperextended lumbar spine and hyperextended knees (see Fig. 7.4). See Table 7.1 for a possible stretching routine to address each postural deviation listed.

STRETCHES FOR FRONTAL PLANE DEVIATIONS

Common postural deviations in the frontal plane may include a laterally leaning head, a scoliotic curve in the thoracic or lumbar spines, an elevated hip, an adducted femur, or an excessively inverted or everted foot. Consider the individual with shortened cervical side-benders on the right, lumbar paraspinals on the left, hip adductors on the left, and ankle evertors on the right (see Fig. 7.5). Table 7.2 lists stretches to address these deviations.

STRETCHES FOR TRANSVERSE PLANE DEVIATIONS

Common postural deviations in the transverse plane may include a rotation of the cervical, thoracic, or lumbar spine, an internally rotated humerus, an internally or externally rotated femur, a pelvic rotation, or an internally rotated tibia and talus, with an excessively pronated foot. Consider the individual with a right rotated cervical spine, internally rotated humeri, a leftward rotated pelvis, externally rotated femurs, and everted and abducted feet (see Fig. 7.6). Table 7.3 lists stretches to address these deviations.

TABLE 7.1 STRETCHES FOR SAGITTAL PLANE DEVIATIONS

Deviation	Stretch (from Chapter 5)
Forward head	Cervical flexors (Fig. 5.2)
Rounded shoulders	Shoulder horizontal adductors (Fig. 5.9)
Hyperextended lumbar spine	Trunk extensors (Fig. 5.20)
	Hip flexors (Fig. 5.24)
Hyperextended knees	Ankle plantarflexors (Fig. 5.33B: soleus)

TABLE 7.2 **STRETCHES FOR FRONTAL PLANE DEVIATIONS**

Deviation	Stretch (from Chapter 5)
Cervical right side-bending	Cervical side-benders (Fig. 5.3): right
Lumbar left side-bending	Trunk side-benders (Fig. 5.22): left
Adducted left hip (possibly higher iliac crest on left)	Hip adductors (Fig. 5.26): left
	Hip abductors (Fig. 5.27): right
	Hip flexors (Fig. 5.24): right
Everted (likely hyper-pronated) right foot	Ankle and foot evertors (Fig. 5.35): right

TABLE 7.3 **STRETCHES FOR TRANSVERSE PLANE DEVIATIONS**

Deviation	Stretch (from Chapter 5)
Cervical right rotation	Cervical rotators (Fig. 5.4): right
Internally rotated humerus	Shoulder internal rotators (Fig. 5.11)
Leftward rotated pelvis	Hip flexors (Fig. 5.24): right
	Trunk rotators (Fig. 5.23): turn trunk left
Externally rotated femurs	Hip external rotators (Fig. 5.29)
Everted and externally rotated feet	Ankle and foot evertors (Fig. 5.35)

SUMMARY

Good posture is essential for optimal function, both in static and dynamic environments. It is, by definition, the position in which the relationship between the various joints allows for optimal function of the musculoskeletal system, and likely the internal organ systems as well. Posture can be affected by many factors, including abnormally shortened or lengthened musculature, joint or skeletal abnormalities, occupation, avocation, lifestyle choices, disease, genetics, or awareness.

Abnormal postures can occur predominantly in the sagittal, frontal, and/or transverse planes; abnormalities, however, almost always occur in a multi-planar environment. Programs to improve posture should be designed after careful assessment of musculoskeletal function in a multi-planar environment. Postures can be modified via education, appropriate strengthening, flexibility and conditioning programs; however, it is unlikely that any of these will be successful without a persistent and determined effort.

Further information regarding posture and body mechanics can be found in Appendix A.

REFERENCES

1. Kendall HO, McCreary EK. Muscle Testing and Function. 3rd ed. Baltimore: Williams and Wilkins, 1993.
2. Kebaetse M, McClure P, Pratt NA. Thoracic position effect on shoulder range of motion, strength, and three-dimensional scapular kinematics. Arch Phys Med Rehabil August 1999;80(8):945–950.
3. Finley MA, Lee RY. Effect of sitting posture on 3-dimensional scapular kinematics measured by skin-mounted electromagnetic tracking sensors. Arch Phys Med Rehabil April 2003;84(4):563–568.
4. Borstad JD, Ludewig PM. The effect of long versus short pectoralis minor resting length on scapular kinematics in healthy individuals. J Orthop Sports Phys Ther April 2005;35(4):227–238.
5. McDonnell MK, Sahrmann SA, Van Dillen L. A specific exercise program and modification of postural alignment for treatment of cervicogenic headache: a case report. J Orthop Sports Phys Ther January 2005;35(1):3–15.
6. Academy of General Dentistry Website. 2007. Available at: http://www.agd.org/consumer/topics/tmj/posture.asp/. Accessed June 1, 2007.

7. Nachemson AL. Disc pressure measurements. Spine January–February 1981;6(1):93–97.

8. Wilke HJ, Neef P, Caimi M, et al. New in vivo measurements of pressures in the intervertebral disc in daily life. Spine April 15, 1999;24(8):755–762.

9. Wilke HJ, Neef P, Hinz B, et al. Intradiscal pressure together with anthropometric data—a data set for the validation of models. Clin Biomech 2001:16(Suppl)1:S111–126.

10. Kera T, Maruyama H. The effect of posture on respiratory activity of the abdominal muscles. J Physiol Anthropol Appl Human Sci July 2005;24(4):259–265.

11. Abe T, Yamada T, Tomita T, et al. Posture effects on timing muscle activity during stimulated ventilation. J Appl Physiol June 1999;86(6):1994–2000.

12. Yamashita H, Hachisuka Y, Kotegawa H, et al. Effects of posture change on the hemodynamics of the liver. Hepatogastroenterology November–December 2004;51(60):1797–1800.

13. Edmonston SJ, Aggerholm M, Eflfving S, et al. Influence of posture on the range of axial rotation and coupled lateral flexion of the thoracic spine. J Manipulative Physiol Ther March–April 2007;30(3):193–199.

14. Li Y, McClure PW, Pratt N. The effect of hamstring muscle stretching on standing posture and on lumbar and hip motions during forward bending. Phys Ther August 1996;76(8)836–845.

15. Hyrsomallis C, Goodman C. A review of resistance exercise and posture realignment. J Strength Cond Res August 2001;15(3):385–390.

16. Wang CH, McClure P, Pratt NE, et al. Stretching and strengthening exercises: their effect on three dimensional scapular kinematics. Arch Phys Med Rehabil August 1999;80(8):923–929.

17. Katzman WB, Sellmeyer DE, Stewart AL, et al. Changes in flexed posture, musculoskeletal impairments, and physical performance after group exercise in community-dwelling older women. Arch Phys Med Rehabil February 2007;88(2):192–199.

18. Falla D, Jull G, Russell T, et al. Effect of neck exercise on sitting posture in patients with chronic neck pain. Phys Ther April 2007;87(4)408–417.

19. Itoi E, Sinaki M. Effect of back-strengthening exercise on posture in healthy women 49 to 65 years of age. Mayo Clin Proc November 1994;69(11):1054–1059.

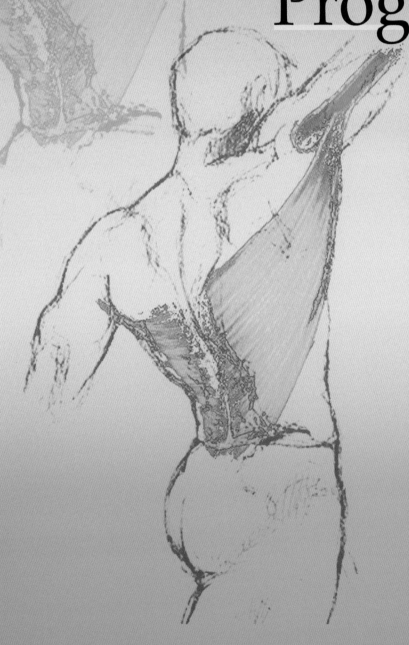

PART THREE

Special Stretches and Stretching Programs

Workplace Stretching Programs

The United States Department of Labor's Occupational Safety and Health Administration reported over four million cases of nonfatal injuries and illnesses in 2005. Of these cases, 503,000 were sprains and strains and over 270,000 were back injuries.[1] Research suggests a relationship between both the postural and biomechanical stresses encountered in the workplace and the rate of worker injury.

The importance of workplace ergonomics should not be underestimated. In fact, the Occupational Safety and Health Administration proposed a multi-step strategy to address the problem, including a national advisory committee on *ergonomics,* a term referring to workplace body mechanics and equipment and environmental design.

Liberty Mutual's 2002 Workplace Safety Index showed the ergonomics-related injuries "overexertion" and "falls" to be the leading cause of workplace injuries, with their percentage contribution to all workplace injuries being 26 and 12.5%, respectively.[2] Injuries due to repetitive motion made up 5.7% of the total. The research of Stuebbe et al on employees at a packaging plant over a 27-month period showed a close relationship between the postural and biomechanical stresses encountered at work and the rate of musculoskeletal injury.[3]

Whether from prolonged sitting, prolonged standing, excessive or repetitive lifting, or the chronic repetition of other tasks, work-related complaints are common. This chapter identifies two basic types of work and the injuries that are most commonly associated with them. It then outlines a general approach to the assessment, education, and treatment of individuals with work-related symptoms. Stretching programs for different types of work are provided, as well as a general, whole-body program for daily workplace stretching.

TYPES OF WORK AND WORK–RELATED INJURIES

Though work environments and challenges are infinitely variable, all forms of work can generally be categorized as either static or dynamic. *Static work* is that which requires extended periods of time in a particular position or positions, such as seated or standing in one place, whereas *dynamic work* requires hours of repetitive movements, such as construction work, certain manufacturing jobs, and massage therapy. Some types of work combine the challenges, and therefore the risks and benefits, of both stasis and movement. For example, a clerk in a store might spend part of the day seated as a cashier and part of the day walking, bending, and lifting while stocking shelves. Or a manufacturing job might require 8 hours a day of repetitive hand movements while in a seated position. Obviously, an attempt to address every type of work individually would be futile. Therefore, the following discussion is limited to a consideration of the pain, dysfunction, and injury that result from the most common types of static or dynamic work.

Static Work Injuries

Static injuries may result from prolonged positions that place excessive stress on particular musculoskeletal tissues. For example, the posterior cervical and thoracic structures experience excessive stress during long periods of sitting, with the head and shoulders forward and rounded. Similar static stresses on different joint structures and soft tissues can result from work environments demanding long periods of time in standing positions.

SITTING

The advance of computer technology over the last two decades has led to a mass migration of workers toward desk jobs. This dramatic change in work habits has brought on a new generation of chronic injuries, particularly of the spine and upper extremities related to prolonged sitting. The ergonomic challenges of work that demand prolonged periods of time in seated positions often result in pain from either chronically stretched or contracted muscles, tense ligaments, or chronically compressed joints.

For example, a computer programmer may sit for 8 to 10 hours a day in front of a computer with his or her head jutting forward, shoulders rounded, and lower back chronically flexed. In this position, posterior cervical, shoulder, thoracic, and lumbar musculature become chronically lengthened to support the body's weight. Also, chronic tension in the tendons and ligaments may contribute to pain and/or dysfunction of the involved tissues. To get an idea of how this might occur in the neck or back, simply extend one of your fingers to the end of its range of motion (ROM) by applying pressure with the fingers of your opposite hand. Initially you will not notice much, but after just a couple of minutes, you will begin to notice pressure and eventually pain in the tissues under tension. Now imagine how overstressed back and neck muscles might feel after several hours of such tension over the course of weeks, months, or years!

STANDING

Standing presents its own unique set of challenges, beginning at the feet and working upward to the head and neck. Gravity imposes the weight of the body on the feet pronating them, causing a lengthening of the plantar structures and a compressive stress on the metatarsal heads. Often hyperextended knees ache from prolonged compression, while the lumbar spine also suffers from hyperextension due to lazy posture and a weak core. Forward head, rounded shoulders, and increased thoracic kyphosis may accompany these lower extremity challenges, leading to stiffness in the neck and shoulders.

Dynamic Work Injuries

Dynamic work injuries occur as the result of movement. The movement may result in injury as a result of excessive load or excessive repetition of an otherwise tolerable load. In both cases, the incidence and severity of the injury may be dependent on the postures under which these loads occur. In most cases, more effective postures and body mechanics will reduce the chances of incurring a dynamic work injury.

REPETITIVE MOVEMENT

In dynamic environments, the worker, or more specifically one or more of the worker's muscles or joints, is subjected to what may be very tolerable loads, but with such frequency that the involved tissues begin to break down, resulting in inflammation and pain. With continuing stress, these symptoms may eventually develop into partial or complete tissue tearing or cartilage destruction.

Many types of work require the worker to perform repetitive tasks that increase the risk of some type of overuse injury. These include factory or assembly line work, cashiering, phone work, and work involving a computer. The Bureau of Labor Statistics recorded over 1.4 million cases of repetitive strain injuries that resulted in one or more days of missed work in 2002.[4] Research also shows a link between repetitive fine-motor tasks (such as using a computer mouse) and increased muscular activity in the neck and shoulders, and research suggests this increased activity may lead to injury.[5,6] Such tasks may be particularly problematic if they involve compromised body mechanics, which are quite common in many work environments.

Those who have jobs that require repetitive lifting, or other repetitive movements may benefit from improved flexibility for a couple of reasons. First, appropriate application of stretching may help reduce muscle spasm, achiness, and pain immediately. Second, the long-term application of stretching shortened muscle groups may allow the use of more safe and efficient postures and improved application of body mechanics.

LIFTING

Lifting is often the source of work-related injuries. Lifting injuries may result from lifting excessive loads or from the repetitive lifting of sub-maximal loads. The incidence of these injuries may be influenced by poor body mechanics, compromised musculoskeletal health, or some combination of the above. Many lifting injuries are avoidable with education, appropriate training in body mechanics, and development of adequate strength and flexibility.

GENERAL APPROACH TO INDIVIDUALS WITH WORK-RELATED PAIN

Individuals who have work-related musculoskeletal injury require both short-term pain relief and long-term strategies for prevention and rehabilitation. Intervention begins with assessment of the individual's case including the specifics of both the ergonomic demands and the individual's physiology.

Most healthcare practitioners would agree that the first step in the approach to work-related injuries is to identify, and then modify or eliminate, the stress or stresses that lead to the injury in the first place. Only after the offending stress has been modified or eliminated can treatment and rehabilitation really begin.

Whether the injuries are the result of work that is static or dynamic in origin, it will be necessary to understand appropriate postures and body mechanics before we can appreciate the excessive static and dynamic stresses placed on the human musculoskeletal system by the force of gravity and other externally applied loads.

Education in body mechanics and injury prevention, combined with the application of the proper strength, conditioning, and flexibility programs, is an essential component in rehabilitating the individual and reducing the chances of re-injury.

Assessment

It is important to develop an understanding of the circumstances that have lead to injury from the perspective of the individual's specific ergonomic challenges, and of his or her individual physiologic makeup. A brief interview between the therapist and client may help reveal specifics of the particular job situation such as physical constraints like work space, expected pace, or repetitive nature of the job. It may also reveal individual challenges such as medical and injury history, height, weight, strength, or flexibility. A working diagnosis should be arrived at via observation of posture and movement, clinical testing, and evaluation of the individual's strength and ROM. In most cases, the diagnosis should be at least initiated by the individual's own physician.

Specific challenges should be addressed as needed. Ergonomic challenges should be undertaken by ergonomic professionals familiar with the specific type of work, and medical challenges should be addressed by the appropriate medical practitioners. We will discuss the general use of body mechanics education, specific strengthening, and flexibility programs below.

In addition to stretching shortened tissues, inappropriately lengthened tissues should be assessed so that the faulty postures and body mechanics promoted by the individual are not exacerbated by aggressive stretching of the already chronically stressed tissues. It is very important, therefore, to assess the antagonist musculature. Chapter 3 explains this recommendation in detail. For example, in prolonged sitting, in addition to assessing the individual for excessive strain at the posterior ligamentous and musculotendinous tissue, one should assess for chronic shortening of the antagonists such as the hip flexors, abdominals, and anterior chest muscles. Any shortened tissues should be stretched aggressively to regain normal length and ROM. Symptomatic and lengthened tissues may be stretched for relief of symptoms, but with reduced tensions and hold times as discussed later in this chapter. The application of stretching exercises should take place only after careful evaluation of ROM needs. (See Chapter 3 for the details of assessment of movement.)

Education in Posture and Body Mechanics

Excessive joint stress and its resulting pain and dysfunction can be mitigated by a more effective distribution of forces throughout the musculoskeletal system. Good body mechanics implies the most efficient movement patterns relative to both the human body and to the given work situation, allowing the performance of the work tasks with minimal stress and strain and maximum overall efficiency. Understanding proper body mechanics allows one to identify modifications to the individual's movement patterns and to the workplace to make more biomechanically advantageous movement patterns possible. With an understanding of effective body mechanics, individuals can begin to move in such a way as to minimize the excessive forces incurred in repetitive or resisted movement.

SITTING

As mentioned above, sitting places increased stress on the neck, shoulders, lower back, and hips. Individuals who sit for prolonged periods of time often succumb to the pressure of gravity by allowing their head to move forward, their shoulders to round, and their cervical, thoracic, and lumbar spine to flex. This posture can result in chronic lengthening of the lower cervical, thoracic, and lumbar extensors and the supporting ligaments. At the same time, this posture gradually places more and more tension on the posterior structures, while allowing the shortening of the anterior (and posterior upper cervical) structures. These include the upper cervical extensor muscles, the anterior chest and shoulder muscles, and the abdominal and hip flexor muscles. Figure 8.1A shows an example of this sitting posture and indicates the shortened versus the lengthened musculature. Figure 8.1B shows a more effective posture.

It is important for the individual to understand and employ proper sitting positions and workstation configurations to decrease the chances of sitting-related injuries.

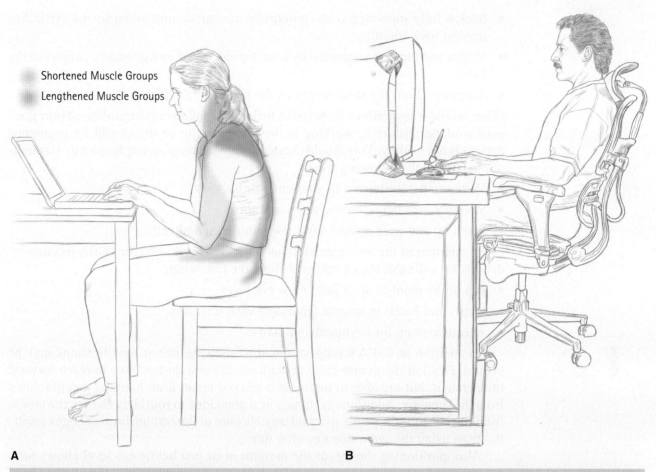

Shortened Muscle Groups
Lengthened Muscle Groups

A   **B**

FIGURE 8.1 Seated posture. A. In this common but poor seated posture, the head is forward, the shoulders rounded, and the back slumped. The drawing highlights lengthened vs. shortened musculature. **B.** In an ergonomically effective posture, the head is aligned above the shoulders, and there is a moderate lordosis in the lumbar and cervical spines.

Marcus et al studied 632 newly hired computer users and related their postures to their incidence of neck and shoulder or arm and hand symptoms and concluded that a significant reduction in the rate of injury might be obtained by using specific seated postures.[7]

In addition to the ergonomic workstation design, specific positioning of the computer screen, keyboard, and mouse are also important factors in the reduction of risk. Though likely an intuitive connection, research can even link the use of the mouse to changes in upper trapezius tone, which may in turn predispose the individual to injury.[6]

The following guidelines for setting up a computer workstation were developed by the Occupational Safety and Health Administration (OSHA 2005). The OSHA website (www.osha.gov/SLTC/etools/computerworkstations/) is an excellent resource with graphics providing more specific and detailed information and examples.

- Hands, wrists, and forearms are straight, in-line (with each other), and roughly parallel to the floor.
- Head is level or bent slightly forward, facing forward, and balanced. Generally it is in line with the torso.
- Shoulders are relaxed and upper arms hang normally at the sides of the body.
- Elbows stay in close to the body and are bent between 90 and 120 degrees.
- Feet are fully supported by floor or footrest.

- Back is fully supported with appropriate lumbar support when sitting vertical or leaning back slightly.
- Thighs and hips are supported by a well-padded seat and generally parallel to the floor.
- Knees are about the same height as the hips with the feet slightly forward.

Other excellent suggestions from OSHA include the following: Regardless of how good your working posture is, working in the same posture or sitting still for prolonged periods is not healthy. You should change your working position frequently throughout the day in the following ways:

- Make small adjustments to your chair or backrest.
- Stretch your fingers, hands, arms, and torso.
- Stand up and walk around for a few minutes periodically.

In addition to the recommendations for seated work, specific OSHA recommendations for sitting at the computer include the following:

- Top of the monitor at or just below eye level
- Wrists and hands in neutral alignment with forearms
- Adequate room for keyboard and mouse

In addition to OSHA's suggestions, the following minor modifications may be helpful. Position the mouse close enough so that you do not have to reach forward to operate it, but are able to maintain a relaxed upper arm, hanging straight down from the shoulder. Additionally, it may be a good idea to routinely change the mouse from the left to right hands to avoid any chronic unilateral postural changes resulting from using the same side day after day.

Also, positioning the top of the monitor at or just below eye level allows for a neutral alignment of the head and neck as long as the actual focus is near the top of the screen. From top to bottom of the screen may be a distance of 10–12 inches, and thus looking at the bottom may cause 20–30 degrees of increased cervical flexion. Individuals should therefore attempt to keep the actual work near the top of the screen.

Experience also suggests that keeping the feet flat on the floor is less important than maintaining an appropriate angle of the thigh. Maintaining the knees at or just below the level of the hip allows for proper positioning of the lumbar (and therefore thoracic and cervical) spine. This may be a particular issue for those with limited lower back and/or hamstring flexibility.

STANDING

Work that requires prolonged periods of standing, particularly in confined areas, places significant stress on the musculoskeletal system. Gravity's effect on the head, neck, and shoulders may be similar to that seen with prolonged sitting, resulting in a forward head and rounded shoulders. However, the effects from the mid-torso inferiorly may be quite different. For example, prolonged standing often causes the worker to relax his or her abdominal muscles and tilt the pelvis anteriorly. Although this position hyperextends the lower back, it is often comfortable in the short term; this is likely because it allows the individual to support the weight of his or her torso on the ligamentous structure in the anterior hips rather than employing the local abdominal musculature. However, overstretching of the abdominal musculature and compression of the lower spinal joints posteriorly make this posture a poor long-term choice. Figure 8.2A shows this posture and highlights both the shortened and the lengthened musculature.

Good standing posture was described in detail in Chapter 7. As you recall, the normal cervical curvature is concave, the thoracic curve is convex, and the lumbar curve is concave (Fig. 8.2B). For optimal function, you should attempt to preserve

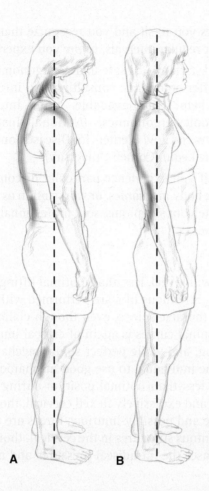

FIGURE 8.2 **Standing posture. A.** In this common poor standing posture, the head is forward, the shoulders rounded, the lordosis is excessive, and the knees locked (hyperextended). **B.** An ergonomically effective standing posture preserves the normal spinal curves.

these curves as you perform static standing work. For example, the standing worker should be encouraged to do the following:

- Stand with feet shoulder-width apart, with the weight evenly balanced between the ball and heel of each foot and knees slightly flexed (unlocked).
- Attempt to balance the head directly over the shoulders, which in turn should be directly over the hip bones, the middle of the knee, and at a point just in front of the ankle.
- Attempt to keep work as close to the body as possible to decrease the tendency to reach forward, rounding head, neck and shoulders, more than necessary to accomplish the given task.
- Consider placing one foot on a slightly elevated surface (3–6″) to reduce the tendency to stand with hyperextension at the lower back.
- Change positions frequently.

REPETITIVE MOVEMENTS

Many workers suffer injuries when they are pressured to work quickly, especially in confined areas with physical barriers. These challenges make it difficult to utilize appropriate body mechanics. However, keeping in mind the basic principles identified below will help reduce the risk of injury. Because it is impossible to consider the postural and movement demands involved in all work situations, we provide the following basic guidelines:

- Be aware of any particular strains placed on your body by the specific demands of your work, and strive to reduce the severity of those strains by modifying your position or movements or by completely changing your position if possible. For example, if your job requires you to sit and you recognize that you are flexed forward, stand up and extend at regular intervals, *before* you experience discomfort or pain.

- Be sure that your workstation is as safe and as ergonomically sound as possible. Your employer may offer ergonomic consulting and intervention as one of your benefits. If in-house help is not available, useful Internet resources include: www.cdc.gov/niosh/topics/ergonomics/ (National Institute of Occupational Safety and Health), www.cdc.gov/ (Centers for Disease Control and Prevention), and www.ergo.human.cornell.edu/ (Cornell University).

- Do not procrastinate. If you experience particular discomfort, address it early by adjusting your posture, body mechanics, or workstation as described earlier. If these changes do not alleviate your symptoms, seek professional help early on, before the problems become serious.

BODY MECHANICS FOR LIFTING

As any construction site will reveal, less-than-optimal lifting mechanics are more the norm than the exception. Strenuous lifts are performed with rounded shoulders and hyperflexed lumbar and thoracic spines, even though claims of bent knees purport safety. Maintaining the spinal curves is again of critical importance in reducing the risk of injury while lifting, and while perfect spinal mechanics may not always be possible, it encourages the individual to use good mechanics whenever possible.

Figure 8.3A shows a less-than-optimal position during a lift. Note the forward head, rounded shoulders, and excessively flexed cervical, thoracic and lumbar spines. In this position, excessive and possibly injurious forces are transferred to the posterior muscular and ligamentous structures in the cervical, thoracic, and lumbar spines. Spinal flexion also increases the intradiscal pressures and may also cause injury to related structures.

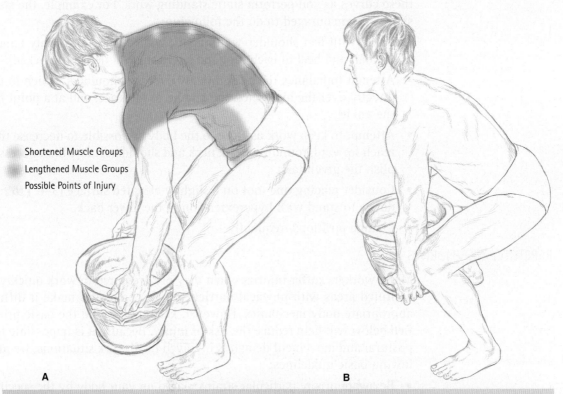

Shortened Muscle Groups
Lengthened Muscle Groups
Possible Points of Injury

A   B

FIGURE 8.3 Lifting posture. A. A less-than-optimal position during a lift. Note the forward head, rounded shoulders, and excessively flexed cervical, thoracic, and lumbar spines. **B.** A better lift with the spine is maintained in neutral.

Some general guidelines to promote safe and effective lifting are provided below. Also, consult Appendix A for further reading suggestions.

- While lifting, maintain the spine's neutral position as much as possible. This is the position in which it is most able to sustain both the intrinsic load of the weight of the rest of the body, as well as any extrinsic load transmitted to the spine by the hands and arms (Fig. 8.3B).

- Use the strength in your legs, not your back, to perform the lift. Most lifting injuries occur at the moment the load is first lifted off the ground or other surface. However, using your legs will be useless in protecting the spine if it is not kept in, or near neutral. You *must* find a way to maintain the spinal curves. You can do so either by bending the knees and flexing forward from the hips (not the spine) as shown in Figure 8.3B or by getting down closer to the load by kneeling on one knee (Fig. 8.4A). This position allows the pelvis to tilt anteriorly (to neutral), which in turn allows the spine to maintain a protective lumbar curve.

- For objects on the floor and/or too wide to fit between the knees, a half-kneeling approach may prove useful. Note how the spine is held in neutral in Figure 8.4A and Figure 8.4B.

- Keep the object close to you. The load on the spine increases dramatically as the length of the lever arm increases. In this case, the lever arm is essentially the perpendicular distance from the object being lifted to the spine. Also keep the weight as close to your center of gravity as possible, which in men is roughly the level of the second lumbar vertebra and in women is about the level of the sacrum. Not only should you carry the load at this level, but you should also move it there before standing up with the load whenever possible. This means bringing

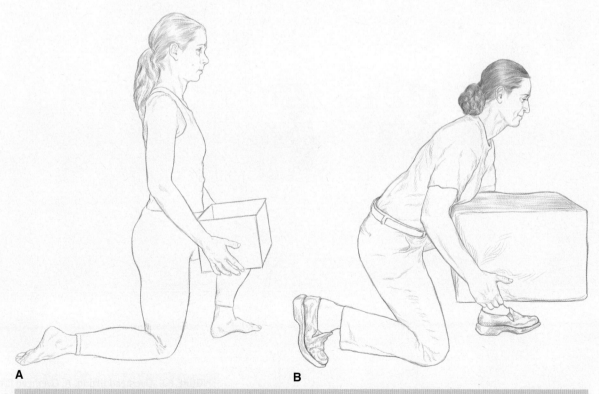

A   B

FIGURE 8.4 **Lifting an object from the floor. A.** Lifting an object from the floor by assuming a half-kneeling position. **B.** Lifting a large object from the floor. Note alignment of spine and bending from the "hips."

the load up to your center of gravity before straightening up from the squatting or kneeling position.

- Move your feet first. When transferring a load, such as carrying a box from one position to another, move your feet first to avoid twisting at the waist.
- When lifting overhead, be careful not to hyperextend your spine. If an overhead lift feels as if it is forcing you to bend backward, think of bending back at your knees while keeping your stomach tight to support your spine and maintain its neutral alignment. Figure 8.5A shows an overhead lift without attention to tightening the abdominals and bending the knees, and Figure 8.5B shows a more effective position.

Conditioning

Understanding and implementing appropriate body mechanics are critical components of injury prevention. Conditioning is also very important in reducing the risk of workplace injuries. Various studies have shown the benefit of improved conditioning in reducing the incidence of injuries in the workplace. Studies by Knapik et al showed decreases in overuse injuries and injuries in general, resulting from physical training program advances in army recruits.[8] Biering-Sorensen's study showed that good isometric endurance of the back musculature may prevent first-time occurrences of lower back trouble, and it also showed reduced flexibility and strength as residual signs in those with recurrent or persistent back trouble.[9] DeWeese showed intervention with a daily stretching program could help reduce the number of reported OSHA recordable injuries in workers in a packaging plant in Macedon, NY.[10] Cady et al con-

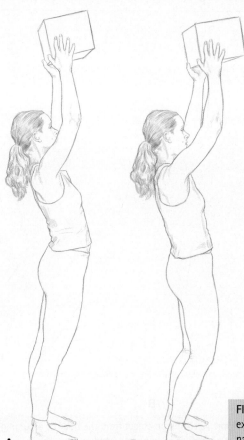

FIGURE 8.5 Overhead lifting. A. Overhead lift with excessive lumbar lordosis. **B.** Overhead lift with abdominal contraction and resultant neutral spine.

A   B

cluded that physical fitness and conditioning in firefighters is preventative of back injuries in the 1,652 firefighters they studied over a 3-year period.[11] Moore concluded that a 36-session stretching intervention produced improved flexibility scores and likely reduced injury rates.[12]

Conditioning includes the development and maintenance of appropriate levels of cardiovascular fitness, physical strength, and endurance and flexibility. Though a detailed discussion is outside the scope of this book, we will address each component below.

CARDIOVASCULAR CONDITIONING

Cardiovascular fitness is important in the maintenance of general health and in the reduction of workplace injuries. Cardiovascular fitness programs should include those for general health and fitness as well as additional training for job-specific demands, should there be any. The basics of cardiovascular conditioning are discussed in Chapter 10.

STRENGTH TRAINING

Developing musculoskeletal strength is also a critical component in reducing the risk of workplace injury and in improving work performance in many cases. Muscular strength should be considered in both general and specific categories. The individual should strive for general strength that includes a balance of upper body, lower body, and core musculature. Core muscles generally refer to those stabilizing the spine and pelvis, including, but not limited to, the abdominals, obliques, lumbar extensors and rotators, and pelvic floor. Specific strengthening should address the specific occupational demands as well as the individual's particular physical challenges. While a detailed discussion is outside the scope of this book, basic strength training principles are covered in Chapter 10.

INCREASING FLEXIBILITY

An understanding of good posture and body mechanics is essential for injury prevention and rehabilitation, but individuals must also have the functional flexibility to be able to achieve effective biomechanics. Stretching will improve your ROM, which may help you assume more effective work postures and to perform tasks more safely, with the best possible body mechanics. Stretching may also help immediately reduce the intensity of pain and stiffness in muscles and joints.

Individuals who wish to achieve permanent changes in muscle length generally need to hold stretches for 30 seconds at a moderate intensity, and perform them daily over several weeks or months. In contrast, individuals can experience immediate, short-term reductions in pain and stiffness with shorter, 5–30 second hold times at a reduced intensity. Bear in mind that permanently lengthening tissues that are already overstretched may exacerbate the very condition that the individual is attempting to alleviate. Take for example the extensors of the cervical spine of an individual who works on a computer for 8 hours a day. Although he or she may be experiencing pain and stiffness in these muscles, the chronic forward head posture may actually be lengthening the lower cervical extensors over the long term. To further lengthen these muscles through an aggressive stretching program would be counterproductive, increasing the imbalance from anterior to posterior and likely worsening the problem. A better solution would be to use a less aggressive approach on the lengthened, painful muscle—that is, shorter hold times and less intensity—and use longer hold times and greater intensity for the shortened, though not painful, anterior musculature.

For this reason, the stretches recommended in the next section of this chapter have two separate categories: one for shortened tissues and one for lengthened tissues. For shortened musculature, follow the general recommendations described in detail in earlier chapters: hold each for 30 seconds at an intensity sufficient to elicit a feeling of strong stretch, not pain. Perform these exercises at least once daily, and at least 4 times each week. For lengthened, stiff, and sore musculature, the goal is moderation or relief of symptoms, not increased length. Therefore, the protocol calls for a reduced intensity, short of a strong stretch, and reduced hold times. Hold times are based on the individual's experience for relief of symptoms and will generally vary between 5 and 30 seconds. These stretches can be used frequently (5–10 times per day) as needed.

Many of the stretches listed in the following sections of this chapter have been selected from Part Two of this book. For a detailed description of how to perform these stretches, please consult the figure numbers cited.

STRETCHES FOR STATIC WORK

The following sections provide basic stretching programs for individuals who do seated work and those who do standing work. When appropriate, one should perform a full assessment of the individual's specific flexibility needs (see Chapter 3) to help design a program specific to his or her needs.

Seated Work

Probably the best recommendation for individuals who perform seated work is to stand up frequently throughout the day. In addition, you should perform as many of the following stretches as possible from a standing position. Below are a few quick stretches that can be used for individuals who sit for long periods of time. Following these quick stretches are more detailed and specific programs carefully chosen from Chapters 5 and 6.

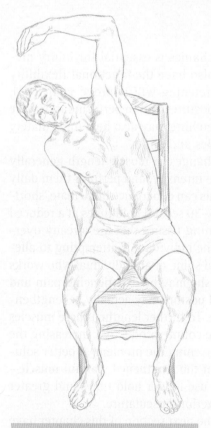

SEATED SIDE BEND

POSITION. Seated

STRETCH. Reach your left hand up as high as possible, then move it in an arc over toward the right, following with your head and neck (Fig. 8.6). You may use your right hand as support on the chair. Repeat to the left.

RESULT. You should feel a stretching sensation along the left side of your neck, underarm and ribcage, and down to your left hip.

FIGURE 8.6 Seated side bend

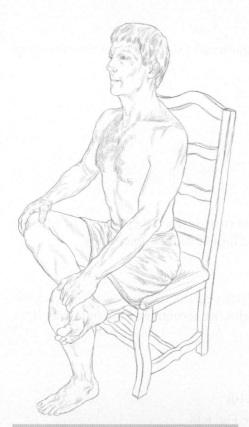

FIGURE 8.7 Seated hip stretch

SEATED HIP STRETCH

POSITION. Seated

STRETCH. Cross your right ankle over your left knee. Place your right hand on your right knee, and use your left hand to grasp your right ankle (Fig. 8.7). Gently press down on your right knee. Lift your chest and shoulders while extending your middle and lower back (push your chest out). Repeat to opposite side.

RESULT. You should feel a stretching sensation from the front to the side (anterior to lateral) right hip.

SEATED ROTATION

POSITION. Seated

STRETCH. Lift your head and shoulders while extending your middle and lower back. Rotate your head and shoulders toward the right and grasp the chair as able, with both hands (Fig. 8.8). Slowly apply an added rotation stretch toward the right, following with your head. Repeat to the left.

RESULT. You should feel a stretching sensation through your lower, to mid and upper back, and neck.

> ⚠ **CAUTION!** You should not feel sharp pain in your neck or lower back. If you do experience pain, you should back off the intensity of the stretch or eliminate it altogether.

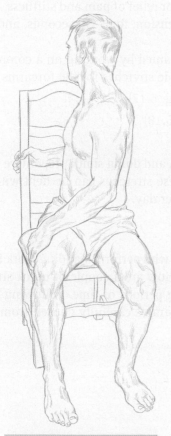

FIGURE 8.8 Seated rotation

GENERAL STRETCHING PROGRAM FOR SHORTENED TISSUES

A general stretching program to address the shortened tissues includes the following:

- Upper cervical extensors (see Fig. 5.1)
- Shoulder horizontal adductors (see Fig. 5.9)
- Shoulder flexors (see Fig. 5.5)
- Spinal flexors (see Fig. 8.10, below)
- Hip flexors (see Fig. 5.24)
- Knee flexors (see Fig. 5.3)
- Ankle dorsiflexors (see Fig. 5.32)

As these stretches are intended to lengthen shortened tissue; they should be held for 30 seconds at a moderate intensity and be performed at least once daily.

GENERAL STRETCHING PROGRAM FOR LENGTHENED TISSUES

To address lengthened tissues and reduce or relieve pain, tension, or stiffness in the posterior cervical, thoracic, and lumbar muscles, we recommend the following light stretching program:

- Lower cervical extensors (see Fig. 5.1)
- Shoulder extensors (see Fig. 5.6)
- Shoulder horizontal abductors (see Fig. 5.10)
- Shoulder internal rotators and flexors (see Fig. 6.6)
- Spinal extensors (see Fig. 4.64A,B)

Again, because these stretches are intended for relief of pain and stiffness, they should be held with gentle rather than aggressive tension, for 5–30 seconds, and performed as often as needed throughout the day.

If the chronic sitting position is accompanied by working on a computer or any other repetitive task, it makes sense to include stretches for the forearms and hands:

- Wrist, finger, and hand extensors (see Fig. 5.17)
- Wrist, finger, and hand flexors (see Fig. 5.18)
- Intrinsic hand muscles (see Fig. 5.19)

Because typing, handling a computer mouse, and doing similar repetitive movements are likely to result in shortened tissues, these stretches can be held with moderate tension for 30 seconds each, at least once per day.

Standing Work

Probably the best recommendation for those who perform standing work is to change positions frequently throughout the day. Below are a couple of quick stretches that can be used for individuals who sit for long periods of time. Following these quick stretches are more detailed and specific programs carefully chosen from Chapters 5 and 6.

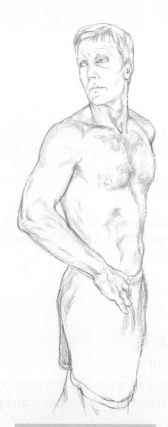

FIGURE 8.9 Neck, upper and middle back, and torso rotation

NECK, UPPER AND MIDDLE BACK, AND TORSO

MOTION AFFECTED. Rotation

POSITION. Standing

STRETCH. Turn your head, then your shoulders, and then your entire back maximally toward the right (Fig. 8.9). You may use your arms to help you rotate. Repeat toward the left.

RESULT. You should feel a stretch in your neck and your upper, middle, and lower back.

STANDING BACK EXTENSION

POSITION. Standing

STRETCH. Place your hands on your hips and carefully bend backward, beginning at the neck and progressing down to the thoracic and lumbar spines (Fig. 8.10). Be careful not to hyperextend at either the cervical (neck) or lumbar spine.

RESULT. You should feel a stretching sensation in the front of your neck, chest, and down to your abdomen and hips.

> ⚠ **CAUTION!** You should *not* feel excessive pressure in your neck or lower back! Be sure to ease off the stretch if you feel pressure in these areas.

As you will see below, many of the stretches recommended for individuals doing seated work are useful for those who work standing up.

GENERAL STRETCHING PROGRAM FOR SHORTENED TISSUES

A general stretching program to address shortened tissues commonly found in those who work standing up include the following:

- Upper cervical extensors (see Fig. 5.1)
- Shoulder horizontal adductors (see Fig. 5.9)
- Shoulder flexors (see Fig. 5.5)

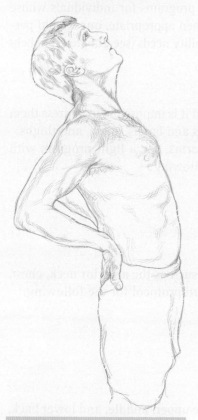

FIGURE 8.10 Standing back extension

- Spinal flexors (see Fig. 8.10)
- Hip flexors (see Fig. 5.24)
- Knee flexors (see Fig. 5.3)
- Ankle plantar flexors (see Fig. 33B,C)
- Ankle dorsiflexors (see Fig. 5.32)

As these stretches are intended to lengthen shortened tissue, they should be held for 30 seconds at a moderate intensity (see Chapter 3 for details) and performed at least once daily.

GENERAL STRETCHING PROGRAM FOR LENGTHENED TISSUES

To address lengthened tissues and reduce or relieve pain, tension, or stiffness in the posterior cervical, thoracic, and lumbar muscles, we recommend the following light stretching program:

- Lower cervical extensors (see Fig. 5.1)
- Shoulder extensors (see Fig. 5.6)
- Shoulder horizontal abductors (see Fig. 5.10)
- Shoulder internal rotators and flexors (see Fig. 6.6)
- Thoracic and lumbar spinal extensors (see Fig. 5.20)

Again, because these stretches are intended for relief of pain and stiffness, they should be held with gentle rather than aggressive tension, for 5–30 seconds, and performed as often as needed throughout the day.

STRETCHES FOR DYNAMIC WORK

The following sections provide some basic stretching programs for individuals whose work requires repetitive movements and/or lifting. When appropriate, one should perform a full assessment of the individual's specific flexibility needs (see Chapter 3) to help design an individualized program.

Work Requiring Repetitive Movements

Obviously, there are many types of repetitive work and it is impossible to address them all, so we will concentrate here on the neck, forearms and hands, spine, and thighs.

To address a strained neck, shoulders, and forearms, use a light program with moderate tensions and 5–30 second holds for the following:

- Lower cervical extensors (see Fig. 5.1)
- Shoulder horizontal abductors (see Fig. 5.10)
- Wrist, finger, and hand extensors (see Fig. 5.17)
- Wrist, finger, and hand flexors (see Fig. 5.18)

To address shortened muscles related to posture such as the anterior neck, chest, and shoulders muscles and hip flexors, use a standard protocol for the following:

- Cervical flexors (see Fig. 5.2)
- Shoulder horizontal adductors (see Fig. 5.9)
- Hip flexors (see Fig. 5.24)

Work Requiring Lifting

As most lifting tasks place particular demands on the upper, middle, and lower back, the thigh muscles, and the shoulder muscles, stretches for these groups are included here. A light program with moderate tensions and 5–30 second holds should be used for the following:

- Shoulder horizontal abductors (see Fig. 5.10)
- Shoulder flexors (see Fig. 5.5)
- Spinal extensors (see Fig. 6.12)
- Knee extensors (see Fig. 5.31)

   To perform lifting tasks adequately, particular attention should be paid to the anterior chest, the abdominals, and the hip flexors. Address shortened tissues with a standard protocol of 30-second holds eliciting a feeling of strong stretch:

- Shoulder flexors/horizontal adductors (see Fig. 5.9)
- Spinal flexors (see Fig. 8.10)
- Hip flexors (see Fig. 5.24)
- Hip external rotators/extensors (see Fig. 5.25)
- Ankle plantarflexors (see Fig. 5.33B)

WHOLE-BODY WORKPLACE STRETCHING PROGRAM

The following is a brief, non-specific stretching program to help individuals address workplace tension throughout the body. Hold each stretch for 30 seconds with moderate tension.

- Neck and Torso Rotation (see Fig. 8.9)
- Spinal Side-bending (see Fig. 6.2)
- Spinal Extension (see Fig. 8.10)
- Back and Shoulders (see Fig. 5.6)
- Wrist and Forearm Flexion (see Fig. 6.16)
- Wrist and Forearm Extension (see Fig. 6.17)
- Hamstrings (see Fig. 5.30A)
- Calves (see Fig. 5.33B)

SUMMARY

Work is challenging enough without the added burden of workplace pain, dysfunction, and injury. Understanding the human musculoskeletal system and its basic interaction with the work environment is a necessary first step in preventing injury and promoting healing. In approaching individuals with work-related pain or stiffness, it makes sense to begin with an interview exploring work environment and required tasks from a biomechanical perspective, and then follow with a thorough assessment of posture, body mechanics, and current ROM. Of course, we must also consider the individual's past injury and overall medical history as well. The data you gather will help you design a more appropriate work environment and create a conditioning program that should help you reduce the risk of injury while enhancing your work performance.

   An appropriately designed flexibility program is an important component of that conditioning program. It should allow for both the immediate, short-term relief of pain and stiffness, and the long-term achievement of appropriate postures and movement patterns, thereby increasing career longevity and reducing the risk of injury, both within and beyond the workplace.

REFERENCES

1. US Department of Labor, Bureau of Labor Statistics Website. 2004. Available at: http://www.bls.gov/iif/oshwc/osh/case/ostb1258.pdf. Accessed June 15, 2007.
2. Liberty Mutual Workplace Safety Index Website. 2007. Available at: http://www.libertymutual.com/omapps/ContentServer?cid=1078439448036&pagename=ResearchCenter%2FDocument%2FShowDoc&c=Document. Accessed June 15, 2007.
3. Stuebbe P, Genaidy A, Karwowski W, et al. The relationships between biomechanical and postural stresses, musculoskeletal injury rates, and perceived body discomfort experienced by industrial workers: a field study. Int J Occup Saf Ergon 2002;8(2):259–280.
4. US Department of Labor, Bureau of Labor Statistics Website. 2007. Available at: http://www.bls.gov/iif/home.htm. Accessed June 15, 2007.
5. Zennaro D, Laubli T, Krebs D, et al. Trapezius muscle motor unit activity in symptomatic participants during finger tapping using properly and improperly adjusted desks. Hum Factors Summer 2004;46(2):252–266.
6. Jensen C, Finsen L, Hansen K, et al. Upper trapezius muscle activity patterns during repetitive manual material handling and work with a computer mouse. J Electromyogr Kinesiol October 1999;9(5):317–325.
7. Marcus M, Gerr F, Monteilh C, et al. A prospective study of computer users: II. Postural risk factors for musculoskeletal symptoms and disorders. Am J Ind Med April 2002;41(4):236–249.
8. Knapik JJ, Hauret KG, Arnold S, et al. Injury and fitness outcomes during implementation of physical readiness training. Int J Sports Med July 2003;24(5):372–381.
9. Biering-Sorensen F. Physical measurements as risk indicators for low-back trouble over a one-year period. Spine 1984;9(2):106–119.
10. DeWeese C. How multiple interventions reduced injuries and costs in one plant. Work 2006;26(3):251–253.
11. Cady LD, Bischoff DP, O'Connell ER, et al. Strength and fitness and subsequent back injuries in firefighters. J Occup Med April 1979;21(4):269–272.
12. Moore TM. A workplace stretching program. Physiologic and perception measurements before and after participation. AAOHN J December 1998;46(12):563–568.

Stretching for Sports

Stretching is an accepted part of most athletic conditioning programs worldwide. However, although most reputable sports programs include some type of stretching in their overall conditioning scheme, the types of stretches and their frequency, duration, intensity, and method of application vary greatly, as do the theories that support their specific use. As noted in Chapter 1, research regarding the usefulness of pre-event stretching is inconclusive. It is therefore very important to carefully consider the motivation, planning, and application of each individual case before implementing a stretching program.

This chapter provides stretching programs for individuals involved in a number of common sports. As with all stretching programs (for which the goal is to increase muscle length) in this book, we advise that individuals hold each stretch for 30 seconds at a moderate intensity, and perform the program 3 or more times per week. Notice that, although this chapter gives you some guidelines for choosing safe and effective stretches, it does not relieve you of the responsibility to seek individual information, via a full flexibility assessment, which will enable you to individualize your prescription. In addition, as all sports differ, it is important to seek sport-specific information from reputable sources regarding flexibility issues for the sport in particular. Stay abreast of the latest information available in the field, including trends in performance, or research into injury that might cause you to adjust an existing flexibility program. Should the stretches be directed at particular muscle groups? Should they be performed at greater or lesser intensity? Duration? Should they be performed before, during, or after training or competition? These are some of the many questions that should be answered in order to ensure that the flexibility program is as safe and effective as possible.

Although this chapter provides stretching programs for a number of popular sports, because of the constraints of space and scope, it does not cover every sport of interest to every individual. If you wish to supplement the programs given below, we encourage you to consult Chapter 5, which details stretching for all major muscle groups. For information on those sports not addressed, or for more detailed information on those we have discussed, we encourage you to consult professionals involved in the particular sport. In many cases, a basic understanding of the movement patterns and musculature involved in a particular sport will allow you to be able to use Chapter 5 to design an effective program. If there are particular injuries associated with a chosen sport, whether it is covered in this chapter or not, you should consult Chapter 10 for information on how to modify the basic stretching program.

The sports covered in this chapter include:

- baseball
- basketball
- bicycling
- football
- golf
- gymnastics
- hiking
- hockey
- in-line skating (see skating)
- kayaking
- rock climbing
- running
- skating
- skiing
- soccer
- swimming
- tennis
- track and field
- volleyball
- weightlifting

The following are stretching programs recommended for each sport listed above. We have tried to emphasize the muscle groups that are most likely to require stretching for the effective performance of that sport. Goals for range of motion (ROM) are best determined on an individual basis and should consider the specific needs of the athlete, and the specific demands of the sport and position. Chapter 3 will help assess individual flexibility needs. A brief discussion of the physical demands of each sport precedes each stretching program.

BASEBALL

Throwing requires strong and flexible shoulders and upper arms, including the rotator cuff. An efficient swing requires a flexible torso, shoulders, forearms, and wrists. Fielding and base-running require sprinting and rapid direction changes that call for flexibility in the hips, knees, ankles, and torso.

Below are stretches recommended for baseball players:

- Shoulder Horizontal Abductors (Fig. 5.10)
- Shoulder Horizontal Adductors (Fig. 5.9)
- Shoulder Adductors (Fig. 5.8)
- Rotator Cuff: Shoulder Internal Rotators (Fig. 5.11), Shoulder External Rotators (Fig. 5.12), and Forearm Supinators (Fig. 5.15)
- Forearm Pronators (Fig. 5.16)
- Wrist and Finger Flexors (Fig. 5.18)
- Wrist and Finger Extensors (Fig. 5.17)

- Torso Rotators (Fig. 5.23)
- Hip Flexors (Fig. 5.24)
- Hip Extensors (Fig. 5.25)
- Hip Abductors (Fig. 5.27)
- Hip Adductors (Fig. 5.26)
- Knee Flexors (Fig. 5.30)
- Knee Extensors (Fig. 5.31)
- Ankle Dorsiflexors (Fig. 5.32)
- Ankle Evertors (Fig. 5.35)
- Ankle Invertors (Fig. 5.34)

BASKETBALL

Quick movements, including rapid pivoting and direction changes from head to toe, plus sprinting, jumping, and landing, all demand flexibility about the spine, hips, knees and ankles, while shooting, dribbling, blocking out, and wrestling for rebounds require upper body flexibility.

Below are stretches recommended for basketball players:
- Cervical Flexors (Fig. 5.2)
- Cervical Extensors (Fig. 5.1)
- Cervical Rotators (Fig. 5.4)
- Spinal Extensors (Fig. 5.20)
- Spinal Flexors (Fig. 5.21)
- Spinal Rotators (Fig. 5.23)
- Hip Flexors (Fig. 5.24)
- Hip Extensors (Fig. 5.25)
- Knee Flexors (Fig. 5.30)
- Knee Extensors (Fig. 5.31)
- Ankle Dorsiflexors (Fig. 5.32)
- Ankle Plantarflexors (Fig. 5.33)
- Ankle Evertors (Fig. 5.35)
- Shoulder Horizontal Adductors (Fig. 5.9)
- Shoulder Flexors (Fig. 5.5)
- Shoulder Extensors (Fig. 5.6)
- Elbow Extensors (Fig. 5.14)
- Wrist and Finger Flexors (Fig. 5.18)
- Wrist and Finger Extensors (Fig. 5.17)

BICYCLING

Though the ROM demands are not great in the legs of a cyclist (as the range is constant and determined by the setup of the bike), there is a need for stretching the neck, upper back, hips, thighs and calves. The constantly flexed upper body and torso may benefit from stretching the abdominals, as well as the front of the chest and shoulders, while supporting the upper body on the handlebars requires use of the upper and lower arms, wrists, and hands.

Below are stretches recommended for cyclists:

- Cervical Rotators (Fig. 5.4)
- Cervical Flexors (Fig. 5.2)
- Cervical Extensors (Fig. 5.1)
- Shoulder Flexors (Fig. 5.5)
- Shoulder Extensors (Fig. 5.6)
- Shoulder Abductors (Fig. 5.7)
- Spinal Extensors (Fig. 5.20)
- Spinal Flexors (Fig. 5.21)
- Hip Flexors (Fig. 5.24)
- Hip Extensors (Fig. 5.25)
- Hip Abductors (Fig. 5.27)
- Hip Adductors (Fig. 5.26)
- Knee Extensors (Fig. 5.31)
- Knee Flexors (Fig. 5.30A)
- Ankle Plantarflexors (Fig. 5.33B)
- Ankle Dorsiflexors (Fig. 5.32)
- Shoulder Extensors (Fig. 5.6)
- Shoulder Horizontal Abductors (Fig. 5.10)
- Elbow Flexors (Fig. 5.13)
- Elbow Extensors (Fig. 5.14)
- Wrist and Finger Flexors (Fig. 5.18)
- Wrist and Finger Extensors (Fig. 5.17)

FOOTBALL

Although the demands vary greatly according to position, most football players will benefit from flexibility in the neck, shoulders, arms, and hands, as well as the torso, hips, thighs, and calves. The tremendous loads incurred via contact with other players make sufficient flexibility critical in these areas.

Below are stretches recommended for football players:

- Cervical Flexors (Fig. 5.2)
- Cervical Extensors (Fig. 5.1)
- Cervical Rotators (Fig. 5.4)
- Cervical Side-benders (Fig. 5.3)
- Shoulder Flexors (Fig. 5.5)
- Shoulder Extensors (Fig. 5.6)
- Shoulder Horizontal Adductors (Fig. 5.9)
- Elbow Flexors (Fig. 5.13)
- Elbow Extensors (Fig. 5.14)
- Wrist and Finger Flexors (Fig. 5.18)
- Wrist and Finger Extensors (Fig. 5.17)
- Spinal Rotators (Fig. 5.23)

- Spinal Flexors (Fig. 5.21)
- Spinal Extensors (Fig. 5.20)
- Spinal Side-benders (Fig. 5.22)
- Hip Flexors (Fig. 5.24)
- Hip Extensors (Fig. 5.25)
- Hip Abductors (Fig. 5.27)
- Hip Adductors (Fig. 5.26)
- Knee Extensors (Fig. 5.31)
- Ankle Plantarflexors (Fig. 5.33B)
- Ankle Dorsiflexors (Fig. 5.32)

GOLF

Golf requires rapid and powerful torso rotation starting at the hips, and following through the torso, to the shoulders, arms, and hands superiorly, and through the knees, feet, and ankles inferiorly. The flexibility of both the accelerators and the decelerators of this motion is important.

Below are stretches recommended for golfers:

- Hip Abductors (Fig. 5.27)
- Hip Adductors (Fig. 5.26)
- Hip Internal Rotators (Fig. 5.28)
- Hip External Rotators (Fig. 5.29)
- Spinal Rotators (Fig. 5.23)
- Shoulder Flexors (Fig. 5.5)
- Shoulder Horizontal Abductors (Fig. 5.10)
- Shoulder Extensors (Fig. 5.6)
- Shoulder Adductors (Fig. 5.8)
- Elbow Flexors (Fig. 5.13)
- Elbow Extensors (Fig. 5.14)
- Forearm Pronators (Fig. 5.16)
- Forearm Supinators (Fig. 5.15)
- Wrist and Finger Flexors (Fig. 5.18)
- Wrist and Finger Extensors (Fig. 5.17)
- Knee Flexors (Fig. 5.30A)
- Ankle Plantarflexors (Fig. 5.33B)
- Ankle Evertors (Fig. 5.35)

GYMNASTICS

Reaching extremes of human motion in most every direction, gymnasts require exceptional ROM at most joints, especially in the shoulders, spine, and hips. Because of this very high level of flexibility, gymnasts might be hopelessly unstable if it were not for their excellent strength and neuromuscular control.

Below are stretches recommended for gymnasts:

- Shoulder Flexors (Fig. 5.5)
- Shoulder Extensors (Fig. 5.6)

- Shoulder Abductors (Fig. 5.7)
- Shoulder Adductors (Fig. 5.8)
- Shoulder Horizontal Adductors (Fig. 5.9)
- Shoulder Internal Rotators (Fig. 5.11)
- Shoulder External Rotators (Fig. 5.12)
- Elbow Flexors (Fig. 5.13)
- Elbow Extensors (Fig. 5.14)
- Forearm Supinators (Fig. 5.15)
- Forearm Pronators (Fig. 5.16)
- Wrist and Finger Flexors (Fig. 5.18)
- Wrist and Finger Extensors (Fig. 5.17)
- Spinal Flexors (Fig. 5.21)
- Spinal Extensors (Fig. 5.20)
- Spinal Rotators (Fig. 5.23)
- Spinal Side-benders (Fig. 5.22)
- Hip Flexors (Fig. 5.24)
- Hip Extensors (Fig. 5.25)
- Hip Abductors (Fig. 5.27)
- Hip Adductors (Fig. 5.26)
- Knee Flexors (Fig. 5.30A)
- Knee Extensors (Fig. 5.31)
- Ankle Plantarflexors (Fig. 5.33B)
- Ankle Dorsiflexors (Fig. 5.32)

HIKING

Ascending and descending moderate to very steep slopes with uneven surfaces place particular demands on lower extremity ROM. Carrying a moderate to heavy pack places extra stress on the shoulders, neck, and thoracic and lumbar spines, while further increasing the load on the legs.

Below are stretches recommended for hikers:

- Spinal Flexors (Fig. 5.21)
- Spinal Extensors (Fig. 5.20)
- Hip Abductors (Fig. 5.27)
- Hip Adductors (Fig. 5.26)
- Hip Flexors (Fig. 5.24)
- Hip Extensors (Fig. 5.25)
- Knee Flexors (Fig. 5.30A)
- Knee Extensors (Fig. 5.31)
- Ankle Dorsiflexors (Fig. 5.32)
- Ankle Plantarflexors (Fig. 5.33B)
- Shoulder Flexors (Fig. 5.5)
- Shoulder Extensors (Fig. 5.6)
- Shoulder Abductors (Fig. 5.7)

- Cervical Flexors (Fig. 5.2)
- Cervical Extensors (Fig. 5.1)
- Cervical Side-benders (Fig. 5.3)
- Spinal Flexors (Fig. 5.21)
- Spinal Extensors (Fig. 5.20)

HOCKEY

Rapid sprints and sharp direction changes make extreme demands on the hips, thighs, knees, and ankles, whereas explosive movements of the upper body and torso require flexibility in the spine, shoulders, arms, and hands.

Below are stretches recommended for hockey players:
- Hip Adductors (Fig. 5.26)
- Hip Abductors (Fig. 5.27)
- Hip Flexors (Fig. 5.24)
- Hip Extensors (Fig. 5.25)
- Knee Extensors (Fig. 5.31)
- Knee Flexors (Fig. 5.30A)
- Ankle Plantarflexors (Fig. 5.33B)
- Ankle Dorsiflexors (Fig. 5.32)
- Spinal Flexors (Fig. 5.21)
- Spinal Extensors (Fig. 5.20)
- Spinal Rotators (Fig. 5.23)
- Spinal Side-benders (Fig. 5.22)
- Shoulder Flexors (Fig. 5.5)
- Shoulder Extensors (Fig. 5.6)
- Shoulder Abductors (Fig. 5.7)
- Shoulder Adductors (Fig. 5.8)
- Shoulder Internal Rotators (Fig. 5.11)
- Shoulder External Rotators (Fig. 5.12)
- Elbow Flexors (Fig. 5.13)
- Elbow Extensors (Fig. 5.14)
- Wrist and Finger Flexors (Fig. 5.18)
- Wrist and Finger Extensors (Fig. 5.17)

KAYAKING

Optimal control of both whitewater and sea kayaks requires maintaining an upright torso with the hips flexed and knees nearly extended. Hip flexibility is critical to allow the upper body to function optimally. Much of the power delivered to the paddles comes from rotation of the torso, with the fine-tuning coming from the arms and hands. Flexibility of the forearms, hands, and fingers is of obvious importance.

Below are stretches recommended for kayakers:
- Hip Flexors (Fig. 5.24)
- Hip Extensors (Fig. 5.25)
- Hip Abductors (Fig. 5.27)

- Hip Adductors (Fig. 5.26)
- Knee Flexors (Fig. 5.30A)
- Knee Extensors (Fig. 5.31)
- Ankle Dorsiflexors (Fig. 5.32)
- Ankle Plantarflexors (Fig. 5.33)
- Spinal Rotators (Fig. 5.23)
- Spinal Side-benders (Fig. 5.22)
- Spinal Extensors (Fig. 5.20)
- Shoulder Flexors (Fig. 5.5)
- Shoulder Extensors (Fig. 5.6)
- Shoulder Abductors (Fig. 5.7)
- Shoulder Adductors (Fig. 5.8)
- Shoulder Internal Rotators (Fig. 5.11)
- Shoulder External Rotators (Fig. 5.12)
- Forearm Supinators (Fig. 5.15)
- Forearm Pronators (Fig. 5.16)
- Wrist and Finger Flexors (Fig. 5.18)
- Wrist and Finger Extensors (Fig. 5.17)

ROCK CLIMBING

Successful rock climbing demands excellent ROM in the spine, shoulders, elbows, wrists, and hands as well as in the hips, knees, feet, and ankles. An infinite variety of challenging moves and resultant body positions may not be possible without very high levels of flexibility.

Below are stretches recommended for rock climbers:

- Cervical Flexors (Fig. 5.2)
- Cervical Extensors (Fig. 5.1)
- Cervical Side-benders (Fig. 5.3)
- Cervical Rotators (Fig. 5.4)
- Spinal Flexors (Fig. 5.21)
- Spinal Side-benders (Fig. 5.22)
- Spinal Rotators (Fig. 5.23)
- Shoulder Extensors (Fig. 5.6)
- Shoulder Abductors (Fig. 5.7)
- Shoulder Horizontal Adductors (Fig. 5.9)
- Shoulder External Rotators (Fig. 5.12)
- Elbow Flexors (Fig. 5.13)
- Elbow Extensors (Fig. 5.14)
- Wrist and Finger Flexors (Fig. 5.18)
- Wrist and Finger Extensors (Fig. 5.17)
- Intrinsic Hand Muscles (Fig. 5.19)
- Hip Flexors (Fig. 5.24)
- Hip Extensors (Fig. 5.25)
- Hip Abductors (Fig. 5.27)

- Hip Adductors (Fig. 5.26)
- Knee Flexors (Fig. 5.30A)
- Knee Extensors (Fig. 5.31)
- Ankle Plantarflexors (Fig. 5.33B)
- Ankle Dorsiflexors (Fig. 5.32)
- Ankle Invertors (Fig. 5.34)
- Ankle Evertors (Fig. 5.35)

RUNNING

Sprinters need torso and upper extremity flexibility in addition to the obvious needs of the hips, knees, ankles, and feet. Distance runners need to maintain flexibility despite the chronic stresses on their hips, knees, ankles, and feet.

Note that a study by Craib et al involving sub-elite male distance runners suggests inflexibility in some muscle groups may actually benefit performance.[1] This information may be consistent with other researchers who have found that stretching muscles, at least immediately prior to participation, may hinder performance in sprinting, jumping, and muscular contraction. The actual ROM necessary for optimal performance remains a matter of debate. We encourage the clinician to keep abreast of the latest research findings relative to his or her particular sport, so that the prescription of stretching, strength training, and conditioning can be as current and valuable as possible. See Chapter 1 for a more detailed discussion of the benefits and limitations of stretching.

Below are stretches recommended for runners:

- Spinal Rotators (Fig. 5.23)
- Spinal Extensors (Fig. 5.20)
- Shoulder Flexors (Fig. 5.5)
- Shoulder Extensors (Fig. 5.6)
- Shoulder Horizontal Adductors (Fig. 5.9)
- Elbow Flexors (Fig. 5.13)
- Hip Flexors (Fig. 5.24)
- Hip Extensors (Fig. 5.25)
- Hip Abductors (Fig. 5.27)
- Hip Adductors (Fig. 5.26)
- Knee Flexors (Fig. 5.30A)
- Knee Extensors (Fig. 5.31)
- Ankle Plantarflexors (Fig. 5.33B)
- Ankle Dorsiflexors (Fig. 5.32)

SKATING

Alternating one-legged stance challenges the hips and thighs, while the additional height of the skate places additional stress on the knees and lower leg. The prolonged flexed position of the torso places extra load on the spinal and hip extensors, while the rhythmic swinging of the shoulders and upper arms contributes to forward momentum.

Below are stretches recommended for skaters:

- Hip Abductors (Fig. 5.27)

- Hip Adductors (Fig. 5.26)
- Hip Flexors (Fig. 5.24)
- Hip Extensors (Fig. 5.25)
- Knee Flexors (Fig. 5.30A)
- Knee Extensors (Fig. 5.31)
- Ankle Plantarflexors (Fig. 5.33B)
- Ankle Invertors (Fig. 5.34)
- Ankle Evertors (Fig. 5.35)
- Spinal Rotators (Fig. 5.23)
- Spinal Flexors (Fig. 5.21)
- Spinal Extensors (Fig. 5.20)
- Shoulder Flexors (Fig. 5.5)
- Shoulder Horizontal Adductors (Fig. 5.9)

SKIING (ALPINE)

Alpine skiing places significant demands on the skier's hips and knees in addition to their torso and lower legs. The variety of turn types, shapes, and diameters, combined with the increased forces generated through these turns, makes flexibility in these areas critical.

Below are stretches recommended for alpine skiers:

- Hip Extensors (Fig. 5.25)
- Hip Flexors (Fig. 5.24)
- Hip Abductors (Fig. 5.27)
- Hip Adductors (Fig. 5.26)
- Hip Internal (Fig. 5.28)
- Hip External Rotators (Fig. 5.29)
- Knee Flexors (Fig. 5.30A)
- Knee Extensors (Fig. 5.31)
- Spinal Extensors (Fig. 5.20)
- Spinal Rotators (Fig. 5.23)
- Spinal Side-benders (Fig. 5.22)
- Ankle Plantarflexors (Fig. 5.33B)
- Ankle Invertors (Fig. 5.34)
- Ankle Evertors (Fig. 5.35)

SKIING (NORDIC)

Both the classic and skating forms of cross-country skiing challenge flexibility throughout lower extremities, particularly in the hips and calves. Propulsion with ski poles places demands on the core and upper extremities, demanding adequate flexibility particularly at the shoulders, arms, and torso.

Below are stretches recommended for Nordic skiers:

- Hip Flexors (Fig. 5.24)
- Hip Extensors (Fig. 5.25)

- Hip Abductors (Fig. 5.27)
- Hip Adductors (Fig. 5.26)
- Hip External Rotators (Fig. 5.29)
- Knee Flexors (Fig. 5.30A)
- Knee Extensors (Fig. 5.31)
- Ankle Plantarflexors (Fig. 5.33B)
- Ankle Dorsiflexors (Fig. 5.32)
- Shoulder Flexors (Fig. 5.5)
- Shoulder Extensors (Fig. 5.6)
- Shoulder Abductors (Fig. 5.7)
- Shoulder Adductors (Fig. 5.8)
- Shoulder Horizontal Adductors (Fig. 5.9)
- Shoulder Internal Rotators (Fig. 5.11)
- Shoulder External Rotators (Fig. 5.12)
- Elbow Extensors (Fig. 5.14)
- Wrist and Finger Flexors (Fig. 5.18)
- Wrist and Finger Extensors (Fig. 5.17)
- Spinal Flexors (Fig. 5.21)
- Spinal Extensors (Fig. 5.20)
- Spinal Rotators (Fig. 5.23)

SNOWBOARDING

Riding goofy or regular requires torso mobility to open the upper body downhill, while flexibility of the hips, knees, and ankles are also very important in allowing for flexion, extension, and rotation of the lower extremities integral to the performance of the turns. Chest and shoulder mobility are important in maintaining a balanced upper body during turn execution.

Below are stretches recommended for snowboarders:

- Spinal Rotators (Fig. 5.23)
- Spinal Side-benders (Fig. 5.22)
- Spinal Flexors (Fig. 5.21)
- Spinal Extensors (Fig. 5.20)
- Hip Extensors (Fig. 5.25)
- Hip Flexors (Fig. 5.24)
- Knee Flexors (Fig. 5.30A)
- Knee Extensors (Fig. 5.31)
- Ankle Plantarflexors (Fig. 5.33B)
- Ankle Dorsiflexors (Fig. 5.32)
- Ankle Evertors (Fig. 5.35)
- Shoulder Flexors (Fig. 5.5)
- Shoulder Horizontal Abductors (Fig. 5.10)
- Shoulder Horizontal Adductors (Fig. 5.9)

SOCCER

Sprinting and rapid direction changes, not to mention explosive kicking movements, make extraordinary demands on the torso, hips, knees, and ankles of the soccer player. Headers and throw-ins make neck and upper extremity ROM also very important.

Below are stretches recommended for soccer players:

- Spinal Rotators (Fig. 5.23)
- Spinal Flexors (Fig. 5.21)
- Spinal Extensors (Fig. 5.20)
- Spinal Side-benders (Fig. 5.22)
- Hip Flexors (Fig. 5.24)
- Hip Extensors (Fig. 5.25)
- Hip Abductors (Fig. 5.27)
- Hip Adductors (Fig. 5.26)
- Hip Internal Rotators (Fig. 5.28)
- Hip External Rotators (Fig. 5.29)
- Knee Flexors (Fig. 5.30A)
- Knee Extensors (Fig. 5.31)
- Ankle Dorsiflexors (Fig. 5.32)
- Ankle Plantarflexors (Fig. 5.33B)
- Ankle Invertors (Fig. 5.34)
- Ankle Evertors (Fig. 5.35)
- Cervical Flexors (Fig. 5.2)
- Cervical Extensors (Fig. 5.1)
- Cervical Rotators (Fig. 5.4)
- Cervical Side-benders (Fig. 5.3)
- Shoulder Flexors (Fig. 5.5)
- Shoulder Extensors (Fig. 5.6)
- Shoulder Adductors (Fig. 5.8)

SWIMMING

Although the precise physical demands vary according to the stroke, the ROM required of the shoulders is typically great, especially in freestyle, backstroke, and butterfly. Much of the power and efficiency in swimming comes from the torso, and much of this would not be accessible without adequate spinal flexibility from the neck to the lower back. Hip and ankle mobility are important for efficient kick.

Below are stretches recommended for swimmers:

- Shoulder Horizontal Adductors (Fig. 5.9)
- Shoulder Extensors (Fig. 5.6)
- Shoulder Adductors (Fig. 5.8)
- Shoulder Flexors (Fig. 5.5)
- Shoulder Internal Rotators (Fig. 5.11)
- Shoulder External Rotators (Fig. 5.12)
- Cervical Flexors (Fig. 5.2)
- Cervical Rotators (Fig. 5.4)

- Spinal Flexors (Fig. 5.21)
- Spinal Extensors (Fig. 5.20)
- Spinal Rotators (Fig. 5.23)
- Hip Flexors (Fig. 5.24)
- Hip Extensors (Fig. 5.25)
- Ankle Dorsiflexors (Fig. 5.32)
- Ankle Plantarflexors (Fig. 5.33B)
- Hip Adductors (Fig. 5.26)

TENNIS

In addition to the obvious need for shoulder, forearm, and wrist mobility, tennis demands particular mobility and strength of the torso. Rapid and repetitive stops, starts, and direction changes stress the lower extremities in all planes of motion, and therefore require adequate flexibility throughout the lower extremities.

Below are stretches recommended for tennis players:
- Shoulder Horizontal Adductors (Fig. 5.9)
- Shoulder Adductors (Fig. 5.8)
- Shoulder External Rotators (Fig. 5.12)
- Shoulder Internal Rotators (Fig. 5.11)
- Shoulder Flexors (Fig. 5.5)
- Wrist and Finger Flexors (Fig. 5.18)
- Wrist and Finger Extensors (Fig. 5.17)
- Forearm Supinators (Fig. 5.15)
- Forearm Pronators (Fig. 5.16)
- Spinal Rotators (Fig. 5.23)
- Spinal Flexors (Fig. 5.21)
- Spinal Extensors (Fig. 5.20)
- Spinal Side-benders (Fig. 5.22)
- Hip Adductors (Fig. 5.26)
- Hip Abductors (Fig. 5.27)
- Hip Flexors (Fig. 5.24)
- Hip Extensors (Fig. 5.25)
- Knee Flexors (Fig. 5.30A)
- Knee Extensors (Fig. 5.31)
- Ankle Plantarflexors (Fig. 5.33B)
- Ankle Dorsiflexors (Fig. 5.32)
- Ankle Invertors (Fig. 5.34)
- Ankle Evertors (Fig. 5.35)

TRACK AND FIELD

From high jump to shot put, hurdles to the mile, the diversity of demands placed on the body by this category of sport are endless. Throwers may need to concentrate on shoulder, wrist, and forearm flexibility, while sprinters and jumpers may concentrate on the hips, thighs, and calves. All track and field athletes should benefit from a flexible spine and torso. As the individual events may have widely varying demands, athletes should seek the specific advice of knowledgeable coach and staff; however, some generally helpful stretches are provided here.

Below are stretches recommended for track and field athletes:

- Shoulder Flexors (Fig. 5.5)
- Shoulder Extensors (Fig. 5.6)
- Shoulder Horizontal Adductors (Fig. 5.9)
- Shoulder Internal Rotators (Fig. 5.11)
- Shoulder External Rotators (Fig. 5.12)
- Wrist and Finger Flexors (Fig. 5.18)
- Wrist and Finger Extensors (Fig. 5.17)
- Forearm Supinators (Fig. 5.15)
- Forearm Pronators (Fig. 5.16)
- Hip Flexors (Fig. 5.24)
- Hip Extensors (Fig. 5.25)
- Hip Abductors (Fig. 5.27)
- Hip Adductors (Fig. 5.26)
- Knee Flexors (Fig. 5.30A)
- Knee Extensors (Fig. 5.31)
- Ankle Plantarflexors (Fig. 5.33B)
- Ankle Dorsiflexors (Fig. 5.32)
- Cervical Flexors (Fig. 5.2)
- Cervical Rotators (Fig. 5.4)
- Cervical Side-benders (Fig. 5.3)
- Spinal Flexors (Fig. 5.21)
- Spinal Extensors (Fig. 5.20)
- Spinal Rotators (Fig. 5.23)
- Spinal Side-benders (Fig. 5.22)

VOLLEYBALL

Ballistic takeoffs and landings, rapid direction changes, and explosive upper extremity movements make whole-body flexibility a must. Particular care should be taken to stretch the muscles of the shoulders, upper and lower forearms, wrists and hands, neck, torso, hips, knees, ankles, and feet.

Below are stretches recommended for volleyball players:

- Shoulder Flexors (Fig. 5.5)
- Shoulder Extensors (Fig. 5.6)
- Shoulder Abductors (Fig. 5.7)
- Shoulder Adductors (Fig. 5.8)
- Shoulder Horizontal Adductors (Fig. 5.9)
- Shoulder Internal Rotators (Fig. 5.11)
- Shoulder External Rotators (Fig. 5.12)
- Elbow Flexors (Fig. 5.13)

- Elbow Extensors (Fig. 5.14)
- Forearm Pronators (Fig. 5.16)
- Forearm Supinators (Fig. 5.15)
- Wrist and Finger Flexors (Fig. 5.18)
- Wrist and Finger Extensors (Fig. 5.17)
- Cervical Flexors (Fig. 5.2)
- Cervical Rotators (Fig. 5.4)
- Spinal Flexors (Fig. 5.21)
- Spinal Extensors (Fig. 5.20)
- Spinal Rotators (Fig. 5.23)
- Hip Flexors (Fig. 5.24)
- Hip Extensors (Fig. 5.25)
- Hip Adductors (Fig. 5.26)
- Hip Abductors (Fig. 5.27)
- Knee Flexors (Fig. 5.30A)
- Knee Extensors (Fig. 5.31)
- Ankle Plantarflexors (Fig. 5.33B)
- Ankle Dorsiflexors (Fig. 5.32)

WEIGHTLIFTING

A balanced weightlifting program requires a balanced flexibility program. The stretching program, as the weightlifting program, should reflect balance between front and back, upper and lower, left and right. It also should be attentive to the individual's postural challenges, such as tight anterior chest and shoulders, which would require additional emphasis on stretching these areas. Individuals whose strengthening programs are heavy on a particular area, say for instance, calves, likely require an increased emphasis on stretching these areas to maintain optimal ROM at the ankle. The stretching program below is generally balanced, but slightly weighted to account for the more common imbalances seen in weightlifting programs. Common imbalances might include tightness in the anterior chest and shoulders, anterior upper arms, anterior torso, anterior thighs, and calves. As most weightlifting involves grip, stretching of the wrist and fingers are important. For information on assessing the individual for specific flexibility needs, consult Chapter 3. Posture is discussed in Chapter 7.

Below are stretches recommended for weight lifters:

- Cervical Flexors (Fig. 5.2)
- Cervical Extensors (Fig. 5.1)
- Cervical Side-benders (Fig. 5.3)
- Spinal Flexors (Fig. 5.21)
- Spinal Extensors (Fig. 5.20)
- Spinal Rotators (Fig. 5.23)
- Spinal Side-benders (Fig. 5.22)
- Shoulder Flexors (Fig. 5.5)
- Shoulder Extensors (Fig. 5.6)
- Shoulder Abductors (Fig. 5.7)

- Shoulder Adductors (Fig. 5.8)
- Shoulder Horizontal Adductors (Fig. 5.9)
- Shoulder Internal Rotators (Fig. 5.11)
- Elbow Flexors (Fig. 5.13)
- Elbow Extensors (Fig. 5.14)
- Forearm Pronators (Fig. 5.16)
- Forearm Supinators (Fig. 5.15)
- Wrist and Finger Flexors (Fig. 5.18)
- Wrist and Finger Extensors (Fig. 5.17)
- Intrinsic Hand Muscles (Fig. 5.19)
- Hip Flexors (Fig. 5.24)
- Hip Extensors (Fig. 5.25)
- Hip Adductors (Fig. 5.26)
- Hip Abductors (Fig. 5.27)
- Hip External Rotators (Fig. 5.29)
- Knee Flexors (Fig. 5.30A)
- Knee Extensors (Fig. 5.31)
- Ankle Plantarflexors (Fig. 5.33B)
- Ankle Dorsiflexors (Fig. 5.32)
- Ankle Invertors (Fig. 5.34)
- Ankle Evertors (Fig. 5.35)

SUMMARY

A specific flexibility program—designed to help the individual achieve optimal ROM, reduce the risk of injury, or restore normal movement following injury—is a very important part of any sports-conditioning program. Program design should consider not only the sport-specific demands, but also the needs of the individual. Individual needs should consider medical history, goals, and details as revealed in a flexibility assessment. Clinicians should keep abreast of a rapidly expanding body of relevant research and question applications of stretching that are not supported by it. After goals are set and the stretching program is implemented, the clinician should monitor the individual's progress so that he or she can make any necessary modifications to enhance the specificity and usefulness of that specific program.

REFERENCES

1. Craib MW, Mitchell VA, Fields KB, et al. The association between flexibility and running economy in sub-elite male distance runners. Med Sci Sports Exerc June 1996;28(6):737–743.

Stretching for Rehabilitation of Injuries

According to the Bureau of Labor Statistics, there were 270, 890 recorded back injuries and 503,530 injuries involving strains, sprains, and tears in the United States in 2005.[1] The cause of these injuries varies from falls and other accidents, childhood play, work-related trauma, assault, and injury during participation in some type of athletic activity. Participation in recreational sports may be a frequent cause of injury, as Requa et al found 475 injuries in 986 adult participants in recreational sports programs over a 12-week period.[2] Injury in team sports such as football and hockey are common; however, running, an activity in which many more Americans are engaged, may produce the most injuries overall. Running, especially that involving higher volumes, such as training for a marathon, is a frequent cause of overuse injuries. Bovens et al studied 73 runners training for a marathon for 18 months and found a staggering 85% of those in the study suffered at least one injury during that period.[3] Maughan et al found that 58% of the 497 respondents incurred some type of injury in their preparation for the marathon.[4] And a recent review by Fredericson et al found articles reporting injuries in nearly 90% of those training for marathons.[5]

Regardless of their cause, many injuries require some type of rehabilitation. We define *rehabilitation* as a regaining of appropriate range of motion (ROM), strength, and function. More traumatic, or severe injuries resulting in significant functional loss, require treatment in professionally managed rehabilitation programs. When the injury is less extensive and produces only mild to moderate dysfunction, opinions regarding the need for and type of professional intervention vary. If there is any question regarding the need for referral, a referral should be made. Generally, it makes most sense to begin with the individual's own primary care provider who may then make a referral to the appropriate rehabilitation provider if necessary. Although many individuals will not require ongoing hands-on therapy, most will benefit from an initial evaluation, and from having the appropriate rehabilitation professional monitor and modify their program at pre-determined intervals.

Prevention is the best medicine. Ultimately, prevention amounts to reducing the amount of risk to which one is exposed. The risk of injury can be reduced through physical conditioning, education in safety and body mechanics, worksite modification, and use of appropriate equipment. Physical conditioning should be directed at improving one's level of flexibility, strength, conditioning, and task-specific skill.

Despite our best efforts, injuries inevitably occur. These injuries warrant appropriate rehabilitation. Successful rehabilitation includes restoration of normal ROM, strength and function. Normal function is generally defined by achieving the skill to perform the task—be it a sport or an activity of daily living—as before the injury. This chapter covers the role of stretching and flexibility in the overall context of rehabilitation.

INITIAL APPROACH TO INJURY

Injuries may be described as originating from repetitive, traumatic, or prolonged static stress. *Repetitive strain injuries,* which often occur as a result of work-related movements and are discussed further in Chapter 8, generally result from excessive repetition involving an otherwise tolerable stress, such as typing on a computer keyboard or running a power drill. In contrast, *traumatic injuries* result from a single bout of excessive force, such as when a person slips and falls on an icy sidewalk. Excessive time spent in one position, such as long haul truck driving, may result in *prolonged static stress injury,* in this case to the driver's lumbar disc or posterior supporting ligaments. In either case, the rehabilitation of these injuries should be considered quite seriously.

Addressing the Mechanism of Injury

The mechanism of injury must be acknowledged and addressed. This advice might seem obvious, especially if the individual's injury results from trauma. But in cases of repetitive or prolonged static injuries, the mechanism of the injury may not be so clear, so determining it may take some investigative work. Tennis might be the cause of an individual's elbow pain, but what aspect of tennis? Is the racket improperly strung? Or is the individual repetitively hitting the ball off-center of the racket face, causing excessive torque at the elbow? Could the size of the grip be the culprit? Or, is the individual simply playing too long or too often, especially if there has been little buildup to this level?

Running injuries may also result from a myriad of factors. Did the injury result from too much, or too rapid, an increase in mileage? Or did the injury result from poor mechanics, placing excessive stresses and strains on particular musculoskeletal, joint, or ligamentous structures? Are the running shoes appropriate for the individual's mechanics? Do they fit properly?

Whatever the cause, the mechanism of injury must be determined and modified or eliminated. Quitting tennis, running, or any other activity for a period of time is an option, but most people would rather continue to participate in their activity while undergoing a treatment intervention. To pursue the most effective intervention, we must first stop and investigate the cause and the mechanism leading to the strain or trauma. Failure to do so can merely delay a much more serious injury.

Once you have determined the mechanism of injury and have made the necessary modifications to the activity to mitigate the excess stress, you can then focus on maintenance or restoration of appropriate levels of ROM, conditioning, and coordination specific to the activity during the rehabilitation process. Appropriate modifications of the causal activity can also be prescribed by knowledgeable coaches or professionals involved in the activity. If this is not possible, or is proving unsuccessful, it is prudent to consult a trusted healthcare provider who is familiar with the activity.

Of course, there are situations in which the best solution is indeed the cessation of the activity in question. In these cases, alternative activities may be substituted, preferably ones that share common movement patterns and muscle groups, yet are different enough to allow participation without any exacerbation of the active symptoms. A good example of this substitution is the use of the elliptical trainer for an injury derived from running. Full weight-bearing use of the legs in a reciprocal motion with limited knee flexion make it a reasonable substitute, but only if it can be performed without aggravating the injury.

More serious injuries may require total cessation of the activity and all related activities. Cessation may need to continue for weeks or months depending on the severity of the injury. Generally, if this is the case, the injured individual will be under his or her own physician's care, and the length of the layoff will be determined by that physician and/or a rehabilitation specialist to which the individual has been referred.

Stretching Injured Tissues

How often have you heard someone explain that they are "stretching out" an injury? Their back hurts and they bend forward and sideways to relieve the tension, or their hamstring is strained and they are bending forward with their leg up on a chair to "stretch it out."

Is stretching in this manner helpful or harmful? As usual, it depends. Our bodies seem to have an intrinsic sense of what is healthful and what is harmful. We all assume positions to relieve stresses on particular joints without being educated to do so. In particular, stretching to relieve tension in particular joints or muscles may be useful in many situations, but it may also delay healing or even exacerbate an injury.

Determining whether or not to recommend stretching out an injury involves consideration of both the timing and mechanism of injury and the individual's report of symptoms. If the individual has sustained a tension-related injury, such as a strain to the hamstring while lifting a box or an ankle sprain while sprinting around the bases, it would make no sense to stretch it to further lengthen the tissue. Instead, the individual's ROM can be maintained, and gradually progressed back to the pre-injury state, by active range of motion exercises. (See "Active Range of Motion" under "Increasing ROM/Flexibility.")

On the other hand, chronic aches and stiffness often respond immediately and appropriately to stretching. Careful stretching of muscles to relieve "aching" or "stiff" muscles or joints to a point at which the symptoms are relieved is appropriate. The stretch should not re-create or exacerbate the pain. As we have emphasized throughout this book, pain is generally a sign that damage is imminent. Chapter 2 provided guidelines for stretching at an effective intensity without placing excessive stress on the muscular, ligamentous, or joint tissues.

Applying Rest Ice Compression Elevation (RICE)

Depending on the severity of the injury, stopping the inflammation may be the first priority. Particularly with traumatic injuries that involve severe pain, obvious swelling, and/or redness, the application of ice is paramount to manage pain and prevent the progression of the injury due to swelling and inflammation. Obviously, immediate medical attention should be instigated for any traumatic injuries that involve severe bleeding, loss of consciousness, seizure, or possible spinal injuries.

For less emergent cases involving trauma or acute overuse injury involving pain and inflammation, most athletic and healthcare providers would recommend the use of *rest, ice, compression,* and *elevation*–RICE.

Use the RICE acronym for Rest Ice Compression Elevation (Fig. 10.1):

- Rest the injury. Depending on severity of the injury the individual may need to stop, or at least modify, the offending activity. In more involved cases, he or she should stop all activity involving the injured tissues. Rest is often the most overlooked aspect of dealing with injured tissues, particularly in athletes or other people who are often reluctant to stop their activity.

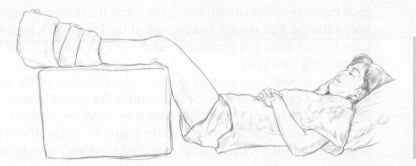

FIGURE 10.1
Applying RICE post-injury. Patient is supine 90/90 with the injured limb elevated and ice applied.

- Ice the injury. Though many variables exist and much research needs to be done, the general consensus confirms the value of ice therapy for the reduction of pain. Hubbard et al reviewed 55 related articles and found that ice consistently reduced pain when used as a modality following injury.[6] Ice may be applied via the use of crushed ice, gel packs, or ice massage. There are also a number of different commercially available icing modalities such as Cryo-Cuff (registered trademark). In reality, the mode of application is much less relevant than the effect of the cold. Cooling the tissue to reduce inflammation is the primary goal. According to MacAuley, the target temperature is a reduction of about 10–15 degrees C (50–60° F).[7]

  It is generally accepted that ice should be applied for 15–20 minutes, though some recent studies suggest icing is more effective if applied intermittently for shorter periods. Bleakley et al showed those subjects treated with an intermittent protocol of 10 minutes on, 10 minutes off, 10 minutes on, repeated every 2 hours showed enhanced pain relief as compared with those using the standard 20-minute protocol, also applied every 2 hours.[8] In a review article, MacAuley concluded that icing in repeated 10-minute applications was also more effective than in the standard protocol.[7]

- Compress the injured tissue. In cases where swelling is present, compression may help moderate or even reduce its severity. Compression may be achieved with the use of an ace wrap or compression stocking. Kraemer et al studied the effects of compression on pain and recovery in muscles subjected to maximal eccentric exercise.[9] They found that compression helped decrease resulting inflammation, decrease perceived pain, lowered levels of creatine kinase (a marker for DOMS), and accelerated recovery of force production in muscles. In addition, more specific or "focal" compression may be more helpful than general compression.[10] An example of focal compression is the use of a horseshoe-shaped pad fitted around the lateral malleolus in the case of an ankle sprain to help the compression form more closely to the shape of the leg.

- Elevate the injury. As inflammation *is* an accumulation of fluid in the injured area, and excessive amounts of fluid may result in increased pain and is counterproductive to healing tissues. Elevation of the injured limb helps reduce the amount of swelling and allows for more optimal healing of the injured tissues.

LONG-TERM REHABILITATION OF INJURY

As noted in the introduction to this chapter, complete rehabilitation requires the restoration of not only the pre-injury levels of strength and ROM, but also of balance, coordination, and task-specific skills. Achieving these goals in a safe and timely fashion is often quite challenging. It is necessary to provide the healing tissues with sufficient physical stimulation to cause related tissues to adapt in the desired manner (i.e., improved strength, ROM, etc.). This physical stimulation may be in the form of tensile or compressive forces generated by stretching or muscular contraction. An inadequate challenge may fail to stimulate healing or promote sufficient adaptation to prepare the body for safe return to activity. Excessive stress in terms of resistance, frequency, or duration may interfere with the healing of tissues or, worse, exacerbate the injury.

Inadequate rehabilitation following injury may prove to be a large factor in re-injury. Many people experience an incomplete return of ROM following a sprained ankle or a fractured bone in the foot or leg. In many cases, the individual may not even be aware of this until it is discovered years later, perhaps during an evaluation for another injury. For example, it is not uncommon for a significant loss of ankle dorsiflexion, or subtalar inversion-eversion, to persist for years after the original injury. This restriction in motion may alter the individual's mechanics and may, over time, lead to knee, hip, or back pain. Incomplete return of appropriate functional strength may also be a factor in injuries occurring months or even years later. Failing to restore sufficient hip abduction strength to an individual whose ankle was immobilized and nonweightbearing for 6 weeks may seem inconsequential in the early return to activity; however, as lower extremity biomechanics may have been altered by the weakness, patello-femoral, hip, or lower back pain may be the long-term result. Often, these individuals were told they needed no therapy or other professional guidance, and that their normal motion and function would return without any further professional intervention.

Some clinicians advocate the complete return of normal ROM before attempting to regain strength. Though opinions vary, each case is individual, and the clinician should pursue the return of flexibility, strength, conditioning, balance, coordination, and functional skills simultaneously, within the constraints imposed on each by the details of the particular injury. Generally, there is no reason strength should not be pursued early on; however, the resistance may be quite limited. In some cases the resistance may be less than the weight of the limb; in such cases, assisted exercise may be necessary, in which some of the weight of the limb is essentially reduced or removed by assistance of an external force such as the individual's un-injured limb, or via the assistance of the clinician. Certainly, there are cases in which no resistance should be applied, but these are generally severe enough to have already required medical intervention. If the injury is obviously severe, or you are unsure as to how to proceed, referral to a physician is prudent.

Increasing Range of Motion and Flexibility

Restoration of ROM is an essential component of rehabilitation. In most cases, the goal of rehabilitation is the return of all of the pre-injury ROM. With serious, traumatic injuries or in post surgical cases, however, the goal may be simply to attain a functional ROM—an ROM that allows the individual to participate safely in the desired activity. For example, a patient who has undergone total knee replacement might be able to regain 120 degrees of knee flexion, enabling the patient to climb stairs (Livingston et al),[11] whereas a return of the "normal" 140 degrees (White et al) of ROM is unlikely.[12]

Before continuing our discussion of ROM, it is important to distinguish between two distinct types of ROM: active range of motion (AROM) and passive (PROM). AROM involves motion created by the muscles producing motion at the particular joint, whereas PROM involves motion driven by forces created outside of the joint.

ACTIVE RANGE OF MOTION

AROM exercise has several benefits. One benefit is that the use of the muscle encourages blood flow, which is essential in healing. This mechanical action of the muscle combined with enhanced blood flow may reduce local inflammation. Another benefit of AROM is its inherent safety factor. The use of active contraction of the injured muscle's antagonist to safely produce motion in the agonist muscle itself establishes both a safe range in which to continue moving and a built-in system of progressing. The use of active contraction of the antagonists to help with rehabilitation of the injured agonist is described in more detail below.

AROM exercise can be started early on in the rehabilitation program as long as the individual pays close attention to sensations in the injured area. If active range is painful with the injured muscle-tendon unit, active motion can be introduced with the antagonist muscles to promote passive movement at the injured tissue. For example, an injured triceps muscle may be too painful to allow active contraction; however, active contraction of the biceps shortens the biceps, bringing the forearm toward the humerus (assuming a standing position). The triceps is thus passively lengthened (Fig. 10.2A). When the biceps is allowed to relax and contract eccentrically, the forearm falls and the triceps is allowed to shorten (Fig. 10.2B). In this manner, the injured triceps can be taken through its available pain-free range with little force requirement from the triceps itself. As the injured tissue heals, more pain-free range will be available, and this daily improvement can be progressed until full range is regained.

Involving the antagonist in AROM is quite simple; however, it does require forethought. The body must be set up in such a way as to allow gravity to resist and lengthen the antagonist muscle. In the example above (see Fig. 10.2A above), the agonist, or triceps, does not have to work against gravity; instead, the biceps does. If the injured muscle were the biceps, this position would have to be changed. In this case, we could raise the straight arm directly overhead, then allow the triceps to relax and the elbow to flex while maintaining the humerus directly overhead. The triceps would be raising and lowering the forearm against gravity, and the biceps would be "going along for the ride."

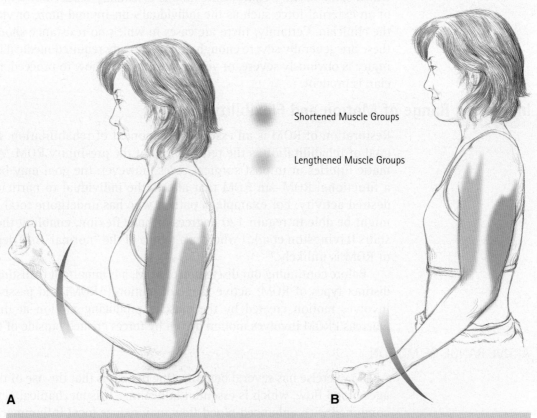

Shortened Muscle Groups

Lengthened Muscle Groups

A   B

FIGURE 10.2 Triceps. **A.** Lengthening with shortening biceps. **B.** Shortening with eccentric lengthening of biceps.

When there is no longer any pain with contraction of the injured muscle, active exercise can be begun to strengthen it. Strengthening should be begun with very low loads and progressed carefully. Strengthening is covered later in this chapter.

> ⚠ **CAUTION!** If no progress in ROM is attained over time, especially if many days or weeks have passed, the individual should be referred to his or her primary care physician.

PASSIVE RANGE OF MOTION AND STATIC STRETCHING

When active ROM is no longer producing results over time, PROM can be introduced. Again, PROM is range attained by the application of external forces, as opposed to that attained by the contraction of the muscles crossing the joint.

The difference between AROM and PROM is shown in the following examples. In Figure 10.3A, active contraction of the individual's quadriceps (AROM) is causing passive lengthening of the hamstrings (PROM). This is as opposed to PROM's use of outside forces, such as the clinician's hands, the force applied by gravity, or by muscles other than those about the joint being targeted. Figure 10.3B shows an example of PROM applied by a clinician, and 10.3C shows PROM applied by the individual, with the lever being the forward leaning trunk.

It is generally considered PROM when a clinician moves a client's joint through a particular ROM without the assistance of that client. As the amount of force and the particular techniques with which these stretching forces are applied vary greatly, they should be performed only by those trained in these techniques. We will consider the use of static stretching, which is a form of PROM, below.

Since static stretching is the application of external forces to produce movement and improve the mobility of (in this case) recovering tissues, it should initially be undertaken very carefully. If the individual does not experience increased pain during or after the stretch, than the stretch can be progressed according to standard stretching protocol. (See Chapters 2 and 3 for details.)

> ⚠ **CAUTION!** Severe or chronic joint pain experienced during any type of PROM should be cause for alarm. Attempt to determine the reason for this pain and modify or eliminate the application of the stretching force. In case of uncertainty, referral to the primary care provider is always the prudent option.

Regaining Strength

Regaining strength means much more than being able to lift the same amount of weight as before the injury. It also means being able to perform specific activities at the pre-injury level of intensity, resistance, and skill. Return of normal strength is critical not only in the performance of the particular sport or activity, but also to help prevent the recurrence of injury. However, in some instances, graded return to activity is possible before complete return of strength.

GOALS OF STRENGTHENING INJURED TISSUES

Exercise for the injured joint and its associated tissues should first be designed to do no harm. It should neither cause further damage nor interfere with the healing process. Next, the exercise should be designed to stimulate healing. This generally means bringing much-needed blood flow to the area. In addition, exercise should appropriately load the cartilage to stimulate growth of new tissue, as well as load the

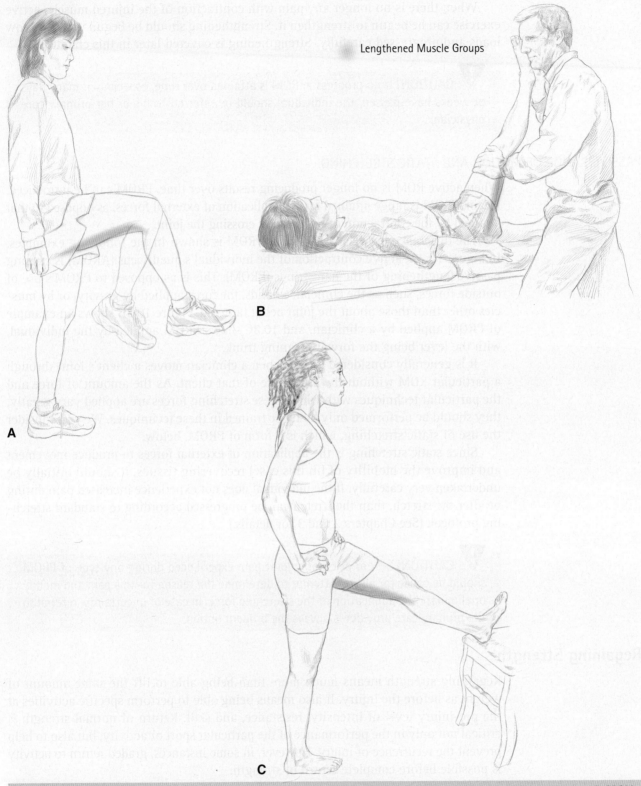

Lengthened Muscle Groups

FIGURE 10.3 Hamstring. **A.** AROM of the hamstring: an individual standing with hip flexed to 90 degrees and knee extending. **B.** PROM of the hamstring: an individual having her hamstring stretched by a clinician. **C.** PROM of the hamstring: an individual stretching her hamstring muscles using static stretching.

tendons in order to encourage the new tissue to be laid down in an orientation appropriate to resist the forces to which it will eventually be subjected.

> ⚠ **CAUTION!** Strengthening exercises should *not* cause pain in the injured tissues. Pain in the injured tissues is generally cause for modification or elimination of the exercise in question. It is for this reason that the clinician and the client should become quite familiar with the various sensations experienced during the performance of exercises. This is true even if the pain experienced is not during the exercise, but even for hours or days following.

EXERCISES FOR STRENGTHENING INJURED TISSUES

Resistance training is generally the preferred method for regaining strength and can be an excellent modality if part of a well-designed program. Various methods of resistance training exist, each having their respective advantages and disadvantages.

Resistance machines offer the benefits of safety and convenience as the individual's movements are guided and limited by the machine itself. This allows the individual to concentrate on the particular movement pattern and decreases the chances of dropping the weight and causing injury. Free weights, on the other hand, require that the individual uses more balance and coordination while performing the lift, necessitating the use of stabilizing muscles in addition to those under primary load. The thoughtful practitioner will be able to combine different modalities to design the most appropriate program for the client undergoing rehabilitation.

As the strengthening program progresses, the exercises can be progressed from general movements to exercises that more accurately approximate the movements demanded by the activity or sport. Sport cords, cable pulleys, surgical tubing, etc. can be incorporated to vary the planes of resistance and further mimic the activity and attack more specific movement weaknesses. Take for example a basketball player whose movement pattern during jumping (weight bearing knee flexion) tends to be excessive hip adduction and internal rotation (Fig. 10.4). To reduce this tendency, we might consider strengthening both the hip abductors and the hip external rotators. To do this, we might have the athlete perform one-legged standing hip abduction with the sport cord attached to the forefoot (Fig. 10.5). In this manner, the sport cord is trying to internally rotate and adduct the femur via the foot and lower leg, necessitating the use of the hip external rotators. The sport cord is also resisting abduction at the hip.

A rehabilitative program includes strength training exercises for the whole body as well as for the injured joint (or joints). Whole-body programs should be balanced and include muscles on both sides of the body—those that flex and those that extend all of the joints. In general, programs can be designed to address opposing joint movements to assure balance in strength development. This can easily be accomplished by planning exercises for antagonistic movements (Fig. 10.6A and B). For example, an exercise involving a "push," such as a seated chest press or bench press, can easily be balanced by a resisted rowing exercise (a "pull"). Likewise, an overhead press can be balanced by a lat pull down; a leg extension exercise by a leg curl; and so on.

RESISTANCE AND REPETITIONS

Exercises involving the injured tissue should be performed cautiously, with relatively low loads and a relatively high frequency In most cases, individuals will not injure themselves with an amount of weight they can lift 20–30 times under control. Therefore, a useful protocol is to exercise the injured joint or muscle with a light weight allowing 25 repetitions without pain, one to two times daily, 4–6 days per week. Pain

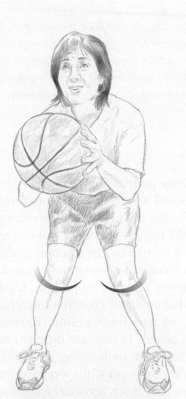

FIGURE 10.4 A basketball player squatting to jump. Shows excessive hip adduction and internal rotation and genu valgum.

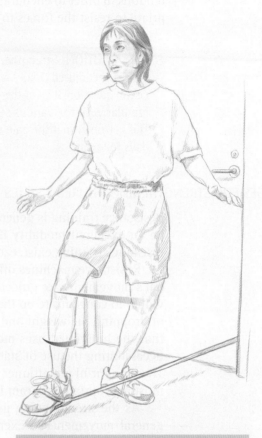

FIGURE 10.5 Athlete performing resisted abduction and external rotation with sport cord.

is not acceptable during or after the exercises, and, if encountered, should cause you to modify or eliminate the exercise. As the injury heals, the resistance may be progressed to eventually meet the pre-injury protocols. The ACSM (Haskell et al) recommends 8–10 exercises at a resistance allowing for 8–12 repetitions performed on two or more nonconsecutive days each week for healthy individuals.[13]

As the individual progresses, adjustments to the resistance can be made to accommodate improved strength and coordination, as well as modified goals. After 4 to 6 weeks, the individual's musculoskeletal system should have adapted to the resistance exercise, and it should be safe to move on to more aggressive programs (i.e., more resistance, lower repetitions, and possibly an increased number of sets), though it is not necessary to do this. Generally, the more strength required during the sport or activity, the greater the resistance and the lower the repetitions should be. For example, weightlifters or football linemen may have programs that include work at near maximal resistance, with multiple sets, at as little as 3–6 repetitions. In contrast, runners or cyclists, who would not benefit from the increased bulk of such a program but want to improve their strength and muscular endurance, might follow programs based around multiple sets of 12–15 repetitions at lower weights.

In general, however, rehabilitation programs should involve more exercises with one or more sets of relatively light resistance. Choosing weights that allow for 20–30 repetitions assures that individuals will not use too much resistance and encourages increased blood flow useful in healing tissues. Using a greater variety of exercises rather than multiple sets assures that the muscles and joints are challenged by a greater

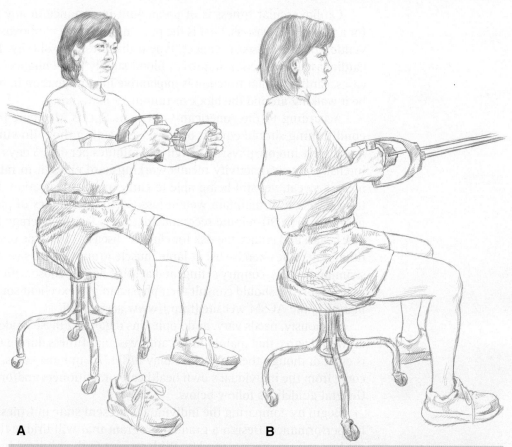

FIGURE 10.6 An exerciser performing **A.** seated chest press and **B.** seated row

variety of stimuli and resistance in a number of planes, which more approximates how the muscles and joints will be used in real life. Such challenges can promote functional strengthening rather than just improved strength in selected directions. Additional information regarding training and conditioning may be found in Appendix A.

FREQUENCY

The recommended frequency appropriate for resistance training varies greatly and may be effected by injury type, stage of rehabilitation, type of resistance training, desired outcomes, and, of course, theory. Generally, the smaller the resistance, the more frequently it may be applied. Patients in the early stages of in-patient rehabilitation may have two physical therapy appointments in the same day, as the loads that they are able to tolerate are relatively very light and do not require significant rest between performances. In contrast, a power lifter may be lifting such extreme relative weights that he or she may only be able to perform the exercise once per week. Most individuals should perform specific rehabilitation-related exercises 4 to 5 times per week and general strengthening exercises 2 to 3 times per week.

Conditioning

Conditioning includes both the cardiovascular system and the musculoskeletal system, as improved cardiovascular function is not possible without specific musculoskeletal changes. Our focus here will be the cardiovascular system, as training for the musculoskeletal system is covered above and the details of adaptations of the musculoskeletal system resulting from cardiovascular loads is beyond the scope of this text.

Cardiovascular fitness is of paramount importance in any rehabilitation program for a number of reasons. First is the proven benefits of cardiovascular fitness in the prevention of heart disease, cancer, type II diabetes, and obesity. Furthermore, enhanced cardiovascular function improves blood supply and enhances healing. And, in most cases, cardiovascular function is imperative in participation in the individual's activity, be it walking around the block or running a marathon.

According to the American College of Sports Medicine (ACSM), cardiovascular conditioning should consist of exercise meeting the following guidelines: Perform moderately intense physical activity 30 minutes per day, 5 days per week.[14] "Moderate-intensity physical activity means working hard enough to raise your heart rate and break a sweat, yet still being able to carry on a conversation. It should be noted that to lose weight or maintain weight loss, 60 to 90 minutes of physical activity may be necessary. The 30-minute recommendation is for the average healthy adult to maintain health and reduce the risk for chronic disease." The type of exercise should be continuous aerobic exercise using large muscle groups such as walking, cycling, running, swimming, cross-country skiing, and aerobic dance. Those with special challenges such as heart disease should consult their physician. An excellent source of additional information is the ACSM website (http://www.acsm.org/).

Obviously, needs vary, as do opinions regarding these guidelines. Most professionals would agree that maintaining cardiovascular fitness during the rehabilitation phase is critical, though their strategies may differ. As in most cases, the best advice should come from the individual's own healthcare practitioners and/or training professionals. General guidelines follow below.

Begin by comparing the individual's present state of fitness with the desired level for performance. Design a gradual program that will bridge this gap, with relatively modest gains occurring weekly. With respect to their injury, individuals should avoid working out "until it hurts," as the programs should be designed so that each successive workout can be achieved at an intensity and duration that is *below the threshold of pain*. The training program should be similar to that which the individual followed before the injury and should consider the guidelines listed above.

For those participating in activities in which performance is not significantly affected by cardiovascular performance, cardiovascular health is still of significant importance. These individuals should consider walking, swimming, or using a bike, elliptical trainer, stair climber, etc. to develop a cardiovascular training program that meets the guidelines just stated.

Development of Functional Skills and Balance

It is not enough to restore normal ROM, strength, and cardiovascular conditioning. All of these components must be developed in such a way as to improve the individual's functional performance. This involves also restoring pre-injury levels of motor control. Motor control may be thought of as the ultimate ability of the body to perform the task; it includes balance, and coordination. It makes use of sufficient strength and ROM.

Balance is affected by input from the visual, vestibular, somatosensory, and proprioceptive systems. *Proprioception* may be defined as the body's ability to sense where its parts are in space. If you close your eyes and bend your elbow, you know it is moving even though you cannot see it. This is possible because of a complex system of neurologic receptors located in your joints, tendons, and ligaments. These receptors collect information about joint position, movement, and movement speed and relay this information to your central nervous system. Injury to tendons and ligaments may disrupt the function of the proprioceptive system and thereby hinder balance and the ultimate performance of the functional task. It is for this reason that functional training should involve proprioceptive/balance challenges, such as unstable surfaces or complex tasks.

Exercises can be performed on wobble boards, foam rolls, etc. to increase the proprioceptive/balance challenge. In this way, the appropriate strengthening task can be modified early on in the rehabilitation process. These exercises should challenge all planes of movement and should continue well into the late stages of rehabilitation.

Strength training in particular should focus on functional movement patterns as early as possible, as gross strength without appropriate balance and coordination will not yield the best performance results. As the rehabilitation progresses, exercises that approximate more nearly the individual's actual activities should command a higher percentage of the workout time. For athletes, a good deal of the advanced training should look like the performance of their sport. For nonathletes, the advanced training should more approximate the activities that were limited because of the injury. For example, an individual who was having difficulty standing up from a chair should eventually perform exercises in which he or she is performing squatting exercises that involve similar movement patterns to that involved in standing from a seated position.

SUMMARY

Injury risk can be reduced through education and appropriate physical conditioning. Education about an individual's particular activity, be it an activity of daily living or a sport, including the physical demands and the inherent risk factors, may help reduce the risk of injury. Specific training programs designed to build the necessary levels strength, cardiovascular conditioning, flexibility, and task-specific skill may help further reduce the risk of injury in these individuals.

Inevitably, injuries occur and their complete rehabilitation is essential not only to return individuals to full and productive life, but also to prevent new or recurrent injuries. A complete rehabilitation program should address ROM, general and specific strength, general and specific conditioning, and return of functional skills, all to at least pre-injury levels. Flexibility training may begin with either active or passive range of motion, depending upon the specifics of the injury, and then later progressed to static stretching as needed. Strength training begins with regaining the ability to move through a full ROM, on to lightly resisted high repetition exercise, and finally toward higher resistances and more specific movement patterns. The recovery of functional skills should begin with exercises resembling the particular sport or activity as early as possible, within the constraints of that particular injury and progressing throughout the rehabilitation program toward actual return to activity.

REFERENCES

1. Bureau of Labor Statistics. Injuries, Illnesses and Fatalities. 2005. Available at: http://www.bls.gov/iif/home.htm. Accessed August 28, 2007.
2. Requa RK, DeAvilla LN, Garrick JG. Injuries in recreational adult fitness activities. Am J Sports 1993;21:461–467
3. Bovens AM, Janssen GME, Vermeer HGW, et al. Occurrence of running injuries in adults following a supervised training program. Int J Sports Med 1989;10:S18.
4. Maughan RJ, Miller JD. Incidence of training-related injuries among marathon runners. Br J Sports Med September 1983;17(3):162–165.
5. Fredericson M, Misra AK. Epidemiology and aetiology of marathon running injuries. Sports Med 2007;37(4–5):437–439.
6. Hubbard TJ, Denegar CR. Does cryotherapy improve outcomes With soft tissue injury? J Athl Train September 2004;39(3):278–279.
7. MacAuley DC. Ice therapy: how good is the evidence? Int J Sports Med July 2001;22(5):379–384.

8. Bleakley CM, McDonough SM, MacAuley DC, et al. Br J Sports Med August 2006;40(8):700–705:discussion 705. Epub 2006 Apr 12.

9. Kraemer WJ, Bush JA, Wickham RB, et al. Influence of compression therapy on symptoms following soft tissue injury from maximal eccentric exercise. J Orthop Sports Phys Ther June 2001;31(6):282–290.

10. Wilkerson GB, Horn-Kingery HM. Treatment of the inversion ankle sprain: comparison of different modes of compression and cryotherapy. J Orthop Sports Phys Ther May 1993;17(5):240–246.

11. Livingston LA, Stevenson JM, Olney SJ. Stair climbing kinematics on stairs of differing dimensions. Arch Phys Med Rehabil May 1991;72(6):398–402.

12. White DJ, Norkin CC. Measurement of Joint Motion. A Guide to Goniometry. 3rd Ed. Philadelphia: FA Davis Company, 2003.

13. Haskell WM, Lee I, Pate RR, et al. Physical Activity and Public Health: Updated Recommendation for Adults from the American College of Sports Medicine and the American Heart Association. Med Sci Sports Ex 2007; Special Reports.

14. American College of Sports Medicine (ACSM). Physical Activity and Public Health Guidelines. 2007. Available at: http://www.acsm.org/AM/Template.cfm?Section=Home_Page&TEMPLATE=/CM/HTMLDisplay.cfm&CONTENTID=7764. Accessed August 29, 2007.

Advanced Stretching

With contributions by Tamara Hlava

When hearing of advanced stretching, many people might imagine the participants stretched into impossibly contorted positions, as in a bad game of "Twister." Fortunately, advanced stretching, as defined here, is not at all complicated and does not require an unusually flexible body. Instead, the word *advanced* implies a form of stretching that can take place easily once the individual has achieved a certain level of body awareness. This in turn is derived from experience, an improved understanding of anatomy and physiology, and an awareness of one's posture, movements, balance, and relative comfort or pain. Developing an improved sense of body awareness empowers the individual to be able to perform a wider variety of stretches and combinations of stretches directed at a greater variety of movement challenges.

Clinicians are often challenged to develop stretches that serve clients' unique needs, whether to enhance the performance of a particular movement through improved range of motion (ROM) or to moderate particular symptoms with stretching exercises. One may be need to create stretching exercises that address two or more joints simultaneously or that stretch nonmuscular structures such as nerve or joint capsular tissue. One might determine that one or more stretching aids, such as a physiotherapy ball or surgical tubing, would be beneficial or may decide to integrate into a traditional stretching program principles from a complementary field such as *hatha yoga* or proprioceptive neuromuscular facilitation (PNF). This chapter provides the information that will help integrate these and other advanced techniques into individualized stretching programs.

COMBINATION STRETCHES

Individuals who achieved a solid understanding of the fundamental principles of stretching, as covered in Chapter 2, and have developed an accurate sense of intensity and related body awareness may derive further benefit from stretching more than one muscle group simultaneously.

> **CAUTION!** As always, the clinician and the client should pay close attention to the sensations experienced during the stretches. Pain in the joint(s) should not be tolerated and the exercise should be modified to eliminate the joint pain. Especially if this joint pain is severe, consultation with the individual's primary care practitioner may be prudent.

Benefits of Combination Stretching

Stretching muscles at more than one joint simultaneously may prove useful in terms of overall function. As most, if not all, activities and sports involve simultaneous movement at one or more joints, it may be beneficial to stretch more than one muscle group at a time. For example, in an individual exhibiting tightness, stretching the ankle plantarflexors and the hip flexors on the same side may benefit an individual's gait because the end range of both dorsiflexion and hip extension are reached at the end of the stance phase (Fig. 11.1). Let's examine this example, and other examples, in further detail below.

Examples of Combination Stretches

Consider a combined hip flexor and ankle plantarflexor stretch. As mentioned above, in normal walking mechanics, end-range ankle dorsiflexion and end-range hip extension occur at the same phase of gait. This phase comes at the completion of the stride (e.g., on the right foot), just before the right heel begins to lift prior to swinging the right foot forward. To stretch both of these movements simultaneously, the individual assumes the position for stretching the gastrocnemius (see Fig. 4.91): standing, with arms outstretched and supported against a wall or by a chairback, taking a step forward with the right (in this case) foot. While keeping the left foot in place, heel down, and knee straight, the individual moves his or her hips forward until a stretching sensation is felt in the right calf area. Now, by tilting the pelvis posteriorly (flattening, or flexing the lumbar spine), this individual may be able to achieve a simultaneous stretch of the psoas (Fig. 11.2).

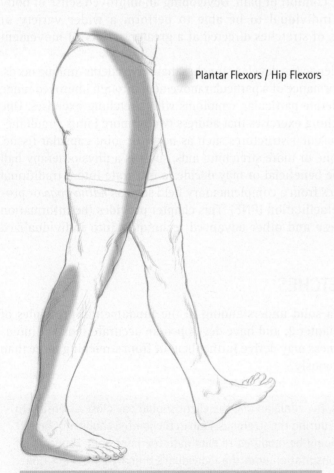

Plantar Flexors / Hip Flexors

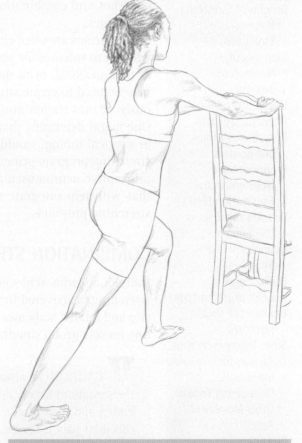

FIGURE 11.1 Right leg reaches end range dorsiflexion and hip extension simultaneously

FIGURE 11.2 Simultaneous stretch of ankle plantar-flexors and hip flexors

It may take a few trials before the individual feels both of these muscle groups stretching simultaneously, but it will become easier with practice and as awareness builds. Because the lumbar spine tends to hyperextend with hip extension, tilting the pelvis posteriorly to achieve a stretch of the psoas poses an additional challenge, which may require additional concentration, coordination, and awareness. Other combination stretches may pose similar biomechanical challenges. Although some individuals find it difficult to isolate movements occurring at separate joints, most succeed with a little focus and practice.

Another example is a "hurdler stretch" (Figure 11.3). Here, the individual, with careful attention, might safely accomplish a stretch of both the hamstrings of the left leg and the adductors of the right leg. Note that this individual has the right foot plantarflexed fully. This avoids the external rotation stress that might be applied at the knee by the tibia. A word of caution is in order here. Because of the possibility of excessive force being directed at the knee of the trailing leg, the individual performing the stretch should remain very aware of the sensations experienced, and the stretch should be modified or discontinued if there is any knee pain or discomfort during the stretch. Professional consultation is recommended whenever there is uncertainty.

With this perspective, you can design exercises primarily to meet the needs of the desired movement pattern. For example, for a pitcher who wishes to improve his or her fastball, you might design a stretch that encompasses not only external rotation at the shoulder, but also horizontal abduction at the shoulder, extension and rotation at the thoracic and lumbar spines, ipsilateral hip extension, and so on (Fig. 11.4).

The number of possible stretching combinations is endless. You may design useful combinations by examining the components of motion necessary for successful performance of the desired task. Carefully applied forces and attention to detail will allow for the creation of safe and useful combination stretches if desired.

STRETCHING NONMUSCULAR STRUCTURES

It is possible to stretch tissues other than muscles, such as the spine or other joints. In fact, stretching will always involve tissues in addition to the intended musculotendinous unit. When we focus stretches on particular muscles or muscle groups, local con-

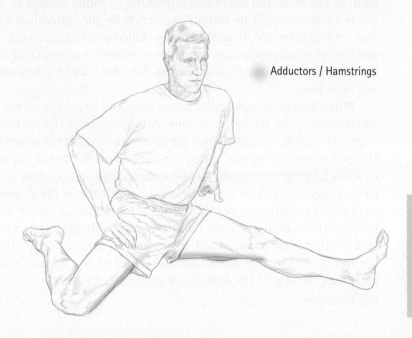

Adductors / Hamstrings

FIGURE 11.3
"Hurdler stretch."
Stretch of adductors
of the right leg and
hamstrings of the
left leg. Note
plantarflexion of
the left foot.

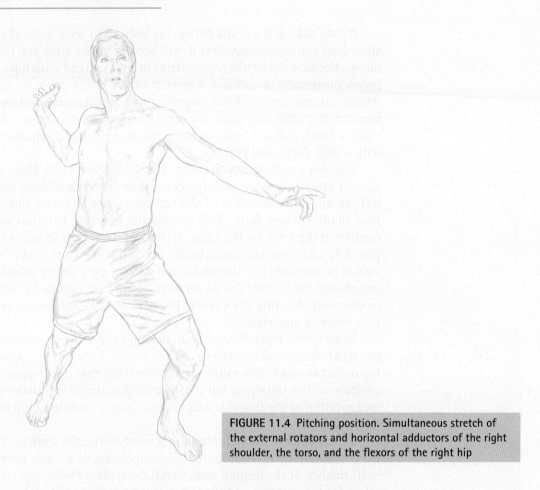

FIGURE 11.4 Pitching position. Simultaneous stretch of the external rotators and horizontal adductors of the right shoulder, the torso, and the flexors of the right hip

nective tissues and other joint structures, such as ligaments, nerves, and blood and lymph vessels, and skin, are also stretched to a certain degree.

We may choose to stretch the back or the neck, the knee or the ankle, rather than a particular muscle group. While successfully stretching the bony tissue is unlikely, stretching the ligamentous or capsular tissue surrounding the joints is possible and can be advantageous in certain circumstances. A clinician may choose to have a client stretch his or her spine to affect posture, or knee to restore normal extension. In any case, the attempted stretching of joints should be considered carefully. Injured joints should be initially screened by the individual's primary care physician and then treated, if necessary, by skilled practitioners such as osteopaths, chiropractors, physical or massage therapists, or athletic trainers. Once these joint restrictions have been treated, or medically cleared, then they can be safely addressed with stretching exercises.

When injury occurs, cases when only the ligament or the muscle involved in isolation are rare. Rather, a variable combination of tissues becomes damaged. The degree to which various tissues are involved in a stretch may be affected by injury. Depending on the type of injury sustained and the tissue involved, the percentage of stretch being attenuated by the muscle-tendon unit may be diminished. A routine example might be a muscle strain resulting in the deposition of scar tissue. In this case the primary resistance to stretching might be the scar tissue rather than the fascial components of the muscle-tendon unit. Another example might be injury to a joint, which might result in the joint capsule and or ligamentous structure becoming the primary restriction and target of any applied stretch. In these examples, lengthening of the scar tissue might be the primary objective of the stretching program.

> ⚠ **CAUTION!** It is again important to discern which tissue is under primary stretch. In the example discussed above, stretching scar tissue may prove quite useful by eliminating related movement restrictions. However, if continued stretching of the "scar" tissue results in continued increases in pain levels (especially if combined with reductions in ROM), the exercise should be modified or eliminated.

Benefits of Stretching Nonmuscular Structures

Stretching of joints such as the back, elbow, or knee may primarily be of benefit to restore normal motion to the respective joint. Often, when an injury occurs to or near a joint structure, the joint may become the primary restriction. Primary joint restriction may also be the long-term consequence of a particular postural problem resulting from poor workplace ergonomics or just plain poor postural habits. Restoration of normal movement may be of obvious importance in those cases where the joint limitation is affecting normal movement, such as a restricted ankle joint causing a limitation in stride length or a lack of knee flexion causing difficulty with ascending or descending stairs. Less obvious but still important might be the improvement or restoration of thoracic spine extension, allowing an improved positioning of the head and a resultant decrease in cervical symptoms.

Focused stretching of neurologic tissues should generally only be performed by professionals trained specifically in these techniques. Properly applied nerve stretching may be useful for the reduction of nerve-related pain or other related dysfunction.

> ⚠ **CAUTION!** Stretching that exacerbates nerve-related pain, especially if it escalates over repeated application, should be modified or eliminated. If unsure as to the nature of the pain, consultation with the individual's primary care practitioner may be prudent.

Examples of Nonmuscular Stretches

Stretching exercises, which in these cases may be applying the primary stress to the joint structures, should be undertaken with acute awareness as to the sensation(s) associated with performance. Individuals should maintain awareness not only of the sensations occurring while performing the exercise, but also of symptoms occurring immediately after the exercise and even during the following 1 or 2 days. Careful attention to the sensations experienced during the stretch will reveal whether the joint, the muscle-tendon unit, the nerve, or other connective tissue is being stretched. Anecdotal evidence suggests that most individuals can generally tell which tissues are under tension or compression. For instance, an individual may say, "That is not a muscle—it feels like nerve pain," or "It feels as if the joint is blocked." Although no one knows exactly what combination of tissues is really being stretched in any given exercise, if it feels as if the stretch is occurring in the joint, then it probably is.

> ⚠ **CAUTION!** Do not tolerate joint pain unless you are very sure of what is happening within the joint and have a very good reason for performing the stretch!

The spine provides a good example of nonmuscular tissues that may benefit from stretching. Many individuals experience movement restrictions of the spine that are attributable, at least in part, to the vertebral joints. While stretching of the actual bones is unlikely, the cartilaginous and ligamentous tissues may be modified with appropriate stretching forces. However, you should bear in mind that any hypomobility at a particular vertebral segment may be accompanied by a hypermobility at another segment. This is true of many joints, not only those of the spine. Because overstretching a hypermobile vertebral (or other) joint could cause further injury or dysfunction, individuals experiencing back, neck, or other joint pain, or who have known joint dysfunction should be referred to their primary healthcare provider.

As a specific example of a spinal stretch, let's consider the thoracic spine, which in many individuals is either excessively flexed or rounded. Chronic postures may, over time, result in structural changes in the joints, such as lengthened capsular and ligamentous structures posteriorly and shortened structures anteriorly. Carefully applied stretching forces may help counter these changes. In this case, extension of the thoracic spine may be accomplished by lying supine over a carefully placed towel, pillow, or therapy ball. Maintaining this position for at least 30 seconds should prove useful in extending the thoracic spine. An example of this stretch performed over a therapy ball is shown below, and described under "Using Stretching Aids" (Fig. 11.5).

A "stiff" ankle proposes another example in which the stretching forces may be focused primarily on joint versus musculotendinous structures. Significant restrictions in ankle dorsiflexion are often related to shortened joint structures. Carefully applied stretching forces with the knee flexed may improve the individual's ankle ROM (Fig. 11.6). Again, stretches like this should not be performed if there is significant pain or known pathology in the joint(s).

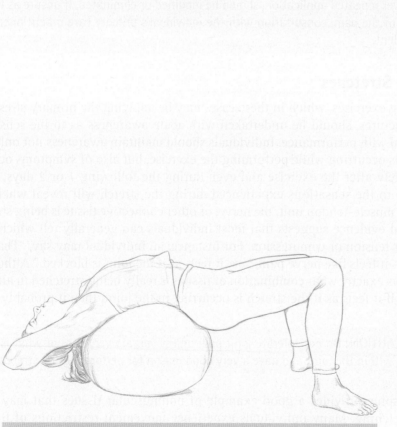

FIGURE 11.5 Thoracic extension over a ball with neutral L/S supporting neck with hands

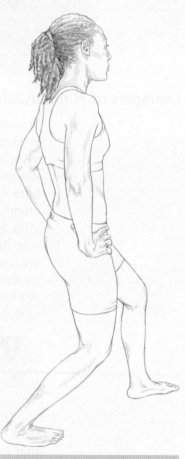

FIGURE 11.6 Soleus stretch

Note: The stretch shown above is the same as that for the soleus (see Chapter 4). In the event of a stiff talo-crural joint, the stretching force will likely be attenuated in that joint before there is enough motion to stretch the soleus muscle.

Improving joint ROM primarily limited by nonmuscular structures is possible with careful, attentive application of forces. As with muscle stretching, however, the stretches are not likely to affect only the target tissues. In other words, except in the early stages of rehabilitation following injury or surgery that require medical management, it is unlikely that one will be able to isolate a stretch to specific joint-related structures. More likely, the stretches will emphasize rather than isolate joint structures. For this reason, one should attempt to develop the movement capabilities of both the musculotendinous structures and the joint structures as a functional unit. After all, the ultimate goal is to attain or restore movement capabilities that allow for optimal function.

USE OF STRETCHING AIDS

Many devices are available to help individuals stretch. There are belts, bands, wedges, and bolsters—devices designed to increase mechanical advantage and improve the ease and the effectiveness of the stretch. Few, if any, of these devices offer stretching opportunities unavailable to those without these devices. Still with careful consideration, some of these aids/devices may be used to the benefit of the stretching individual.

> ⚠ **CAUTION!** As always, pay attention to the sensations experienced as some devices may prove more risky than helpful.

When using these devices, it is important to keep in mind that the basic stretching principles in Chapter 2 still apply. Important considerations include:

- Basic parameters such as frequency, duration, and intensity still hold true when using assistive devices. This is especially true regarding attention to the sensations occurring during the exercises.
- Many devices enhance stretching forces by using a type of mechanical advantage. The user should be well aware of the distribution and location of these enhanced forces.
- It is important to consider the forces applied at the "target" muscles as well as any possible forces applied to secondary or unintended joints or muscles. It should be possible to safely use most devices with careful attention and application. As with any exercise, discontinue use and seek professional help if there is pain associated with the use of the device. This is especially true if the pain or discomfort is in an area other than the area of intended stretch.

Physiotherapy Ball

Of all of the assistive devices available, one of the safest, most versatile, and reasonably priced is the physiotherapy ball. The use of the *physiotherapy ball* (also called a *physioball, therapy ball,* or *gym ball*) is no longer restricted to the worlds of personal or athletic training and physical therapy programs. This simple device is now also considered an excellent adjunct to flexibility training as well as functional strength and balance training.

For flexibility training, the physiotherapy ball affords a gradual contour over which stretches can be performed. This may be particularly useful when trying to stretch out the spine. When attempting to stretch out the thoracic spine to improve extension for

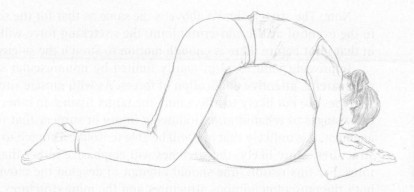

FIGURE 11.7
Prone over ball, elbows on the floor

example, it offers a gradual curve over which to stretch, providing support for the spine while guarding against possibly harmful hyperextensions or fulcrums (Fig. 11.5). The individual lies supine over the ball, supporting the head and neck with the hands. He or she should be advised to tighten the abdominals to avoid hyperextending the lumbar spine, while relaxing the thoracic spine and allowing it to extend over the ball. This position should be held for at least 30 seconds to achieve a useful stretch.

Another useful spinal stretch with the therapy ball is a stretch for thoracic and lumbar flexion (Fig. 11.7). The stretch may be performed by lying prone over the ball, allowing relaxation and a gentle stretch to occur in the neck, upper and midback, and shoulders. From this position, the individual may move slightly forward over the ball until feeling a gentle stretch in the lower back. The individual's knees may come slightly off the floor. Again, hold this position for at least 30 seconds.

Stretching on the therapy ball to improve side-bending of the thoracic and lumbar spine can be achieved by the individual lying on his or her side over the ball with one leg forward and the other leg reaching backward to achieve stability (Fig. 11.8). Once balance is attained, the individual should reach the upper arm directly overhead and allow the body to relax over the ball. Hold the stretch for at least 30 seconds.

This stretch can be varied to improve thoracic and lumbar rotation. The individual keeps the feet in place as before, then rotates the body either forward by reaching the upper arm overhead and anteriorly, or backward (Fig. 11.9) by reaching the upper arm overhead and posteriorly. Do not allow the hyperextension of the lumbar spine in any of these stretches. This can be avoided by tightening the abdominals, slightly tilting the pelvis posteriorly (flattening the lower back).

The *physioball* also has many attributes as an adjunct for functional strength training. If used properly, it calls on many stabilizing muscles in addition to the primary movers involved in the exercise, often significantly improving the useful qualities of the particular exercise. While functional strength training is obviously the subject of another book, an example is provided below. A simple example is a bridge (Fig. 11.10)

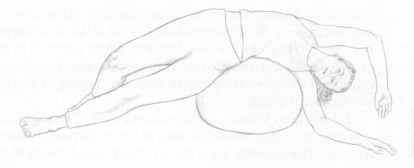

FIGURE 11.8
Side-bend over a ball

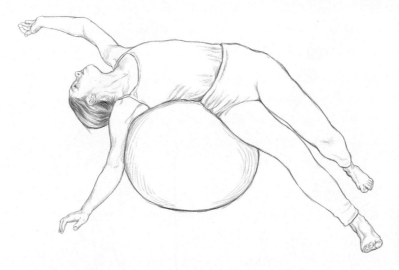

FIGURE 11.9 Side-bend over a ball with rotation, to the right

performed on the ball, versus on the floor. Bridging exercises involve the gluteals, the lumbar extensors and the quadriceps muscles. Performing these exercises on a physioball adds the additional challenge of "rolling off of the ball" which quickly calls into action other stabilizing muscles such as the obliques, the short rotators of the spine, and the stabilizers of the hip, knee, foot, and ankle.

Belts, Bands, Straps, and Bolsters

Many commercially available stretching aids may assist in helping the individual safely perform stretches that might be difficult without these devices. In most cases, however, an inexpensive belt, strap, or band may work equally as well. Two examples of the use of a band are shown below.

Stretching the quadriceps (the rectus femoris in particular) may pose a particular challenge for individuals having very tight quadriceps. The individual shown in Figure 11.11A, is hyperextending her lumbar spine in order to attempt a quadriceps stretch. Using a belt or flexible band allows her to effectively stretch the quadriceps without hyperextending the lumbar spine (Fig. 11.11B).

Stretching the hamstrings may be more easily accomplished using a belt or band for assistance (Fig. 11.12).

Stretching the shoulder internal rotators on the left and the external rotators on the right (Fig. 11.13).

Stretching the thoracic spine to help improve extension may be accomplished by the use of a simple towel roll as shown in Figure 11.14 (though there are numerous commercially available devices such as wedges and bolsters which may or may not allow for a more effective or specific application of the stretching force).

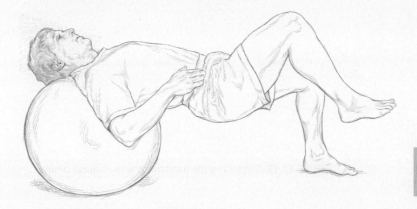

FIGURE 11.10 Bridge march on a therapy ball

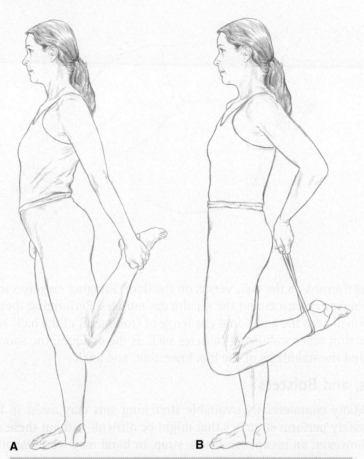

A   **B**

FIGURE 11.11 Quad stretch. A. No assistive device, obvious hyperextension of the lumbar spine. **B.** Using band, neutral lumbar spine.

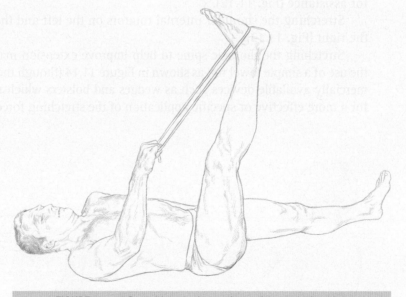

FIGURE 11.12 Stretching the hamstrings with surgical tubing

PROPRIOCEPTIVE NEUROMUSCULAR FACILITATION (PNF)

PNF stretching is an effective means to stretch muscle and improve ROM. Though these methods have been shown to be effective in producing gains in ROM,[1-3] the mechanisms by which these changes take place are still the subject of some debate. PNF techniques are thought to take advantage of the reflex relaxation brought on by the stimulation of one or more neuromuscular reflexes. These reflexes are stimulated by a muscular contraction before and/or during the actual performance of the stretch itself.

Although there are numerous techniques, one of the most popular involves a maximal muscular contraction of the muscle that will undergo stretch, immediately followed by the application of the stretching force. Theoretically, the maximal contraction of the muscle causes a reflex relaxation of that muscle via stimulation of the golgi tendon organs. More recent research has challenged the efficacy of this explanation. Chalmers and Mitchell et al suggest that an increased tolerance to stretch may be a more likely mechanism.[4,5]

These techniques generally involve a clinician or partner who offers both the resistance to the contraction and the stretching force. There remains debate as to whether or not it is as effective as static stretching, as some research has shown PNF stretching to be superior to static stretching,[6,7] while more recent research disagrees. Davis et al showed static stretching to be more effective than PNF stretching at the end of the 4-week study period.[8]

As PNF is a widely used and recognized stretching technique, we offer a brief discussion below. As there are numerous books describing PNF stretching in detail, we discuss the basic concepts rather than specific stretches. Suggested readings can be found in Appendix A.

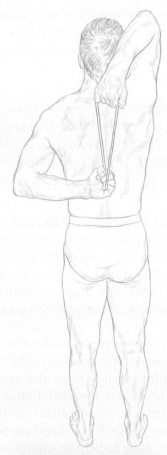

FIGURE 11.13 Stretching the shoulder internal rotators (L) and external rotators (R)

Benefits and Risks of PNF Stretching

PNF stretching has been shown to produce improvements in ROM and may offer an alternative to static stretching in cases where insufficient progress is being made.

PNF stretching generally requires a partner or clinician, both to apply the resistance to muscular contraction and to apply the stretching force. Therefore, we must consider the experience and skill of that individual in terms of both the effectiveness of the technique and the risk of injury. Because of its relative complexity and the maximal isometric contractions involved, the risk of injury may be higher in performing PNF than in static stretching exercises. Because the clinician (or partner)

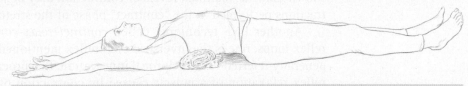

FIGURE 11.14 Lying supine over a towel roll: thoracic extension

cannot feel the stretching force, communication between the clinician and the individual being stretched is very important. Other concerns include increased blood pressure,[3] and the possibility of causing injury due to the use of excessive force or improper technique.

> **CAUTION!** Pain should not be tolerated in the muscle, tendon, nerve, or joint. This is especially true of stretching techniques in which the force is being applied by someone other than the individual undergoing the stretch. A clinician should be sure to educate clients about appropriate and inappropriate sensations and have them give feedback.

As with static stretching, some performance variables may be hindered by PNF stretching. Chapter 2 discusses these challenges in relationship to static stretching in some detail. Bradley et al showed a decrease in vertical jump height for both the static and PNF stretching groups.[9] Careful consideration should prevent the use of this, or any other stretching protocol, in situations in which it might actually hinder the performance of activity. Check the latest research regarding stretching and the specific application in which you are interested.

In the hands of skilled clinicians, PNF stretching deserves consideration, especially in cases where static stretching seems to be making little headway. PNF techniques may prove particularly useful when dealing with injured or otherwise dysfunctional joints and or musculotendinous structures. In these cases, the limitation in ROM may be due to a complex combination of neurologic, musculoskeletal, and/or fascial influences. As the predominance of stretching research has been carried out on healthy populations, much research needs to be done to help us understand the relative usefulness of various stretching techniques as they apply to various "injured" or "abnormal" populations.

Examples of PNF Stretches

PNF stretching utilizes a basic understanding of specialized reflexes to design stretching protocols that take advantage of the resulting muscular relaxation. For example, a PNF technique referred to as *contract-relax* capitalizes on the reflex relaxation following a maximal muscle contraction. This *inverse stretch reflex* is a reflex relaxation of muscle caused by stimulation of receptors in the tendon called golgi tendon organs (see discussion above). These receptors cause relaxation of the muscle in response to the development of excessive tension in the muscle-tendon unit as a protective mechanism. Therefore, a stretch performed immediately after a maximal end-range isometric contraction might allow a more effective lengthening of the muscle than the same stretch performed independently. An example of a *contract-relax* stretch to improve shoulder external rotation is shown below. Figure 11.15A shows the starting position during which the client is attempting to internally rotate the humerus against the clinician's resistance. In Figure 11.15B, the client has relaxed and the clinician is moving the client's humerus further into external rotation. Please note that new research has shown that sub-maximal levels of contraction may be just effective as maximal contractions performed in the "contract" phase of the stretch.[10]

Another PNF technique, called *contract-relax-contract,* utilizes two different reflex loops: one is the inverse stretch reflex mentioned above and another is a loop generally referred to as reciprocal innervation. Reciprocal innervation is basically the reflex relaxation of a muscle caused by contraction of its antagonist. In this technique the clinician moves the client's limb into a position that places the muscle to be stretched at its end range. At this point, the client contracts the agonist against

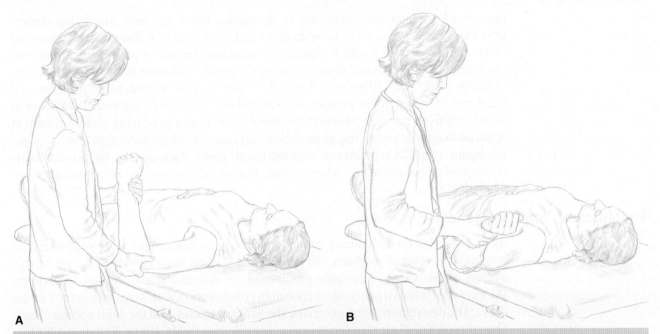

FIGURE 11.15 **External rotator stretch. A.** Resistive phase: clinician resists IR. **B.** Stretch phase: clinician moving client's arm into new ER range.

the resistance of the clinician. Following a 3- to 5-second hold, the client relaxes the agonist and contracts the antagonist, while the clinician moves the limb further into the new range. The difference here is that this passive stretch of the agonist is concurrent with an active contraction of the antagonist, which theoretically causes further relaxation of the target muscle. Sharmann et al suggests that this technique is superior to *contract-relax* and to other stretching techniques.[11]

An example of *contract-relax-contract* stretch might be exemplified by the previous figure, the difference being that the client is actively contracting the external rotators as the clinician is apply the stretching force (Fig. 11.15B).

Although we are primarily discussing flexibility here, other PNF techniques are widely used to treat clinical weakness and functional loss due to injury or disease. These techniques are beyond the scope of this text, but readers with further interest might consult *Proprioceptive Neuromuscular Facilitation* by Voss, Ionta, and Meyers.[12] A more user-friendly guide to PNF stretching is *Facilitated Stretching* by Robert McAtee, which generally describes partner (or clinician) stretches as well their equivalent self stretches.[13]

HATHA YOGA

According to Wikipedia, yoga is "a group of ancient spiritual practices originating in India. Outside of India, yoga is mostly associated with the practice of *asanas* (postures) of Hatha Yoga or as a form of exercise, although it has influenced the entire Indian religions family and other spiritual practices throughout the world." The word *yoga* is a general term indicating a path to union with the divine. Hatha yoga is specifically the physical form of yoga. We will consider *Hatha yoga* here, as it offers a valuable means of improving both flexibility and strength. It may offer individuals an organized and beneficial exercise program promoting flexibility, strength, and awareness.

Benefits of Hatha Yoga

Hatha yoga is used in the West to help improve flexibility, strength, muscular endurance, respiration, and body awareness. Yoga may be also be beneficial for reducing lower back pain, decreasing stress, decreasing blood pressure, improving cholesterol measures, decreasing risk for diabetes and cardiovascular disease, and improving mood. Williams et al found a significant reduction in use of pain medications and improvements in functional disability scores in people with back pain who participated in Hatha yoga.[14] McCaffrey et al found decreases in stress scores, blood pressure, and heart rate in hypertensive persons in Thailand in those practicing yoga.[15] Lavey et al found improved mood in psychiatric patients who began practicing yoga.[16] Bijlani et al found that those practicing yoga showed decreases in total cholesterol and low-density lipoprotein (LDL) cholesterol, and increased "good" high-density lipoprotein (HDL) cholesterol versus controls.[17] Many people also use Hatha yoga to help improve mental clarity.

Examples of Yoga Stretches

Having assessed the individual, you may decide to include one or more yoga exercises into his or her overall program. We have included a few yoga exercises that we believe address a wide variety of muscle groups and are safe and relatively easy to perform. The exercises (*asanas*) below were chosen in collaboration with yoga instructor Tamara Hlava. The description of the exercises, the Sanskrit names, and the short section "Some Thoughts on Yoga" are also the generous contribution of Ms. Hlava. References for further study are listed in Appendix A if a more inclusive program is desired.

DOWNWARD–FACING DOG (BENT KNEES VARIATION), *ADHO MUKHA SVANASANA*

With hands shoulder distance apart on floor, step back keeping knees bent deeply to allow spine to extend and straighten while breathing (Fig. 11.16). Slowly let knees begin to straighten and see if you have given the back and shoulders a little more opening.

DOWNWARD–FACING DOG, *ADHO MUKHA SVANASANA*

Press strongly into the base knuckles of hands with fingers spread wide (middle fingers are parallel with sides of mat). Feet are parallel and hip distance or wider apart. Pedal feet for a few rounds, pressing weight alternatively toward each heel. Let head and neck release, then gaze toward feet.

TRIANGLE POSE, *UTTIHITA TRIKONASANA*

Stand with feet spread apart about 3 feet (Fig. 11.17). Raise arms out to the side to shoulder height, with palms facing down. Turn the left foot 90 degrees to the left and the right foot toward the left, so that the toes of the right foot are turned in slightly. Inhale as you begin to reach the left hand further to the left, beginning to bend to the left, at the waist. Exhale and continue to bend left at the waist as you place your left hand on your left shin. Stretch the right arm up in line with the shoulder, palm facing forward. Chest, hips, and legs should be in the same plane. Repeat pose with opposite side.

EAGLE POSE (CROSSED LEG VARIATION), *GARUDASANA*

Stand with feet hip distance apart. Bend knees into a high squat. Extend right leg out to the side with toes on floor. Extend both arms out to sides at shoulder height. Cross right leg over the bent left, resting lightly on lower thigh of left leg. Dorsiflex right ankle (Fig. 11.18A). Cross right arm over left in front of chest. Bend both elbows and raise them to shoulder height. Attempt to place palms together. Repeat pose with opposite side (Fig. 11.18B).

Variation: Assisted Balance. Place buttocks against a wall and come into the pose. Practice finding a focal point for the eyes to work toward improving balance.

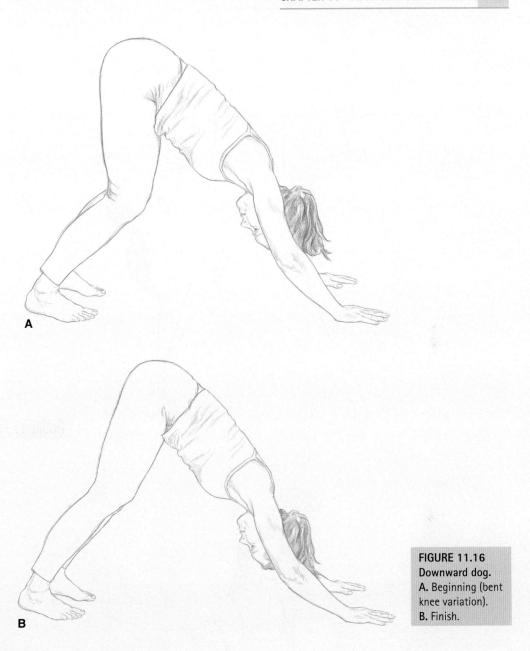

**FIGURE 11.16
Downward dog.
A.** Beginning (bent knee variation).
B. Finish.

COBBLER POSE (BLOCK VARIATION), *BADDHA KONASANA*

Sit on a foam block or folded blanket/towel (Fig. 11.19). Bend knees and place soles of feet together. Sit upright with shoulders relaxed and reach the hands to hold the lower legs. Allow knees to slowly open and move closer to floor. Try moving feet closer to groin. As an alternative, move feet 12–20 inches away from groin.

PIGEON (BLOCK VARIATION), *KAPOTASANA*

Sit on floor with legs extended in front (Fig. 11.20). Place block next to hips on the left side. Begin to bend left leg as you lift and shift left hip bone/buttocks onto the block. Left foot moves into the right groin area, but is likely not touching. Be sure that the left foot is pointed (ankle plantarflexed) to avoid torque at the left knee. Extend right leg to the back. Check to see that the right leg extends straight out, and that the right foot is not sideways (plantarflex right ankle). Move upper body weight onto elbows and let head and neck relax toward the floor. Repeat pose with opposite side.

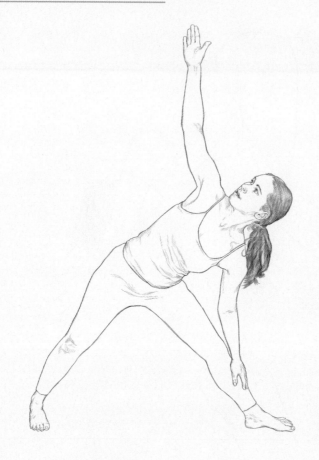

FIGURE 11.17 Triangle pose

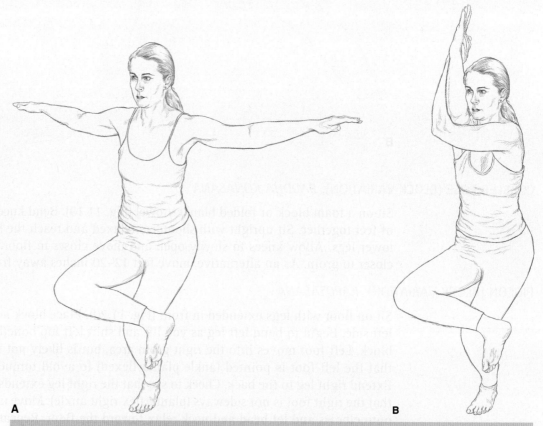

FIGURE 11.18 Eagle pose. A. Beginning. B. Finish.

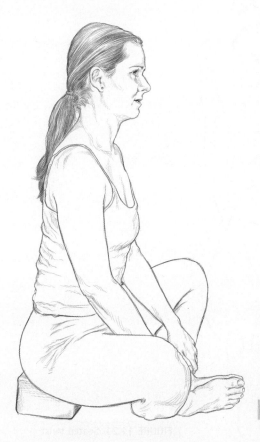

FIGURE 11.19 Cobbler pose

SEATED TWIST (STRAIGHT LEG VARIATION), *MARICHYASANA III*

Sit on floor with legs extended in front (Fig. 11.21). Cross left leg over right at mid-thigh and place left foot onto floor. Exert pressure into left foot so that it feels like you could stand on the foot. Place left palm on the floor behind lower back. Inhale as you raise your right arm over your head and exhale as you cross the right arm in front of chest and place the right elbow on the outside of the left knee. Extend palm and face it toward the left. Repeat pose with opposite side.

Some Thoughts on Yoga

Yoga comes from the Sanskrit word that means to "yoke" or "to join together." Many practitioners of yoga take this to mean "to end the separation between yourself internally and externally and seek to find a better balance between yourself and the world."

Yoga techniques vary from lineage or from teacher to teacher. Some practices are done in heated rooms with specific sequences and are intensely aerobic and strengthening. Others use straps and blocks, and each movement is aligned with a specific breathing sequence.

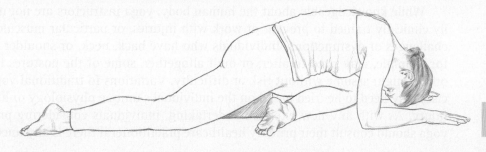

FIGURE 11.20
Pigeon pose

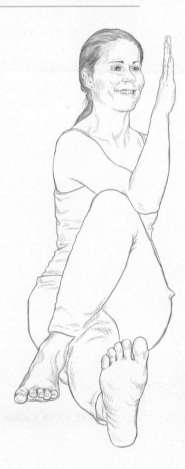

FIGURE 11.21 Seated twist

It is very important to keep your breath flowing steady and evenly in your yoga practice. You can explore how movement and breath may work together in your practice and help keep your balance and concentration in a pose steady and comfortable.

Yoga is not a religion, but it does provide many people with an increased ability to meditate and sit for long periods of time in a deep silence. Whether this is a spiritual practice or a relaxation practice is up to an individual's goals and experience.

There are numerous places to find more information on yoga. Some recommendations are:

- American Yoga Association Beginner's Manual
  http://www.americanyogaassociation.org/contents.html
- Light on Yoga, B.K.S. Iyengar
- The Heart of Yoga, T.K.V. Desikachar

NOTE

While knowledgeable about the human body, yoga instructors are not necessarily clinically trained to prevent or work with injuries, or particular musculoskeletal challenges or dysfunctions. Individuals who have back, neck, or shoulder injuries, for example, may need to alter, or omit altogether, some of the postures in which others might assume without risk or difficulty. Variations to traditional yoga exercises may need to be tried based on the individual's unique physiology or history of injury. As with any new exercise undertaking, individuals considering practicing yoga should consult their primary healthcare practitioner if there is any uncertainty.

This is especially true if the individual has a significant history of back or neck pain or injury.

Guidelines for Individuals Considering Yoga or Other Movement Arts

Clinicians may encounter individuals who follow any of a wide variety of movement-based methodologies. Many of these methodologies purport to improve the individual's flexibility, strength, coordination, and general physical and mental health. As it would be impossible to address all of the types of practices you might encounter, we offer some general guidelines below.

- Check the instructor's references. Certificates of training or certification are often readily available; if not, ask. Next, check with friends or acquaintances who have taken the class or workshop you are considering. What were their experiences and results?

- Research the methodology. It is generally quite simple to search the Internet for information regarding the type of exercise you are considering and, likely, the specific classes and schools as well.

- Let pain be your guide. Regardless of the type of exercise, if it hurts, you probably shouldn't be doing it. Your technique may require some modification, or the exercise may be inappropriate for you and should be completely discontinued.

- Start slowly. This may mean beginning at low intensities, initially shortened durations, and reduced frequencies (sessions per week).

- Start cautiously. Be aware of any sensations you experience in your muscles and joints throughout the exercise sessions. Set goals and track your results. It may help first to think about what you wish to accomplish with these endeavors, and then periodically check to see if these goals are being met.

SUMMARY

An understanding of the basic principles involved in stretching and flexibility along with a developing skill in body awareness, combined with experience performing basic exercises, should allow interested individuals to safely move into the world of advanced stretching. Advanced stretching might mean stretching multiple joints simultaneously, stretching restricted joints, using assistive stretching devices, or using alternative protocols or movement methodologies.

Improved awareness and skill will allow the stretching of multiple joints simultaneously to improve movement "patterns," which may be useful for particular sports or activities. Stretching joints or other nonmuscular tissues to improve ROM in joints whose restriction is not primarily musculotendinous becomes safely possible with these improved stretching skills.

Improved skill and awareness also allow individuals to take advantage of mechanical aids, such as straps, flexible bands, physiotherapy balls, or other products, to improve the effectiveness of individual stretches. Incorporating assistive stretching devices into stretching programs can make them not only more interesting, challenging, and motivating, but also more specific and useful for the individual.

Improved skill and awareness also allow the individual to consider alternatives to "static" stretching. Of the numerous alternatives, proprioceptive neuromuscular facilitation stretching is widely accepted and shown to be effective. One may decide that PNF stretching is indeed a valuable intervention. With an understanding of one's needs and limitations, an individual might also consider other alternatives, such as yoga or other movement arts.

REFERENCES

1. Decicco PV, Fischer MM. The effects of proprioceptive neuromuscular facilitation stretching on shoulder range of motion in overhand athletes. J Sports Med Phys Fitness June 2005;45(2)183–187.

2. Bonnar BP, Deivert RG, Gould TE. The relationship between isometric contraction durations during hold-relax stretching and improvement in hamstring flexibility. J Sports Med Phys Fitness September 2004;44(3)258–261.

3. Cornelius WL, Jensen RL, Odell ME. Effects of PNF stretching on acute arterial blood pressure. Can J Appl Physiol June 1995;20(2)222–229.

4. Chalmers G. Re-examination of the possible role of Golgi tendon organ and muscle spindle reflexes in proprioceptive neuromuscular facilitation muscle stretching. Sports Biomech January 2004;3(1): 159–183.

5. Mitchell UH, Myrer JW, Hopkins JT, et al. Acute stretch perception alteration contributes to success of the PNF "contract-relax" stretch. J Sport Rehabil May 2007;16(2):85–92.

6. Sady SP, Wortman M, Blanke D. Flexibility training: ballistic, static or proprioceptive neuromuscular facilitation? Arch Phys Med Rehabil June 1982;63(6):261–263.

7. Etnyre BR, Abraham LD. Gains in range of ankle dorsiflexion using three popular stretching techniques. Am J Phys Med August 1986;65(4):189–196.

8. Davis DS, Ashby PE, McCale KL, et al. The effectiveness of 3 stretching techniques on hamstring flexibility using consistent stretching parameters. J Strength Cond Res February 2005;19(1):27–32.

9. Bradley PS, Olsen PD, Portas MD. The effect of static, ballistic, and proprioceptive neuromuscular facilitation stretching on vertical jump performance. J Strength Cond Res February 2007;21(1):223–226.

10. Feland JB, Marin HN. Effect of submaximal contraction intensity in contract-relax proprioceptive neuromuscular facilitation stretching. Br J Sports Med August 2004;38(4):E18.

11. Sharman MJ, Cresswell AG, Riek S. Proprioceptive neuromuscular facilitation stretching: mechanisms and clinical implications. Sports Med 2006;36(11):929–939.

12. Voss DE, Ionta MK, Meyers BJ. Proprioceptive Neuromuscular Facilitation. 3rd Ed. Baltimore: Lippincott Williams and Wilkins, 1985:370.

13. McAtee R, Charland J. Facilitated Stretching. 3rd Ed. Human Kinetics Publishers, 2007:193.

14. Williams KA, Petronis J, Smith D, et al. Effect of Iyengar yoga therapy for chronic low back pain. Pain May 2005;115(1–2):107–117.

15. McCaffrey R, Ruknui P, Hatthakit U, et al. The effects of yoga on hypertensive persons in Thailand. Holist Nurs Pract July–August 2005;19(4):173–180.

16. Lavey R, Sherman T, Mueser KT, et al. The effects of yoga on mood in psychiatric inpatients. Psychiatr Rehabil J Spring 2005;28(4):399–402.

17. Bijlani RL, Vempate RP, Yadav RK, et al. A brief but comprehensive lifestyle education program based on yoga reduces risk factors for cardiovascular disease and diabetes mellitus. J Altern Complement Med April 2005;11(2):267–274.

18. Magnusson P, Simonsen E, Aagaard P, et al. Biomechanical responses to repeated stretches in human hamstring muscle in vivo. Am J Sports Med. 1996;24(5):622–628.

19. Rees SS, Murphy AJ, Watsford ML, McLachlan KA, Coutts AJ. Effects of proprioceptive neuromuscular facilitation stiffness and force-producing characteristics of the ankle in women. J Strength Cond Res. 2007 May;21(2):572–577.

Recommended Resources

T his appendix is an attempt to pass along not only the references used in the development of *Stretching for Functional Flexibility,* but also to offer suggestions for further reading regarding stretching and related topics. Included are recommended texts and websites that I have found useful and that the reader might use as a stepping stone to pursue related topics of interest in more detail. All references used in this text are included in each chapter's bibliography.

TOPICS

Anatomy and Physiology
Athletic Training
Biomechanics
Cardiovascular Conditioning
Chiropractic
Ergonomics
Exercise Physiology
Fitness
Human Physiology
Joint Mechanics and Function
Kinesiology
Massage Therapy
Medical Dictionary
Medicine
Occupational Health and Safety
Physical Examination
Physical Therapy
Posture
Proprioceptive Neuromuscular Facilitation
Range of Motion
Sports Injuries
Strength Training
Stretching
Workstation Design
Yoga

ANATOMY AND PHYSIOLOGY

Agur AM, Dalley AF. Grant's Atlas of Anatomy. 11th Ed. Baltimore: Lippincott Williams & Wilkins, 2004:848.
Ganong WF. Review of Medical Physiology. 15th Ed. Norwalk: Appleton and Lange, 1991:754.
Netter FH. Atlas of Human Anatomy. Summit: CIBA-GEIGY Corporation, 1989;551.
Pratt NE. Clinical Musculoskeletal Anatomy. Philadelphia: J. B. Lippincott Company, 1991:333.
Rohen JW, Yokochi C, Lutjen-Drecoll E. Color Atlas of Anatomy. 5th Ed. Baltimore: Lippincott Williams & Wilkins, 2002:500.

Electronic Media

Primal Pictures. Available at: http://www.primalpictures.com/index.aspx.

ATHLETIC TRAINING

Electronic Media

Available at: http://www.nata.org/.

BIOMECHANICS

Nordin M, Frankel VH. Basic Biomechanics of the Musculoskeletal System. 3rd Ed. Baltimore: Lippincott Williams & Wilkins, 2001:496.
Valmassy RL. Clinical Biomechanics of the Lower Extremities. St. Louis: Mosby-Year Book, 1996:510.

CHIROPRACTIC

Electronic Media

American Chiropractic Association. Available at: http://www.amerchiro.org/.

ERGONOMICS

Kromer KH, Kromer HB, Kroemer-Elbert KE. Ergonomics: How to Design for Ease and Efficiency. 2nd Ed. Upper Saddle River: Prentice Hall, 2000:720.

Electronic Media

Centers for Disease Control and Prevention. Available at: http://www.cdc.gov/.

National Institute of Cornell University. Cornell University Ergonomics Web. Available at: http://www.ergo.human.cornell.edu/.

National Institute of Occupational Safety and Health. Available at: http://www.cdc.gov/niosh/topics/ergonomics/.

EXERCISE PHYSIOLOGY

Lamb DR. Physiology of Exercise: Responses and Adaptations. 2nd Ed. New York: Macmillan Publishing Company, 1984:489.

McArdle WD, Katch FI, Katch VL. Essentials of Exercise Physiology. 2nd Ed. Baltimore: Lippincott Williams & Wilkins: 2000:679.

FITNESS

Electronic Media

American College Sports Medicine. Available at: http://www.acsm.org//AM/Template.cfm?Section=Home_Page.

American Council On Exercise. Available at: http://www.acefitness.org/.

National Strength and Conditioning Association. Available at: http://www.nsca-lift.org/.

JOINT MECHANICS AND FUNCTION

Kapandji IA. The Physiology of the Joints; Annotated Diagrams of the Mechanics of the Human Joints, vol 1 Upper Limb. Edinburgh: Churchill Livingstone, 1982:283.

Kapandji IA. The Physiology of the Joints; Annotated Diagrams of the Mechanics of the Human Joints, vol 2 Lower Limb. Edinburgh: Churchill Livingstone, 1987:242.

Kapandji IA. The Physiology of the Joints; Annotated Diagrams of the Mechanics of the Human Joints, vol 3 Trunk and the Vertebral Column. Edinburgh: Churchill Livingstone, 1974:283.

Norkin CC, Levangie PK. Joint Structure and Function. 2nd Ed. Philadelphia: FA Davis Company, 1992:512.

Kinesiology

Lehmkuhl LD, Smith LK. Brunnstrom's Clinical Kinesiology. 4th Ed. Philadelphia: FA Davis Company, 1983: 453.

MASSAGE THERAPY

Braun MB, Simonson S. Introduction to Massage Therapy. Baltimore: Lippincott Williams & Wilkins, 2005:490.

Clay JH, Pounds DM. Basic Clinical Massage Therapy: Integrating Anatomy and Treatment. Baltimore: Lippincott, Williams & Wilkins, 2003:412.

Electronic Media

American Massage Therapy Association. Available at: http://www.amtamassage.org/.

MEDICAL DICTIONARY

Venes D, Thomas CL, Taver CW. Taber's Cyclopedic Medical Dictionary. 19th Ed. Philadelphia: FA Davis and Company, 2001:2439.

MEDICINE

Electronic Media

American Medical Association. Available at: http://www.ama-assn.org/.

MUSCLE TESTING

Kendall FP, McCreary EK, Provance PG. Muscles, Testing and Function. 4th Ed. Baltimore: Williams and Wilkins, 1993:450.

OCCUPATIONAL HEALTH AND SAFETY

Electronic Media

Occupational Health and Safety Administration. Available at: http://www.osha.gov/.

OUTDOOR FITNESS

Musnick D, Pierce M. Conditioning for Outdoor Fitness. Seattle: The Mountaineers, 1999:318.

PHYSICAL EXAMINATION

Hoppenfeld S. Physical Examination of the Spine and Extremities. London: Prentice Hall, 1976:276.

Magee DJ. Orthopedic Physical Assessment. Philadelphia: W. B. Saunders Company, 1992:655.

PHYSICAL THERAPY

Evjenth O, Hamberg J. Muscle Stretching in Manual Therapy: A Clinical Manual. 4th Ed. Milan: New Intherlotho Spa, 1998:175.

Hertling D, Kessler RM. Management of Common Musculoskeletal Disorders: Physical Therapy Principles and Methods. 2nd Ed. Philadelphia: J. B. Lippincott Company, 1990:679.

Electronic Media

American Physical Therapy Association. Available at: http://www.apta.com.

Posture

Kendall FP, McCreary EK, Provance PG. Muscles, Testing and Function. 4th Ed. Baltimore: Williams and Wilkins, 1993:450.

PROPRIOCEPTIVE NEUROMUSCULAR FACILITATION

McAtee RE, Charland J. Facilitated Stretching. 3rd Ed. Champaign: Human Kinetics Publishers, 2007:192.

Voss DE, Ionta MK, Myers BJ. Proprioceptive Neuromuscular Facilitation: Patterns and Techniques. 3rd Ed. Philadelphia: Lippincott Williams & Wilkins, 1985;370.

RANGE OF MOTION

Norkin CC, White DJ. Measurement of Joint Motion: A Guide to Goniometry. 3rd Ed. Philadelphia: FA Davis Company, 1985:404.

SPORTS INJURIES

Roy S, Irvin R. Sports Medicine: Prevention, Evaluation, Management, and Rehabilitation. Englewood Cliffs: Prentice-Hall, 1983:540.

STRENGTH TRAINING

Bompa TO, Cornacchia LJ. Serious Strength Training: Periodization for Building Muscle Power and Mass. Champaign: Human Kinetics Publishing, 1998:301.

STRETCHING

Alter MJ. Science of Flexibility. 2nd Ed. Champaign: Human Kinetics Publishing, 1996:373.

WORKSTATION DESIGN

Electronic Media

U.S. Department of Labor Occupational Safety & Health Administration. Available at: http://www.osha.gov/SLTC/etools/computerworkstations/components.html

YOGA

Austin M. Yoga for Wimps. New York: Sterling Publishing Company, 2000:108.

Iyengar BK. Light on Yoga. Schocken Books, 1995:544.

Christensen A. American Yoga Association Beginner's Manual. Forest City: Fireside Books, 1987:208.

Desikachar TK. The Heart of Yoga: Developing a Personal Practice. Rochester: Inner Traditions International, 1995:272.

Electronic Media

American Yoga Association. Available at http://www.americanyogaassociation.org/.

Index

Page numbers in *italics* denote figures; page numbers followed by *t* indicate tables.